Consumer Drug Digest

Consumer Drug Digest

American Society of
Hospital Pharmacists

Facts On File, Inc.
460 Park Avenue South
New York, N.Y. 10016

Consumer Drug Digest

Library of Congress Cataloging in Publication Data
Main entry under title:
Consumer drug digest.
    Includes index.
    1. Drugs—Popular works.   I. American Society of Hospital
Pharmacists.
RM301.15.C66   615'.1   81-12499
ISBN 0-87196-554-2   AACR2
ISBN 0-87196-686-7(pbk.)

Printed in the United States of America
10 9 8 7 6 5 4 3 2 1

CONTENTS

Introduction

Many people want—and need—more information about medicines. The CONSUMER DRUG DIGEST is an authoritative handbook on drugs, written in language that's accessible to lay readers. The purpose of this book is to help consumers, as patients, understand the medications they take and learn what they can do to help their doctors prescribe the most beneficial drug therapy. It should help patients become responsible participants in their own health care.

This book is both a general source for information about drugs and a quick reference handbook for patients who want to supplement the information provided by doctors and others involved in the care of their health. It is *not*, however, intended as a do-it-yourself handbook or as a substitute for doctors' recommendations. Nor is it intended to help patients "second-guess" their doctors. The guiding assumptions of this book are that its readers have faith in their doctors and the others who are participating in their health care, and that they want to help assure that their drug therapy contributes to their overall good health.

The CONSUMER DRUG DIGEST concentrates on the rational use of legitimate drugs in the treatment of properly diagnosed medical problems. It does not discuss the abuse of prescription drugs, illegally obtained drugs or "street drugs." It includes entries on over 200 of the most frequently prescribed prescription drugs, comprising over 1,000 brand-name products. Selected nonprescription products are also included. The index includes the generic and brand names of all of the drugs covered in the book. *You must know either the generic or brand name of the drug you are taking to look it up in this book.* Simply find the name in the index and turn to the entry on the page to which you are directed. Only some of the many brand names of drug products are included. The brand names included here were selected according to the frequency with which they are prescribed. If you know the generic name of the drug you are taking, but can't find the brand name, the information in the entry on that generic drug will still apply.

Similarly, only a few of the many products that contain more than one drug (called combination products) are included here. If you know the names of the individual drugs in your combination, you can read about those drugs by looking them up in the index.

No attempt has been made to provide *complete* information on any drug or to cover all drug products. Entire volumes have been written about many of the drugs in this book. The information provided here is intended to help consumers take commonly prescribed medicines in a responsible manner. This book will provide answers to some of your general questions about the drugs you are taking and offer suggestions concerning their proper use. It is not intended as a substitute for your doctor's judgment about your individual medical condition. Always share with your doctor everything you know about your general health and medical problems. It will help him direct your health care. Drugs act differently in different people, and only your doctor can prescribe and direct your drug therapy effectively. Frequent suggestions are made to "contact your doctor for more information." Always follow your doctor's advice and the instructions on your prescription label, even if they are different from what you read here.

As indicated above, drugs act differently in different people. This is especially true in children and in old or debilitated patients. Many drugs have not been tested or used extensively in children. Generally speaking, someone younger than 12 is considered a "child"; depending, however, on his or her physical maturity, a "child" could be up to 16 years old. Sometimes a drug's effects on children may be very different from its effects on adults; some drugs should not be given to children under any circumstances. These precautions are noted in the entries on those drugs. No general precautions are made concerning the use of drugs in children, but it is always a good idea to discuss thoroughly with your doctor the use of any drug to treat your child.

Similarly, changes that occur as part of the aging process can affect the way one responds to drugs. Drugs may act quite differently in elderly patients than in younger ones. It is not possible to pinpoint a specific age at which this may begin to occur, but you should be aware that more frequent adjustments of dosages—and more frequent undesired effects—can be expected as the aging process advances. This precaution is not noted in the entries on individual drugs; in general, it applies to all drugs.

While medicine—and drug therapy—are precise sciences, they are also arts. "Always" or "never" situations rarely occur. It must be emphasized again that this book is a guide for you as a patient, and that your doctor must remain the one primarily in charge of your drug therapy. In an entry on a specific drug here you may be advised, for example, that "large doses" of that drug may produce a particular undesirable effect or that the drug may have such an effect "when taken over a long period of time." There are, however, no absolute answers to the questions "how large" or "for how long." Only your doctor, who knows your individual medical condition, can make that judgment. The information in this book can help you to help your doctor in monitoring your therapy and can bring to your attention questions you may wish to discuss with him.

While, in general, the language in this book can be understood by the average reader, some medical and technical terms are used. This occurs primarily in the section of each entry entitled "Precautions," where it is suggested that you tell your doctor if you have certain medical conditions—diabetes, porphyria or lupus erythematosus, for example—before you begin taking the medication in question. These terms describe chronic or inherited diseases; if you suffer from them, you have almost certainly undergone extensive diagnostic investigation or treatment for them in the past, perhaps by doctors other than the one you are now seeing. Thus, while these are technical medical terms, it is assumed that if you have any of these conditions, you know it. "Translations" of these terms into ones more readily understood by other users of this book have consequently been avoided. (Other technical terms are defined, as appropriate, in the Glossary.) The important point is that you must always give your doctor a complete medical history, telling him about any major illnesses you have suffered in the past and any chronic or inherited diseases you may have.

Drugs are grouped in this book according to the major body systems whose ailments they are designed to combat. It is of course impossible to include here every disease. Many drugs are used to treat many different diseases or conditions. To make this book less cumbersome, drugs are described under only one medical condition. For example, prednisone is a "steroid" or cortisone-like drug used to treat many illnesses. It is described in this book under arthritis. If you are taking prednisone for asthma, however, you can use the index to find the entry on prednisone under arthritis; the information in that entry will apply equally to your prescription.

Brief descriptions of some diseases are also included in this book. These descriptions are intended to offer some background information that will help you understand your drug therapy. Again, your physician should be your main source of information about your disease or medical problem.

How Drugs Act

Drugs are chemical compounds that modify the body's characteristic natural chemical reactions. In many cases, drugs do not cure the disease they have been prescribed to treat—they merely ensure that the body's chemical processes take place normally for as long as they are used. Drugs alone are often insufficient to restore normal function. The body's natural ability to recuperate is often at least equally important. For example, many antibiotics do not actually kill bacteria; they merely retard their growth so that the body's normal defense mechanisms can eliminate the infection.

Most drugs are not naturally occurring substances. After they have been at work in the body for a certain period of time, they are gradually eliminated, just like waste products. The exact path that specific drugs follow varies a great deal. Some drugs are broken down into other compounds by the liver before they are eliminated, while others remain unchanged. Ultimately, most drugs (or their by-products) are excreted in the urine, feces, sweat or tears. Some drugs are even eliminated through the lungs—alcohol, for example.

The length of time that it takes for different drugs to be absorbed, exert their intended effect and be eliminated varies considerably. This is why dosage schedules are different for each drug.

Dosage Forms and Routes of Administration

Oral dosage is the most common and convenient route of drug administration. Tablets, capsules and various liquids are common forms in which drugs may be administered orally. Some medications are available in the form of chewable tablets, particularly those that are commonly prescribed for children; certain medications are available as long-acting tablets or capsules. It is important that long-acting tablets and capsules be swallowed whole. If they are chewed, the medication may be released all at once rather than over an extended time.

Syrups, suspensions, solutions and tinctures are various liquid forms in which drugs may be administered. *Syrups* are liquids that contain sugar; they are usually thick. Many cough medications are available as syrups. *Suspensions* are liquids that contain large amounts of solid material that is suspended rather than dissolved. The medication in a suspension will settle to the bottom rather quickly, so it is important to shake a suspension thoroughly before pouring each dose. Most liquid antacid preparations are suspensions. *Solutions* and *tinctures* are clear liquids containing dissolved medication. Some special oral dosage forms are powders, granules or effervescent tablets that are mixed with or dissolved in water before use.

A special form in which some drugs are taken orally is the sublingual tablet. These tablets are *not* swallowed—they are placed under the tongue and allowed to dissolve slowly. The medication is absorbed directly into the bloodstream through the blood vessels under the tongue. This route of administration is useful when a rapid effect is desired, as is often the case in heart patients.

Inflammations or infections of the skin, eyes or ears are frequently treated by means of topical dosage—that is, the application of ointments, creams, solutions, lotions or dusting powders directly to the site of the problem. In some cases—when the skin is severely infected, for example—an antibiotic ointment may be used in conjunction with an oral antibiotic.

Injectable medications may be used when a very rapid effect is required, when a drug is ineffective if taken orally or when the presence or likelihood of nausea or vomiting precludes oral administration. Usually injectable medications are administered by nurses or physicians, unless the patient or a member of his or her family has been specially trained to administer injections.

Some drugs are administered by rectal suppository or enema, particularly in patients who are unable to take oral medication. For example, some anti-nausea medications are available as suppositories. Enemas are commonly used to treat constipation, but may also be used to treat bowel inflammations such as colitis.

TOXICITY

Most drugs are relatively free from toxic effects, but any drug can produce unwanted effects under certain circumstances.

Undesirable drug effects can be classified as follows:

Pharmacologic Effects Unwanted effects due to a drug's pharmacologic actions (side effects) are predictable and, therefore, somewhat controllable. The action of most drugs depends on the size of each dose. If too much of a drug is taken, the drug's action may be stronger than necessary and unwanted effects may occur. In addition, most drugs exert more than one kind of action. Those actions that are unrelated to the intended effect may also cause undesirable symptoms. In some cases, these symptoms can be eliminated or minimized by adjusting the dose; in other cases, the unwanted symptoms may decrease or disappear after the patient's body adjusts to the medication.

Undesirable drug effects are more likely to occur in those whose bodily functions are impaired. Age is an important factor, since the function of certain organ systems may be impaired in the very young and the very old. For example, kidney and liver functions are not well developed in the newborn; these same functions tend to deteriorate in the elderly. As a result, young or old patients may metabolize and excrete certain drugs at a relatively slow rate, causing the drug in question to build up in the bloodstream and, perhaps, to produce undesirable effects.

Other medical conditions can also increase the chances of adverse drug effects. Be sure to tell your doctor about any medical condition you may have, even if it seems unrelated to your current problem.

Allergic Reactions Allergic reactions are unrelated to the pharmacologic action of a drug or to dosage. Such reactions are unpredictable. Practically any drug has the potential to cause an allergic reaction if it is given to a susceptible individual. It is difficult to predict whether a person will be allergic to a particular drug, although, in general, people with hay fever or other allergies are more likely to develop allergies to drugs.

Drugs that are chemically related to a drug to which a person is allergic may also produce in him or her an allergic reaction. For example, a patient who develops an allergy to one particular sulfa drug will probably also be allergic to many other sulfas.

Allergic reactions may involve many different types of symptoms; such symptoms may appear immediately, or not until several weeks after the patient has begun to take a drug. Skin disturbances are the most common symptom. These range from mild redness and itching to severe swelling and skin destruction. Other, less common symptoms of allergic reactions include fever, jaundice and blood reactions, such as certain types of anemia.

The most dangerous type of allergic reaction is anaphylaxis. This life-threatening condition involves a decrease in blood pressure and spasm of the breathing passages. This reaction occurs, if at all, immediately after the administration of a drug and is most common when the drug is given by injection.

Any type of allergic reaction is treated by discontinuing the use of the medication immediately. If symptoms are severe, antihistamines or steroids may be used to help relieve them. Anaphylactic reactions require immediate treatment at a hospital.

To minimize the chance of developing an allergic reaction, it is important to tell your doctor if you have a history of any type of allergy, including hay fever or asthma. This information may provide useful clues to drugs that you should avoid.

It is also important that you tell your doctor about any unusual symptoms that develop after you begin to take a medication.

Drug Interactions A drug interaction results when two or more drugs that are used concurrently affect each other's actions in some way. One or both drugs may become more or less effective, or undesirable effects may occur. Drug interactions are not necessarily bad; in fact, some are brought about intentionally to increase the therapeutic effect of certain drugs. The mechanisms through which drugs can interact are complex and involve changes in the ways that each is absorbed, metabolized and excreted.

Alcohol, because of its widespread use, is probably responsible for more interactions than any other drug. The drowsiness caused by many common medications (antihistamines, tranquilizers, sedatives, pain relievers) may be increased by even small amounts of alcohol.

It is important to note that many liquid medications such as cough syrups contain enough alcohol to produce this effect. If you have questions about the alcohol content of any medications you are taking, ask your pharmacist or check the label.

The important point about drug interactions is that they may occur any time you are taking more than one drug, including nonprescription drugs. Be sure to tell your doctor about all the medications you are taking before beginning to take a new medication, and always check with your doctor or pharmacist before using nonprescription medications.

TERATOGENICITY

The abnormal development of a fetus as a result of events that take place in the mother's body during pregnancy is known as teratogenesis. Known teratogens include X rays, certain diseases (for example, rubella or German measles) and some drugs. The first trimester of pregnancy (from conception to 90 days after conception) is the period during which malformations are most likely to occur.

A few drugs are known to cause teratogenic effects, but the vast majority have not been adequately evaluated for possible teratogenic effects. As a result, the safest course is to avoid taking *any* unnecessary medication during pregnancy, particularly during the first trimester. Be sure to tell your doctor if you are pregnant or if you are planning to become pregnant while taking medication.

HOW DRUGS REACH THE MARKET

Federal regulations require that a new drug cannot be marketed—that is, made available for general use by physicians throughout the country—unless it has been shown to be both safe and effective. In other words, a company that wishes to sell a drug must prove that it is safe for use in humans and, further, that it actually produces the intended effect. (You should realize that "safe" is a relative term; no drug is totally safe, and a physician must decide whether the benefits of a specific drug outweigh the dangers it may pose to the patient.)

To show that a drug is safe and effective, its manufacturer must carry out proper scientific studies, first in animals and then in humans. The drug will be given to animals, usually mice, rats and dogs, and information on its activity, potential usefulness in people, dosage and toxicity will be collected. If, after considering the results of these studies, the company feels the drug is promising, it will cautiously (starting with very low doses) give the drug to a small number of healthy human volunteers. These studies are aimed primarily at finding out how the drug acts in humans; that is, how long a dose remains effective, whether it can be taken by mouth, what side effects can be expected and so on.

If the drug is found to be safe, the question "Is it effective?" must be answered. A large number of patients (up to several thousand) are thus carefully treated with the drug. These patients are closely watched for signs of improvement in their illness and for the appearance of side effects. Over time, a complete picture of how well the drug works and how it is best used will develop.

If at this stage (usually several years, at least, after the drug's development) its manufacturers believe it is safe and effective, they will ask that they be allowed to market it. The Food and Drug Administration (FDA) is the branch of the federal government that makes this decision. The FDA will review the results of all research on the drug (actually, it will already have reviewed the research at several points as it was taking place) and decide whether the drug can be placed in general use or whether more study is necessary.

Patients who receive an experimental drug (referred to as an "investigational drug") are given complete information about its intended use, its expected side effects and how it compares with other treatments already in general use. These patients must voluntarily agree to have an investigational drug prescribed for them. Once patients have been informed about such drugs, their voluntary consent to receive them is known as "informed consent." It is required in all research studies involving human subjects.

Sometimes, a severe side effect may be observed only after the drug has been marketed and used to treat many thousands of patients. Such a side effect may occur in only one out of every 10,000 patients; therefore, it may not have occurred in the comparatively few patients who were given the drug before it was marketed. If the side effect is excessively severe in comparison with the benefits of the drug (or with the side effects of other, similar drugs), the drug will be *recalled*—removed from the market. Drug recalls are rare, but they do happen. If you hear that a drug you are taking has been recalled, ask your doctor or pharmacist what to do. Sometimes only a particular batch of drug or form of the drug is recalled; therefore, don't stop taking it until you have contacted your doctor or pharmacist.

OVER-THE-COUNTER VS PRESCRIPTION DRUGS

A wide variety of medications are available without a doctor's prescription. These so-called "over-the-counter" drugs can be safely used to treat minor illnesses that do not require medical supervision. The primary distinction between prescription and "over-the-counter" drugs is that the latter have a wider margin of safety. They have fewer and milder side effects and little or no potential for addiction. In many cases, a drug will be available only as a prescription drug until experience shows that it is suitable for use by the general public.

This does not mean that "over-the-counter" drugs are harmless. They can and do cause problems if they are not used according to instructions on the labels or when they are used to treat conditions that should be evaluated by a physician. "Over-the-counter" drugs may also affect the way your body responds to other medicines you may be taking. For this reason, you should always check with your pharmacist before beginning to use an "over-the-counter" product if you are already taking medication for another condition.

In contrast to "over-the-counter" drugs, prescription drugs are potent drugs that should only be used after thorough evaluation of a medical problem. They are more likely to cause unwanted side effects and, therefore, can only be used safely under the supervision of your physician.

UNDERSTANDING THE PRESCRIPTION

Prescriptions are usually written in a format similar to the one illustrated below.

John Jones, M.D.
125 Main Street
Cornstalk, NB 10123

Name: Joe Smith
Address: 41 S First Street

R_x

Ampicillin 250 mg
#20
Sig: 1 tid

Do not refill
Refill 1 times

BNDD 10123644
Date   11/13/81

Although the exact placement of information may vary, the following information should appear:

1. The patient's name and address.
2. The superscription—the "R_x" symbol is the heading for the prescribed medication. The origin of this symbol is uncertain. It may have developed either from an abbreviation of the Latin word for recipe or from the sign of Jupiter, which was included on ancient prescriptions in order to invoke the god's blessing. In any case, the symbol has become a standard notation.
3. The name and strength of the drug.
4. Quantity.
5. Directions for use—the notation "Sig." precedes the directions for the use of the medication. The actual directions are usually abbreviated in Latin notation. The most commonly used abbreviations are:

    qd—every day   q_h—every _ hours
    BID—twice a day   ac—before meals

TID—three times a day   pc—after meals
QID—four times a day   prn—when needed.

6. Refill information.
7. Date.
8. The prescriber's name, address and registry (BNDD) number.
9. The prescriber's signature.

In many cases, a physician will transmit the prescription to the pharmacist via telephone. This cannot be done, however, with prescriptions for controlled substances (narcotics, stimulants, etc.). The law requires that pharmacists dispense these medications only upon receipt of a written prescription signed by the physician.

Refill Laws Regulations on refilling prescriptions vary from state to state. Federal law, however, stipulates that prescriptions for Class II controlled drugs may not be refilled and that prescriptions for Class III, IV and V drugs are valid for only six months. A maximum of five refills are allowed during the six-month period. (For an explanation of the differences among different classes of drugs, see the Glossary.)

Pharmacists exercise considerable judgment in determining whether or not to contact a physician regarding refills. Any time that there is a question about the advisability of refilling a prescription, the pharmacist will check with your physician to be sure that he wants you to continue taking that medication. In the event that the pharmacist is unable to reach your doctor for a refill authorization, he may dispense a small quantity to tide you over until he can reach your doctor.

EXPENDITURES FOR DRUGS

The prices of drugs, like those of almost all consumer products, are affected by our general economy. In recent years, these prices have climbed, and many consumers now shop for the "best buy" in their prescriptions, just as they shop for the best buy in a TV set. Prices for identical medications do vary greatly; the reasons for this are numerous.

The price of a prescription must obviously cover the cost of the ingredients, the container used, labor, professional services, overhead and a reasonable level of profit. Different pharmacies have different expenses, which are reflected in the prices you pay. Moreover, some pharmacists calculate their fees and profits in relation to the cost of the ingredients in each prescription, while others have set standard fees that they apply to all of their prescriptions.

But when you think of the prices you pay, more than the prescription itself should be considered. A discount pharmacy may offer a cost savings, but it is unlikely that the pharmacist there will inform you about how to take your prescription, warn you about side effects, keep a patient profile on all of the medications you are taking and answer your questions. This type of care and expenditure of time are built into the price charged for the same drug at another pharmacy. In addition to price, such factors as the convenience of the location, the hours the store is open and the availability of delivery service will obviously affect your selection of a pharmacy.

Generic vs Brand-Name Prescriptions Generic drugs are often less expensive than brand-name products. The generic name is the official name given to a drug, while the brand name is the registered trade name given to a drug by its manufacturer. Since the manufacturer of a specific drug has a large investment in research and advertising, the cost of brand-name products must cover these expenses. For example, a brand-name anti-anxiety agent might cost twice as much as its generic equivalent, chlordiazepoxide. Consumers concerned about costs should discuss this question with their doctors so that prescriptions are written for the least expensive form of a specific drug. And they should ask their pharmacists for help in selecting generic "over the counter" drugs, as opposed to more expensive brand-name products. Some drugs, however, are not available under generic labels because the 17-year patents obtained by their original manufacturers have not yet expired. Furthermore, some brand-name items are priced so low that they don't cost much more than the generics.

Drug Prices in Hospitals Among hospitals, the charges made to patients for drugs also vary widely. Some hospitals simply add a specific percentage to the cost of acquiring the medication. Others charge a dispensing fee, which is calculated according to the cost of acquiring the medication, operating expenses, a profit margin and the number of units that are dispensed. Still other hospitals price their drugs by a markup fee system, which combines features of each of the other two systems. The most recent pricing method tried by hospitals is the per diem system; a uniform drug charge is made per day to each type of patient.

Consumer Drug Digest

HEART DISEASES AND DISEASES OF THE CIRCULATORY SYSTEM

HEART DISEASES AND DISEASES OF THE CIRCULATORY SYSTEM

HEART ATTACK AND STROKE

HEART ATTACK

A heart attack is an acute illness that damages a portion of the heart muscle. "Myocardial infarction," "coronary occlusion" and "coronary thrombosis" are other terms used to describe a heart attack.

A heart attack usually occurs when a blood clot appears in one of the blood vessels of the heart. The clot may have formed slowly or rapidly. Typically a person who suffers a heart attack has a history of heart pain, but many heart victims have never experienced any symptoms of heart problems.

Once a heart attack has occurred, immediate treatment is required. The goal of treatment is to keep damage to the heart muscle at a minimum and to keep the patient alive until the damaged heart muscle can heal. The victim of a heart attack must rest and his or her pain must be relieved promptly. Drugs and other measures, including surgery, are used to help restore normal circulation through the heart and to return the heart to a more normal beat.

Early treatment in the hospital involves a variety of drugs, which are often given by injection. Drug therapy, along with a properly managed exercise program and diet, continues to be very important when a heart attack victim is on the way to recovery.

Drugs given to patients following a heart attack include those used to treat and prevent a variety of heart diseases, any of which may occur once a heart has been damaged by a heart attack.

STROKE

A stroke occurs when a portion of the brain is damaged by bleeding in the brain, which is usually caused by a ruptured blood vessel. Strokes can also occur when blood circulation to the brain is reduced severely because of the presence of blood clots within the vessels in the brain. Other terms used to describe a stroke include "cerebral vascular accident," "intracranial hemorrhage," "cerebral thrombosis," "cerebral embolism" and "apoplexy."

Recovery from a stroke generally requires a long period of time; sometimes permanent damage to the brain occurs, and a full recovery is impossible. A stroke victim may suffer paralysis on one or both sides of the body, speech impairment or the loss or impairment of other body functions. A rehabilitation program which includes massage, exercise, physical therapy or speech training is often necessary.

Following a stroke, the aim of drug therapy is to control high blood pressure and prevent blood clots.

Congestive Heart Failure

This condition, in which a weakened heart cannot do its work as well as it should, is described in many ways. The medical term is "congestive heart failure." To say that the heart is "failing" does not mean that it will stop beating, only that it is not working as efficiently as it should. The term "congestive" refers to a backup or slowdown in the movement of blood and fluids through the circulatory system. "Dropsy" is an old-fashioned term for congestive heart failure that is seldom used today; it refers to the fluid that accumulates in the abdomen and legs of someone suffering from congestive heart failure.

Congestive heart failure occurs when the heart's ability to pump blood has been reduced by congenital heart disease, rheumatic heart disease, high blood pressure, narrowing of the arteries by atherosclerosis, coronary artery disease or heart attack. The heart muscle lacks sufficient strength to keep the blood circulating normally throughout the body. As a result, the flow of blood is inadequate to meet all the body's needs. The heart goes on working, but not as strongly as it should to maintain good health.

To understand what happens when heart failure occurs it is necessary to know something about how the heart works as a pump. The heart is a hollow, muscular organ that pumps blood through the body. An adult's heart is about the size of a man's clenched fist and is shaped like an egg. It is located slightly to the left of the center of the chest and is protected by the breastbone and the rib cage.

In an adult, the heart normally beats between 60 and 90 times per minute, or about 100,000 times a day. It pumps blood, which carries nourishment and oxygen to billions of body cells and removes waste from these cells, through the arteries. The veins then carry blood back to the heart for recirculation. The heart's job is to keep just exactly the right amount of blood flowing to all parts of the body.

The amount of blood pumped by the heart varies with the body's activity. Sometimes a considerable flow of blood is needed, sometimes less. The heart and blood vessels normally have the power to adjust the flow of blood to meet the body's needs.

Most of the time the heart does not work as hard as it is capable of doing. Sitting, standing, walking and other moderate activities place only slight demands upon the heart. But during more strenuous activity the heart must pump harder. The body needs more blood than usual to climb a flight of stairs, and much more to run or exercise vigorously. During some illnesses, and when a fever is present, the heart must also work harder. Normally, the heart has great reserves of strength to call upon and can adjust to meet the body's needs.

When the heart is weakened by a heart attack, rheumatic fever, lengthy periods of high blood pressure, gradual narrowing of the body's arteries or any other abnormal condition, the heart does not pump efficiently. When this happens, the flow of blood slows down and the body's workings are impaired. Blood which is returning to the heart through the veins tends to back up. As the blood fails to circulate sufficiently quickly, some of the fluid in the blood is forced out through the thin blood vessel walls into surrounding tissue.

There the fluid backs up or "congests." The result is swelling or "edema," which can occur in many parts of the body, but is seen most commonly in the legs or ankles. Sometimes fluid collects in the lungs, making a person short of breath.

Heart failure also affects the ability of the kidneys to dispose of salt and water. Salt which is normally eliminated in the urine stays in the body and holds water in the body. The fluid retained in this way aggravates the edema.

Only a physician can determine the treatment for someone suffering from congestive heart failure. Treating the underlying cause of congestive heart failure is often an important part of therapy. For instance, if high blood pressure is placing strain on the heart, it can often be reduced or controlled by drugs and a restricted diet. Or when defective heart valves are causing heart failure, they can often be corrected by surgery.

In general, congestive heart failure requires more than one kind of therapy. The successful treatment of this disorder requires the patient's clear understanding of his or her responsibility and role in treatment. Rest, drugs and a modified diet and daily activity may all be prescribed—and all doctors' instructions should be followed to the letter.

Many patients need rest. Strict bed rest may be necessary, either in the hospital or at home. Physical activity should usually increase only gradually. To avoid strain on the heart, some patients may have to adjust to a slower pace and take things a bit easier.

A sodium-restricted diet is almost always necessary in the treatment of congestive heart failure to prevent or reduce edema or fluid accumulation. Sodium is a mineral essential to life, but ordinarily we get more than we need from the food we eat. Because table salt contains a large amount of sodium, a diet designed to reduce the amount of sodium and fluid in the body restricts the use of table salt and may also require abstaining from certain foods that contain a high amount of sodium. Salt substitutes are available, which makes this task much easier.

Several medications may be prescribed for the treatment of fluid accumulation. One may be a drug called a diuretic or "water pill," which increases the amount and frequency of urination. A diuretic helps the kidneys get rid of excess water and sodium. This not only relieves edema but may also help in controlling high blood pressure.

The most common drugs given orally to patients with congestive heart failure are digitoxin, digoxin, lanatoside C and gitalin, which are all called digitalis glycosides. These drugs can also be used to treat other disorders of the heart, including atrial fibrillation, in which part of the heart has a fast, irregular rhythm or an otherwise irregular heartbeat pattern (these are called "arrhythmias").

Digitalis Drugs
(di ji tal' is)

Brand names for Digitoxin: Crystodigin, Purodigin
Brand name for Digoxin: Lanoxin
Brand name for Gitalin: Gitaligin
Brand name for Lanatoside C: Cedilanid
Brand names for a mixture of chemicals from the digitalis plant: Digifortis, Digiglusin, Pil-Digis

All drugs in the digitalis group act on the body to produce the same effects, both beneficial and otherwise. They are prescribed for patients suffering from congestive heart failure and other heart diseases. A prescription may thus be for digitalis, digitoxin (Crystodigin, Purodigin) or digoxin (Lanoxin), the most commonly-prescribed drugs in the group, or for lanatoside C (Cedilanid) or gitalin (Gitaligin). All of the digitalis drugs are sufficiently similar that they can be discussed as a group. The term "digitalis" is used here to refer to any drug in the group.

Digitalis helps an injured or weakened heart do the very best job that it is capable of doing. Digitalis acts directly on the heart muscle to strengthen the force of the heart muscle's contractions. This sends more blood through the body and makes the heart's action more efficient.

By improving the circulation of blood, digitalis helps remove excess water from the tissues and relieves symptoms of heart failure such as edema (swelling, usually of the lower legs or ankles) and shortness of breath. Digitalis alone will, however, rarely relieve these symptoms completely; doctors may prescribe a diuretic (water pill) in combination with the digitalis. (See the section on **diuretics**, page 9, for more information.) They may also recommend a diet low in salt, because salt holds water in the body and makes diuretics less effective in removing excess water.

Digitalis also slows the heart rate and helps restore a normal, steady rhythm. It can be used alone or in combination with other medications that help regulate the heart beat. (See the section on **irregular heartbeat or arrhythmia**, page 35, for further information.)

UNDESIRED EFFECTS
Digitalis is a strong and effective drug. Patients must work closely with their doctors to find the dosage that works best without producing unwanted effects. If digitalis is prescribed for you, you will probably have to take it for a long time—possibly for the rest of your life.

When you first start to take digitalis, your doctor will probably prescribe a large dose; the dosage will be reduced later on. It is important that you cooperate with your doctor by always taking the exact amount he prescribes and by telling him if you think you are suffering any bad effects from this medication.

Contact your doctor immediately if you experience loss of appetite, excessive salivation, nausea, vomiting or diarrhea; changes in vision such as blurring, color changes (usually in yellow-green vision) or seeing spots or halos; headache, confusion or depression; irregular heartbeats or changes in pulse rate. These could be signs that you are taking too much digitalis; your doctor needs to know about them to adjust the dosage or change the drug.

It is possible to have more digitalis in the body than is needed; having too little can also be a problem. Difficulty in breathing and swelling in the legs and ankles are the most common signs of this. If normal activity causes shortness of breath, or if shortness of breath makes you awaken frequently during the night, tell your doctor.

Once you and your doctor have determined the dosage that is right for you, you will not usually experience side effects as long as you take digitalis exactly as prescribed.

PRECAUTIONS

Digitalis can cause the body to lose potassium, an important mineral or electrolyte, especially if you are also taking a diuretic (water pill). Your doctor may prescribe a potassium replacement. You should also ask for a list of foods that are high in potassium and emphasize them in a well-balanced diet. (See **potassium supplements**, page 54, for more information.)

Before you start to take digitalis, tell your doctor if you are taking any nonprescription drugs, such as laxatives, antacids or cough, cold or allergy medication. These medications can decrease the effect of digitalis or increase it to a potentially dangerous level.

Also tell your doctor about any other prescription drugs you are taking, especially drugs which increase the production of urine (diuretics or water pills) or other drugs for your heart condition. If you do not know the names of the drugs you are taking or what they are prescribed for, take the labeled containers to your doctor or pharmacist.

Be sure your doctor knows if you have ever taken digitalis in the past. Tell him what reaction you had to this medication. (Allergies can occur, although they are uncommon.) Your general state of health can affect the way digitalis acts on you. Tell your doctor everything you can about your health, including especially thyroid, kidney or liver problems.

If you develop an illness other than your heart disease, vomiting and diarrhea can affect the amount of digitalis reaching your heart. If you go to another doctor for such an illness, be sure to tell him that you are taking digitalis. You may wish to carry a card indicating you are taking digitalis so that your doctors will know in the event of an accident that renders you unconscious.

If you are pregnant or plan to become pregnant or are nursing a baby, tell your doctor before you start to take digitalis.

Do not stop taking digitalis unless you have your doctor's permission. Do not take any new drugs without checking first with your doctor.

DOSAGE AND STORAGE

The digitalis drugs come in tablets, capsules and liquid form, and should be used only under the close supervision of a doctor. *It is very important that digitalis be taken on a regular schedule.*

You may be instructed to take a large dose at first and reduce it after a few days. The continuing or maintenance dosage may vary from time to time, depending on your response to the drug. Do not be alarmed if your doctor makes occasional changes in the dosage, especially at the beginning of treatment. Carefully follow the instructions on your prescription label, and ask your doctor or pharmacist to explain any instructions you do not understand.

If your doctor tells you to take digitalis once a day, take it at the same time every day. Taking your medication at the same time you do something else every day, such as brushing your teeth in the morning or going to bed at night, may help you remember to take it.

If you forget a dose, do not take the missed dose when you remember it. Omit that dose and take only the next scheduled dose at the next scheduled time. *Do not take a double dose.* If you forget to take two or more doses in a row, contact your doctor or pharmacist for instructions.

Your doctor may recommend a low-salt or low-sodium diet. Follow his recommendation, because it will help your medication to work as it should. He may also suggest that you stop smoking cigarettes, which can make the heart muscle more sensitive to digitalis. Ask your doctor about use of alcohol and caffeine. He will probably tell you that both are safe in moderation.

While you are taking digitalis, your doctor may ask you to check your pulse every day. He will tell you how to do this, and how rapid your pulse should be. If your pulse is slower than your doctor has told you it should be, contact him to find out whether you should continue taking digitalis.

Your doctor may perform certain tests to determine the effect of digitalis on your body, including blood counts, tests to determine the levels of certain electrolytes (especially sodium and potassium) in your blood and electrocardiograms. *Keep all appointments with your doctor and with laboratories.*

It is important that you keep digitalis out of the reach of children. It has been a frequent cause of accidental poisoning in children. Keep digitalis in the container it came in and do not allow anyone else to take it.

Note: The drugs in this "digitalis group" are all similar but are *not* interchangeable. The body metabolizes each of them differently, and therefore dosage is not the same for all of them.

Diuretics

Diuretics are also used in the treatment of congestive heart failure. (See the sections on **diuretics**, page 9; **thiazide diuretics**, page 11; and discussions of individual drugs under **high blood pressure or hypertension**, page 9.)

High Blood Pressure or Hypertension

High blood pressure or hypertension may be present for many years, unaccompanied by any symptoms other than tiredness, nervousness, dizziness or headaches. Your blood pressure should be checked every time you visit a doctor, for whatever reason, so that high blood pressure can be detected as early as possible. You should have your blood pressure checked annually, even if you have no symptoms of high blood pressure and have not visited a doctor for any other reason.

High blood pressure can be treated easily with a proper diet, moderate lifestyle and drug therapy. If high blood pressure remains untreated, it can lead to much more serious health problems, including congestive heart failure, heart attacks, strokes and serious kidney disease.

High blood pressure occurs when the blood vessels constrict or narrow, causing resistance to the flow of blood. The causes of high blood pressure are many; they include abnormalities in the heart, kidneys or nervous control of the blood vessels.

The drugs used to treat high blood pressure may act on the heart, the nervous system or the kidneys, individually or in any combination. Frequently more than one drug is used.

Thiazide diuretics are considered the most useful drugs in the initial treatment of high blood pressure. If a diuretic alone does not effectively control blood pressure, other drugs discussed in this section and generally referred to as antihypertensive drugs are added to the treatment.

DIURETICS

Diuretics are commonly referred to as "water pills." They act on the kidneys, causing them to eliminate excess water and salt from the body through the urine. For almost 20 years oral diuretics have been a mainstay of treatment for high blood pressure. They help control high blood pressure while keeping the amount of medication prescribed—and the number of undesired effects—at a minimum. Diuretics can help control high blood pressure, but do not cure it. Diuretics are also used to treat the retention of fluid in the body caused by a number of different illnesses, such as heart, liver or kidney disease. Some other drugs, such as steroids or estrogens, can cause your body to retain water; diuretics can be used to relieve this side effect of drug therapy.

THIAZIDE DIURETICS

Thiazide and thiazidelike diuretics are a "family" of drugs that are very closely related in chemical structure and in their action in the body. Their pressure-lowering effects and undesired effects are very similar, but they may differ somewhat in the duration of their diuretic action. Your doctor will choose the one best suited for you and for your lifestyle. Included in the "family" of thiazide diuretics and discussed later in this chapter are chlorothiazide (Chlorulan, Diuril), hydrochlorothiazide (Esidrix, Hydrodiuril, Oretic, Thiuretic), hydroflumethiazide (Diucardin, Saluron), methyclothiazide (Aquatensen, Enduron) and chlorthalidone (Hygroton). Anything written here about thiazide diuretics holds true for all of these individual drugs.

Thiazide diuretics reduce blood pressure by acting on both the kidneys and the blood vessels. In the kidneys, these drugs prevent salt and water from returning to other body tissues. Urine production and the frequency of urination are increased, and an increased amount of salt and water is eliminated from the body. Thus the volume of fluid in the body is reduced, and the amount of salt (whose most important component is sodium) in body tissues is similarly reduced.

At the same time, thiazides act on the small blood vessels, causing the walls of the vessels to relax—the blood vessels consequently expand, and the space available for the circulation of blood is increased. The combined effect of reduced volume of fluid and expanded space is a reduction in blood pressure. Thiazide diuretics, when given alone for mild high blood pressure, will often reduce the pressure to a normal range. They are usually considered the drugs of choice for the initial treatment of high blood pressure when there is no underlying kidney disease. *Unless your doctor tells you to stop, you should continue to take your diuretic even if you feel good.* If you have edema or high blood pressure, you will usually have to take a diuretic, and possibly other drugs, for the rest of your life.

UNDESIRED EFFECTS

Side effects may occur during the first week you take a thiazide diuretic, but they often go away within another week. While you are taking a thiazide diuretic, the levels of minerals or electrolytes such as potassium in your body can get too low. If you begin to suffer from muscle cramps, nausea or weakness, excessive thirst, drowsiness or restlessness or a rapid pulse, call your doctor right away. You may need to eat foods rich in potassium (e.g., bananas, oranges and other fruits) or to take a potassium supplement. (See **potassium supplements**, page 54, for more information.) Sometimes you can take a thiazide diuretic in combination with certain other diuretic drugs to avoid excessive loss of potassium.

PRECAUTIONS

Before starting to take any diuretic, discuss your general health and medical history with your doctor. Be sure to tell him if you have or have ever had liver disease, since the loss of salts and water caused by diuretics can worsen liver disease. Similarly, diuretics can increase blood sugar levels, so if you are diabetic or have a tendency toward diabetes, a change in diet and/or medication for diabetes may be needed. Diuretics can cause a gout attack in patients with a history of gout. Rarely, diuretics can worsen or activate lupus erythematosus. Since these drugs act on the kidneys, your doctor should be told if you have ever had kidney disease or trouble with your kidneys. If your kidneys are not working properly, the amount and type of drug you take may need to be changed.

Most diuretics are chemically similar to the "sulfa drugs" (sulfonamide anti-infectives) and to some of the drugs taken orally for the treatment of diabetes. If you have ever had an allergic reaction to sulfas, to a diabetes-treatment drug or to any diuretic, be sure your doctor knows about it before you begin to take a thiazide or other diuretic.

Also, your doctor must know about any other drugs you are taking, especially cortisone-type drugs or steroids, digitalis heart medicines, lithium carbonate or diabetic drugs. The effects of these drugs may change when you begin taking a diuretic.

Taking a diuretic may make you need to urinate more often—these drugs are designed to remove excess water from your body. Unless your doctor tells you otherwise, take your diuretic in the morning. If you have to take the drug more than once a day, take the second dose before 6:00 p.m. to avoid having to urinate after you have gone to bed.

While taking any diuretic, avoid excessive heat; sweating can cause the loss of too much water and salt from your body.

DOSAGE
Thiazide diuretics may be taken alone or in combination with other drugs used to treat high blood pressure. Different people's responses to thiazides can vary, depending on their diseases, the efficiency of their hearts, their levels of physical activity, their diets and what other drugs they are taking at the same time.

THIAZIDE DIURETICS
Chlorothiazide
(klor oh thye'a zide)

Brand names: Chlorulan, Diuril
(Read the paragraphs on **diuretics** and **thiazide diuretics**, pages 9 and 10.)
Chlorothiazide begins to act as a diuretic, increasing excretion of water and salt, about two hours after it is taken and goes on working for six to 12 hours. No effect on blood pressure may be seen for two to three weeks.

UNDESIRED EFFECTS
Chlorothiazide causes frequent urination, which should decrease after you have been taking it for a few weeks. Because chlorothiazide removes potassium as well as salt from the body, you may experience muscle weakness, cramps,

dizziness or lightheadedness, especially when you stand up or when you arise from a lying position. If your doctor has prescribed a potassium supplement for you, take it as prescribed. Contact your doctor if he has not prescribed supplemental potassium or if these side effects persist in spite of the fact that you are taking a potassium supplement. Allergic reactions such as skin rash or hives, nausea, vomiting, reduced appetite, stomach cramps, diarrhea, headache or blurred vision may also occur.

While you are taking chlorothiazide, you run an increased risk of sunburn. Limit the amount of time you spend in the sun or under a sunlamp. Wear sunglasses and be sure your body is covered by clothing or protected by a sunscreen preparation when you go out in the sun.

If you experience a sore throat or easy bruising, contact your doctor. If you have an illness that causes vomiting or diarrhea, the fluid balance in your body may be upset. Discontinue taking chlorothiazide and contact your doctor.

PRECAUTIONS

Laboratory tests for kidney and liver function, blood counts and tests to determine the levels of sodium, potassium, sugar and uric acid in your blood will probably be done periodically while you are taking chlorothiazide. *Be sure to keep all appointments with your doctor and at the laboratory*.

Before taking chlorothiazide, inform the doctor of other prescription or non-prescription drugs you are taking. If you do not know the names of the drugs or what they were prescribed for, take the labeled containers to your doctor or pharmacist.

Alcoholic beverages may exaggerate the degree to which chlorothiazide lowers blood pressure, causing lightheadedness or dizziness.

If you become pregnant while taking chlorothiazide, contact your doctor before continuing to take it.

DOSAGE AND STORAGE

Chlorothiazide comes in tablets and liquid and is taken orally. Your prescription label tells you specifically how much to take and how often to take it. Follow the instructions carefully and contact your doctor or pharmacist if you have any questions. *Do not take more of this drug than your doctor prescribes* because excessive loss of water and salt from your body can cause unpleasant side effects.

If you are to take this medication twice a day, it is best to take it once in the morning and again in the middle of the afternoon so that you will not have to urinate during the night.

Chlorothiazide should be taken right after meals or with a snack. The liquid should first be thoroughly shaken.

If you forget to take a dose, do not take the missed dose when you remember it. Omit that dose and take your regular dose at the next scheduled time.

Your doctor may recommend that you eat a low-salt or low-sodium diet, take a potassium supplement or increase the amount of potassium-rich foods in your diet (such as bananas and orange juice). Follow his recommendations; the medication will work better and you will feel better.

Keep this medication in the container it came in and out of the reach of children. Do not allow anyone else to take it.

Chlorthalidone

(klor thal' i doan)

Brand name: Hygroton

(Read the paragraphs on **diuretics** and **thiazide diuretics**, pages 9 and 10.)

Chlorthalidone, while not truly a thiazide in chemical makeup, is very similar to the thiazides in structure and in the way it acts on the body. Chlorthalidone is a long-acting diuretic. It begins to work as a diuretic, increasing elimination of water and salt, about two hours after it is taken, and goes on working for 24 to 72 hours. You will have to take chlorthalidone for two or three weeks before you will know if it is going to be effective in lowering your blood pressure.

UNDESIRED EFFECTS

A common effect of chlorthalidone is frequent urination. This tends to disappear after you have been taking the medication for a few weeks. Dry mouth will also disappear after a few weeks, but in the meantime, it can be relieved by chewing gum, sucking on hard candy or drinking fluids.

Because this drug removes potassium as well as salt from the body, you may experience muscle weakness or cramps, or dizziness or lightheadedness, especially on arising from a sitting or lying position. Contact your doctor if you experience these effects. If your doctor prescribes a potassium supplement, be sure to take it as instructed. If you were not given a potassium supplement or if you continue to experience muscle weakness or cramps while taking the supplements, contact your doctor.

While taking chlorthalidone you run an increased risk of sunburn. Limit the amount of time you spend in sunlight or under a sunlamp. When you go out in the sun, wear sunglasses and be sure your body is covered with clothing or protected by a sunscreen preparation.

If you experience a sore throat or easy bruising, contact your doctor. Stomach upsets can be relieved by taking chlorthalidone with meals or a snack. If you have an illness that causes vomiting or diarrhea, the fluid balance in your body may be upset. Stop taking chlorthalidone and contact your doctor.

PRECAUTIONS

Laboratory tests of kidney and liver function, of blood levels of sodium, potassium, sugar and uric acid and blood counts will probably be done periodically while you are taking chlorthalidone. *Be sure to keep all appointments with your doctor and at the laboratory.*

Inform your doctor of all the prescription and nonprescription drugs you are taking. If you do not know the names of the drugs or what they were prescribed for, take the labeled containers to your doctor or pharmacist.

Alcoholic beverages may exaggerate the effect of chlorthalidone in lowering your blood pressure and cause lightheadedness or dizziness.

Chlorthalidone should not be taken during pregnancy except for the treatment of some serious complications of pregnancy. If you become pregnant while taking chlorthalidone, contact your doctor before continuing to take it.

DOSAGE AND STORAGE

Chlorthalidone tablets are usually taken once a day or once every other day. Your prescription label specifies how much to take and when to take each dose. Follow the instructions carefully and contact your doctor or pharmacist if you have any questions. *Do not take more of this drug than your doctor prescribes* because excessive loss of water and salt from your body can cause unpleasant side effects.

It is a good idea to take this medication in the morning with your breakfast so that you will not have to urinate during the night.

If you forget to take a dose, take it when you remember if this is at least 12 hours before your next dose. If it is less than 12 hours to the next scheduled dose, skip the forgotten dose and take only your next scheduled dose at the regularly scheduled time.

Your doctor may recommend certain dietary changes such as a low-salt or low-sodium diet, taking a potassium supplement or increasing the amount of potassium-rich foods (such as bananas and orange juice) in your diet. Follow his recommendations; the medication will work better and you will feel better.

Keep chlorthalidone in the container it came in, and out of the reach of children. Do not allow anyone else to take this medication.

Hydrochlorothiazide
(hye droe klor oh thye'a zide)

Brand names: Esidrix, Hydrodiuril, Oretic, Thiuretic and others

(Read the paragraphs on **diuretics** and **thiazide diuretics**, pages 9 and 10.)

Hydrochlorothiazide begins to work as a diuretic, increasing elimination of water and salt, about two hours after it is taken and goes on working for six to 12 hours. You will have to take this drug for two or three weeks before you will know if it is going to be effective in lowering blood pressure.

UNDESIRED EFFECTS

Frequent urination, a common effect of hydrochlorothiazide, should disappear after you have been taking it for a few weeks.

You may experience muscle weakness or cramps or lightheadedness on standing or arising from a lying position. If your doctor prescribes a potassium supplement, be sure to take it as instructed. If you were not given a potassium supplement, if you experience muscle weakness or cramps or if these symptoms continue in spite of your taking potassium, contact your doctor. Allergic reactions such as skin rash or hives, nausea and vomiting, reduced appetite, stomach cramps, diarrhea, headache or blurred vision may also occur.

You run an increased risk of sunburn while you are taking hydrochlorothiazide. Limit the amount of time you spend in the sun or under a sunlamp. When you go out in the sun, wear sunglasses and be sure your body is covered with clothing or protected by a sunscreen preparation.

Contact your doctor if you experience a sore throat or easy bruising. If you have an illness that causes vomiting or diarrhea, the fluid balance in your body may be upset. Stop taking hydrochlorothiazide and contact your doctor.

PRECAUTIONS

Laboratory tests for kidney and liver function, tests of the levels of sodium, potassium, sugar and uric acid in your blood and blood counts will probably be done periodically while you are taking this drug. *Keep all appointments with your doctor and at the laboratory.*

Inform your doctor of all other prescription and nonprescription drugs you are taking. If you do not know the names of the drugs or what they were prescribed for, take the labeled containers to your doctor or pharmacist.

Alcoholic beverages may exaggerate the effect of hydrochlorothiazide in lowering your blood pressure and cause lightheadedness or dizziness.

Hydrochlorothiazide should not be taken during pregnancy except for the treatment of some serious complications of pregnancy. If you become pregnant while taking hydrochlorothiazide, contact your doctor before continuing to take it.

DOSAGE AND STORAGE

Hydrochlorothiazide comes in tablets and is taken orally. Your prescription label tells specifically how much to take and how often to take it. Follow the instructions carefully and contact your doctor or pharmacist if you have any questions. *Do not take more of this drug than your doctor prescribes* because excessive loss of water and salt from your body can cause unpleasant side effects.

If you are to take this medication twice a day, it is a good idea to take it once in the morning and once in the middle of the afternoon so that you will not have to urinate during the night. Hydrochlorothiazide should be taken right after meals or with a snack.

If you forget to take a dose, do not take the missed dose when you remember it. Omit that dose and take your regular dose at the next scheduled time.

Be sure to follow any dietary recommendations made by your doctor. These may include eating a low-salt or low-sodium diet, taking a potassium supplement or increasing the amount of potassium-rich foods (such as bananas and orange juice) in your diet. The medication will work better and you will feel better.

Keep this medication in the container it came in and out of the reach of children. Do not allow anyone else to take this medication.

Hydroflumethiazide
(hye droe flume eh thye′a zide)

Brand names: Diucardin, Saluron

(Read the paragraphs on **diuretics** and **thiazide diuretics**, pages 9 and 10.)

Hydroflumethiazide begins to eliminate excess water and salt from the system about two hours after it is taken and goes on working for 12 to 24 hours. No effect on blood pressure may be seen for two to three weeks.

UNDESIRED EFFECTS

Hydroflumethiazide causes frequent urination, which should decrease after you have been taking it for a few weeks.

Because hydroflumethiazide removes potassium as well as salt from the body, you may experience muscle weakness, cramps or dizziness, especially when you stand up or when you arise from a lying position. Contact your doctor if these side effects persist. Allergic reactions such as skin rash or hives, headache, blurred vision, reduced appetite, nausea, vomiting and diarrhea may also occur. Be sure to take a potassium supplement if one has been prescribed for you.

While you are taking hydroflumethiazide you run an increased risk of sunburn. Limit the amount of time you spend in sunlight or under a sunlamp. Wear sunglasses and be sure your body is covered by clothing or protected by a sunscreen preparation when you are in sunlight.

If you experience a sore throat or easy bruising, contact your doctor. The fluid balance in your body can be upset by vomiting or diarrhea, so if you have an illness that causes vomiting or diarrhea, stop taking hydroflumethiazide and contact your doctor.

PRECAUTIONS

Keep all appointments for checkups and laboratory tests. Laboratory tests for kidney and liver function, blood counts and tests to determine the levels of sodium, potassium, sugar and uric acid in your blood will probably be done periodically while you are taking hydroflumethiazide.

Before taking hydroflumethiazide, inform your doctor of any other prescription or nonprescription drugs you are taking. If you do not know the names of the drugs or what they were prescribed for, take the labeled containers to your doctor or pharmacist.

Alcoholic beverages may exaggerate the degree to which hydroflumethiazide lowers blood pressure, causing lightheadedness or dizziness.

If you become pregnant while taking hydroflumethiazide, contact your doctor before continuing to take it.

DOSAGE AND STORAGE

Hydroflumethiazide comes in tablets and is taken orally. Your prescription label tells you specifically how much to take and how often to take it. Follow the instructions carefully and contact your doctor or pharmacist if you have any questions. *Do not take more of this drug than your doctor prescribes* because excessive loss of water and salt from your body can cause unpleasant side effects.

If you are to take this medication twice a day, it is best to take it once in the morning and again in the middle of the afternoon so that you will not have to urinate during the night. This medication should be taken right after meals or with a snack.

If you forget to take a dose, omit that dose and take your regular dose at the next scheduled time.

Your doctor may recommend that you eat a low-salt or low-sodium diet, take a potassium supplement or increase the amount of potassium-rich foods (such as bananas and orange juice) in your diet. Follow his recommendations; the medication will work better and you will feel better.

Keep this medication in the container it came in, and keep it out of the reach of children. Do not allow anyone else to take it.

Methyclothiazide
(meth i kloe thye′a zide)

Brand names: Aquatensen, Enduron
(Read the paragraphs on **diuretics** and **thiazide diuretics**, pages 9 and 10.)

Methyclothiazide is the most potent of the thiazide diuretics. Methyclothiazide begins to work as a diuretic, increasing excretion of water and salt, about two hours after it is taken and goes on working for about 24 hours. No effect on blood pressure may be seen for two to three weeks.

UNDESIRED EFFECTS
Frequent urination, a common effect of methyclothiazide, should decrease after you have taken it for a few weeks. Another effect is dry mouth; this effect will disappear after a few weeks. In the meantime, dry mouth can be relieved by chewing gum, sucking on hard candy or drinking fluids.

You may experience muscle weakness, cramps or dizziness because this drug removes body potassium as well as salt. Contact your doctor if these side effects persist. Allergic reactions such as skin rash or hives, nausea and vomiting, reduced appetite, stomach cramps, diarrhea, headache or blurred vision may also occur. Be sure to take your potassium supplement as instructed if one has been prescribed for you.

While taking methyclothiazide you run an increased risk of sunburn. Limit the amount of time you spend in sunlight or under a sunlamp. When you are in sunlight, wear sunglasses and be sure your body is covered with clothing or protected by a sunscreen preparation.

Contact your doctor if you experience a sore throat, easy bruising or a skin rash. If you have an illness that causes vomiting or diarrhea, the fluid balance in your body may be upset. Stop taking methyclothiazide and contact your doctor.

PRECAUTIONS
Laboratory tests for kidney and liver function, blood counts and tests to

determine the levels of sodium, potassium, sugar and uric acid in your blood will probably be done periodically while you are taking this drug. *Keep all appointments with your doctor and at the laboratory.*

Inform your doctor of all prescription or nonprescription drugs you are taking. If you do not know the names of the drugs or what they were prescribed for, take the labeled containers to your doctor or pharmacist.

Alcoholic beverages may exaggerate the degree to which methyclothiazide lowers blood pressure, causing lightheadedness or dizziness.

Methyclothiazide should not be taken during pregnancy except for treatment of some serious complications of pregnancy. If you become pregnant while taking methyclothiazide, contact your doctor before continuing to take it.

DOSAGE AND STORAGE

Your prescription label specifies how much methyclothiazide to take and how often to take the tablets. Follow the instructions carefully and contact your doctor or pharmacist if you have any questions. *Do not take more than your doctor has prescribed.* Excessive loss of water and salt can cause unpleasant side effects.

If you are to take this medication once a day, take it in the morning so you will not have to urinate during the night. Methyclothiazide may be taken after breakfast or lunch or with a midmorning snack.

If you forget to take a dose but remember it on the day you are to take it, take the missed dose. Then take your next regular dose at the scheduled time.

Be sure to follow any dietary recommendations of your doctor. These may include eating a low-salt or low-sodium diet, taking a potassium supplement or increasing the amount of potassium-rich foods (such as bananas and orange juice) in your diet. If you follow your doctor's dietary recommendations, the medication will work better and you will feel better.

Keep this medication in the container it came in, and keep it out of the reach of children. Do not allow anyone else to take it.

OTHER DIURETICS
Ethacrynic Acid
(eth a krin' ik ass id)

Brand name: Edecrin
(Read the paragraph on **diuretics**, page 9.)

Ethacrynic acid causes the kidneys to excrete unneeded salt and water in the urine. Ethacrynic acid is one of the "loop" diuretics because it acts on the loops of the tiny filtering tubes in the kidneys. It is a strong and effective diuretic used to treat high blood pressure and the swelling and water retention caused by a number of medical problems including heart disease and certain diseases of the kidney and liver.

This medication begins to work as a diuretic about 30 minutes after it is taken, and it keeps on working for six to eight hours. Ethacrynic acid may be useful in treating conditions that have not responded to other diuretics or when kidney function is decreased. You may have to take ethacrynic acid for a week or two before you will know if it lowers your blood pressure.

UNDESIRED EFFECTS

Frequent urination commonly occurs when you begin to take ethacrynic acid but usually decreases after you have been taking it for a few weeks.

Ethacrynic acid can cause nausea or loss of appetite. These effects should be lessened if you take this medication with meals or immediately after eating. Contact your doctor if these problems continue. If you have any illness that causes vomiting or diarrhea, the fluid balance in your body may be upset; stop taking ethacrynic acid and contact your doctor.

If your doctor prescribes a potassium supplement for you, be sure to take it exactly as instructed. If you were not given a potassium supplement, or if you experience muscle weakness or cramps, or if these symptoms continue in spite of your use of the supplement, contact your doctor.

Report to your doctor any unusual bleeding or bruising, sore throat, fever, skin rash or yellow skin discoloration. If you experience ringing in the ears or decreased hearing, contact your doctor.

PRECAUTIONS

Because ethacrynic acid is a powerful medication, your doctor will want to monitor your response to it carefully. Among the laboratory tests that will probably be performed while you are taking ethacrynic acid are tests for liver and kidney function, complete blood counts and tests to determine the levels of sodium, potassium, sugar and uric acid in your blood. Keep in touch with your doctor while you are taking ethacrynic acid, and *keep all your appointments for checkups and laboratory tests*.

Ethacrynic acid should not be taken by people taking certain other drugs. Before you begin to take ethacrynic acid, tell your doctor what other prescription or nonprescription drugs you are taking. If you do not know the names of the drugs or what they were prescribed for, take the labeled containers to your doctor or pharmacist.

Alcoholic beverages may exaggerate the degree to which ethacrynic acid lowers blood pressure, causing lightheadedness or dizziness.

Pregnant women and nursing mothers should not take ethacrynic acid.

DOSAGE AND STORAGE

Ethacrynic acid tablets are usually taken once or twice a day. Carefully follow the instructions on your prescription label. Ask your doctor or pharmacist to explain any part you do not understand. *Do not take more of this drug than your doctor has prescribed* because excessive loss of water and salt from your body can cause unpleasant side effects.

This medication should be taken with meals or immediately after eating.

If you forget to take a dose, omit that dose and take only your regular dose at the next scheduled time. *Never take a double dose*.

Your doctor may recommend that you increase the amount of potassium-rich foods (such as bananas and orange juice) in your diet. Be sure to follow his recommendations.

Keep this medication in the container it came in, and keep it out of the reach of children. Do not allow anyone else to take it.

Furosemide

(fur oh' se mide)

Brand name: Lasix

(Read the paragraph on **diuretics**, page 9.)

Furosemide is a "loop" diuretic that acts on the loops of the tiny filtering tubes in the kidneys. It prevents salt from returning to body tissues and excretes unneeded salt and water in the urine. Furosemide is a strong and effective diuretic that is used to treat high blood pressure and the swelling and water retention caused by a number of medical problems, including heart disease and certain diseases of the kidney and liver.

Furosemide begins to work as a diuretic about one hour after you take it, and it keeps on working for four to eight hours. It may be useful in treating people who have not responded to other diuretics or whose kidney function is not normal. You may have to take furosemide for a week or two before you know if it is going to be effective in lowering your blood pressure.

UNDESIRED EFFECTS

Frequent urination commonly occurs when you begin taking furosemide but usually decreases after you have been taking it for a few weeks.

The principal undesirable effects of furosemide are weakness or cramps of the muscles, lightheadedness and dizziness. If you experience any of these effects, contact your doctor. If you have any illness that causes vomiting or diarrhea, the fluid balance in your body may be upset; stop taking furosemide and contact your doctor.

If your doctor prescribes a potassium supplement, be sure to take it exactly as instructed. If you were not given a potassium supplement, or if you experience muscle weakness or cramps, or if these symptoms continue in spite of your use of the supplement, contact your doctor.

PRECAUTIONS

Because furosemide is a strong medication, your doctor will want to check your response to it carefully. Laboratory tests for liver and kidney function, blood counts and tests to determine the levels of sodium, potassium, sugar and uric acid in your blood will probably be done periodically while you are taking furosemide. Keep in touch with your doctor while you are taking it, and *keep all your appointments for checkups and laboratory tests.*

Weigh yourself at least every day or every other day. If you begin to gain weight rapidly or if your hands and feet begin to get puffy, contact your doctor. If you can pinch the skin on the top of your hand and it remains puckered after you let go, contact your doctor.

This drug should not be taken by people who are already taking certain other drugs. Before you begin to take furosemide, tell your doctor what other prescription or nonprescription drugs you are taking. If you do not know the names of the drugs or what they were prescribed for, take the labeled containers to your doctor or pharmacist.

Alcoholic beverages may exaggerate the degree to which furosemide lowers blood pressure, causing lightheadedness or dizziness.

Your doctor may recommend that you increase the amount of potassium-rich foods (such as bananas and orange juice) in your diet. Be sure to follow this recommendation.

Generally, pregnant women, women who might become pregnant during treatment and nursing mothers should not take furosemide.

DOSAGE AND STORAGE

Furosemide tablets are usually taken once or twice a day. Your prescription label gives specific instructions as to how much furosemide to take and how often to take it. Follow these instructions carefully and ask your doctor or pharmacist if you do not understand any part of them. *Do not take more of this drug than your doctor has prescribed* because excessive loss of water and salt from your body can cause unpleasant side effects.

If you are to take furosemide twice a day, take one dose in the morning and one in the middle of the afternoon so you can avoid having to urinate during the night.

If you forget to take a dose, take a missed dose as soon as you remember it. *But do not take two doses at one time to make up for the missed dose.*

Keep this medication in the container it came in. Do not be concerned if your furosemide tablets turn dark after you have had them for a while. This change in color does not make them less effective.

Keep this medication out of the reach of children. Do not allow anyone else to take it.

Spironolactone
(speer on oh lak′ tone)

Brand name: Aldactone
(Read the paragraph on **diuretics**, page 9.)

Spironolactone is used alone or in combination with other drugs to treat high blood pressure and the water retention caused by such conditions as heart disease, liver disease and lung problems. Its action on the kidneys causes them to eliminate unneeded salt and water from the body in the urine.

Although spironolactone's diuretic effect is less rapid and perhaps less effective than that of other diuretics, it removes much less body potassium than these drugs. Therefore, spironolactone is often prescribed in combination with other diuretics and other drugs taken to lower blood pressure when the aim is to reduce potassium loss and increase the lowering of blood pressure. The diuretic effect of spironolactone may not occur until three to five days after the drug is taken. The lowering of blood pressure takes two to four weeks to become evident. Spironolactone may also be useful in treating high blood pressure in those people who have gout or diabetes, two conditions that can be made worse by use of the thiazide diuretics.

UNDESIRED EFFECTS

Spironolactone can cause rapid weight gain and puffiness of the hands or feet. Weigh yourself every day or every other day, and contact your doctor if you begin to gain weight rapidly or notice puffiness in the hands or feet. If you have any illness that causes vomiting or diarrhea, the fluid balance in your body may be upset; stop taking spironolactone and contact your doctor.

Frequent urination is a common effect when spironolactone is first taken. Urination probably will be normal or close to normal after you have taken this drug for a few weeks.

If you experience soreness of the breasts or an increase in their size after you have taken spironolactone, contact your doctor.

PRECAUTIONS

Certain medications and foods should be avoided by people who are taking spironolactone. *Do not use salt substitutes unless your doctor has given you specific instructions for their use. Do not consume grapefruit juice, orange juice, tomato juice, bananas, apricots, coconut, dates, figs, peaches or prunes.* These fruits and juices are high in potassium and could give you more potassium than you need. *Consume these foods only with your doctor's permission.*

Do not take aspirin while you are taking spironolactone. If you need something to relieve minor pain or fever, ask your doctor or pharmacist to recommend an aspirin substitute for you. Inform your doctor of any other medication you are taking. If you do not know the names of these drugs or what they were prescribed for, take the labeled containers to your doctor or pharmacist.

Alcoholic beverages may exaggerate the degree to which spironolactone lowers blood pressure, causing lightheadedness or dizziness.

Your doctor will want to monitor carefully your response to this medication, especially kidney function and levels of sodium, potassium and chloride in your blood. Keep in touch with your doctor while you are taking spironolactone, and *keep all your appointments for checkups and laboratory tests.*

DOSAGE AND STORAGE

Your doctor has determined how often you should take spironolactone tablets, and your prescription label gives specific instructions as to how much you should take at each dose. Follow these instructions carefully and ask your doctor or pharmacist to explain any part you do not fully understand. *Do not take more of this drug than has been prescribed* by your doctor because excessive loss of water and salt from your body can cause unpleasant side effects.

Safe dosages of spironolactone for pregnant women have not been established.

Spironolactone should be taken with meals or immediately after eating. If you forget a dose, take the missed dose as soon as you remember it. *Do not take two doses at once to make up for the missed dose.*

Keep this medication in the container it came in, and keep it out of the reach of children. Do not allow anyone else to take it.

Triamterene

(trye am' ter een)

Brand name: Dyrenium

Triamterene is used to treat water retention caused by such conditions as heart disease, liver disease and lung problems. When used alone it has little if any effect on blood pressure, but it is used in combination with another diuretic or other drugs to treat high blood pressure.

Triamterene acts on the kidneys, causing them to eliminate unneeded salt and water with a much smaller loss of body potassium than most other diuretics cause. Triamterene begins to work as a diuretic about two to four hours after it is taken and continues to work for about 24 hours. It may take up to three weeks for triamterene to have any effect on blood pressure.

UNDESIRED EFFECTS

Frequent urination commonly occurs when you begin taking triamterene but usually decreases after you have been taking it for a few weeks.

If you experience nausea, take triamterene with meals or immediately after eating. Contact your doctor if triamterene causes vomiting or diarrhea, since these effects can upset the fluid balance in your body.

Triamterene can cause skin rash, headache, weakness or dizziness. If you experience any of these effects, contact your doctor.

Weigh yourself every day or every other day and contact your doctor if you begin to gain weight rapidly.

PRECAUTIONS

Certain medications and foods should be avoided by people taking triamterene. *Do not use salt substitutes and do not consume grapefruit juice, orange juice, tomato juice, bananas, apricots, coconut, dates, figs, peaches or prunes.* These are high in potassium and could give you more potassium than you need. *Consume these foods only with your doctor's permission.*

Before taking triamterene, inform your doctor of any other medication you are taking. If you do not know the names of the drugs or what they were prescribed for, take the labeled containers to your doctor or pharmacist.

Alcoholic beverages may exaggerate the degree to which triamterene lowers blood pressure, causing lightheadedness or dizziness.

Your doctor will want to monitor carefully your response to this medication and will probably ask you to have laboratory tests for kidney and liver function, complete blood counts and tests to determine the levels of sodium, potassium and chloride in your blood. Keep in touch with your doctor while you are taking triamterene, and *keep all your appointments for checkups and laboratory tests.*

DOSAGE AND STORAGE

Your doctor has determined how often you should take triamterene capsules, and your prescription label gives specific instructions as to how much you should take at each dose. Follow these instructions carefully and ask your doctor or pharmacist to explain any part you do not fully understand. Do not take more of this drug than your doctor has prescribed because excessive loss of water and salt or excessive retention of potassium in your body can cause extremely unpleasant side effects.

Safe dosages of triamterene for pregnant women have not been established.

Triamterene should be taken with meals or immediately after eating. If you forget a dose, take the missed dose as soon as you remember it. *Do not take two doses at once to make up for the missed dose.*

Keep this medication in the container it came in, and keep it out of the reach of children. Do not allow anyone else to take it.

ANTIHYPERTENSIVES
Clonidine
(kloe′ ni deen)

Brand name: Catapres

The nerves that control the blood vessels and are responsible for contracting and expanding the blood vessels are governed by a collection of nerve cells in the brain called the vasomotor center. Clonidine acts on the vasomotor center and helps keep the blood pressure normal by preventing the nerves from allowing the blood vessels to contract or narrow too much. The vessels remain more relaxed and open, and blood flows more smoothly through the body. This drug works very quickly, causing a decrease in blood pressure usually within an hour.

While clonidine alone may reduce blood pressure, this drug appears to be more effective when prescribed with a diuretic—a water pill. (See the section on **diuretics**, page 9, for more information.) Clonidine is also used with other medications that lower blood pressure, which often makes it possible to reduce the amount of each drug given.

Clonidine is sometimes prescribed for people who have experienced severe dizziness with other medications taken to lower blood pressure.

UNDESIRED EFFECTS

Clonidine makes many people drowsy or less alert than usual when they begin to take it. Do not drive a car or operate dangerous machinery until you know how this drug will affect you.

Some of the common side effects of clonidine are dry nose, mouth and throat, headache and constipation. These effects tend to disappear as treatment continues. However, if they continue or are bothersome, tell your doctor at your next regular visit.

Contact your doctor if you experience swelling of the feet and lower legs, weight gain, depression, insomnia or nightmares. Although these effects do not occur very often, they may require medical attention.

PRECAUTIONS

Before starting to take clonidine, tell your doctor if you have heart or blood vessel disease or kidney disease. He needs this information before he selects the best treatment for you.

Do not drink alcoholic beverages, particularly at the start of treatment. They exaggerate the side effects of clonidine, especially drowsiness.

If you take medications for depression while you are taking clonidine, the effect of clonidine on blood pressure may be decreased. Other drugs may increase clonidine's effect on blood pressure, causing it to go too low. Some of these drugs are antihistamines for hay fever or other allergies, cold remedies, sleeping pills, tranquilizers, and drugs for seizures. Be sure to inform your doctor if you are taking any other prescription or nonprescription drugs. If you do not know what medications you are taking or what they were prescribed for, take the labeled containers to your doctor or pharmacist.

If your doctor recommends a low-salt or low-sodium diet, it is important for you to follow his recommendation. Restricting the intake of salt helps clonidine to work as it should. Be careful about exposure to cold because it can cause paleness and pain in your fingers and toes.

Women who are pregnant or think they may be should tell their doctors before beginning to take clonidine. Nursing mothers should ask their doctor's advice about continuing to nurse if they are to take clonidine.

DOSAGE AND STORAGE

Clonidine tablets are usually taken twice a day. Your prescription label tells you how many tablets to take and when to take them. Follow the label instructions carefully. If you have any questions about the instructions, contact your doctor or pharmacist.

If you forget to take a dose, take it as soon as you remember. However, if you remember a missed dose at the time you are to take another, take only one dose. *Do not take a double dose to make up for the missed one.*

It is important that you take this drug regularly. When your supply of tablets is getting low, contact your doctor or pharmacist about refilling the prescription. Make sure you have enough medication on hand. Check your supply before vacations, holidays and other occasions when you may be unable to get a refill. *Do not stop taking clonidine unless you get permission to do this from your doctor.* If you stop taking clonidine your blood pressure may "rebound" or go up to a dangerously high level.

Keep this medication in the container it came in, tightly closed and away from moisture. Keep it out of the reach of children. Do not allow anyone else to take it.

Guanethidine
(gwahn eth′ i deen)

Brand name: Ismelin

Guanethidine is a powerful and effective drug that lowers blood pressure. It reduces the supply of certain body chemicals that stimulate the nerves of the blood vessels and cause those vessels to contract or narrow. When these chemicals do not reach the nerves, the blood vessels relax, blood flows more easily through the open vessels, and the blood pressure becomes more normal.

Guanethidine is usually prescribed with a diuretic—a water pill. (See the section on **diuretics**, page 9, for more information.) It may also be used with other medications that lower blood pressure.

UNDESIRED EFFECTS

Guanethidine frequently causes lightheadedness, dizziness or fainting, particularly when you get out of bed or rise from a chair. It may help if you get up slowly to give your body time to adjust to the change in position. However, if this problem continues to gets worse, contact your doctor.

These effects are more likely to occur when you drink alcohol, stand in one position too long, or exercise suddenly or too long or when the weather is hot. While you take guanethidine, use alcohol sparingly and avoid strenuous exercise and a hot environment. All of these can increase the undesired effects.

If you become dizzy or weak while urinating or shaving, do these sitting down. Dizziness is usually worse when you first start to take this medication.

Frequent bowel movements and diarrhea are other common side effects when you take this medication. Contact your doctor or pharmacist about such problems. Occasionally, males may be impotent or have difficulty ejaculating when they take guanethidine.

Guanethidine occasionally will cause blood problems that require immediate medical attention. Symptoms of these blood problems are chills, fever, sore throat, difficulty in swallowing and sores in the mouth. If you experience any of these, contact your doctor. Do not stop taking the medication until your doctor advises you to do so.

If you experience swelling of the feet, ankles or lower legs with weight gain, chest pains or difficulty in breathing, contact your doctor. Although these effects do not occur very often, they may require medical attention. They may indicate that the drug is having a bad effect on your heart; your doctor probably will want to change your medication.

PRECAUTIONS

Before taking guanethidine, inform your doctor if you have a history of asthma, heart disease, stroke, diabetes, ulcers or chronic indigestion. Guanethidine may worsen these conditions.

Certain prescription drugs, particularly those given for depression, other forms of mental illness and weight reduction, can lessen or stop the effectiveness of guanethidine. Oral contraceptives may also interfere with the lowering of blood pressure. Before taking guanethidine, tell your doctor if you are taking any other prescription or nonprescription drugs. If you do not know what medications you are taking or what they were prescribed for, take the labeled containers to your doctor or pharmacist.

If your doctor prescribes a low-salt or low-sodium diet or tells you to stop smoking, *follow his instructions.*

Keep all appointments with your doctor so he can perform tests (such as a blood count) to determine how you react to this medication.

DOSAGE AND STORAGE
Guanethidine tablets are usually taken once a day. Follow the instructions on your prescription label and ask your doctor or pharmacist to explain anything you do not understand.

It is important to take this medication regularly on the schedule your doctor prescribes. Take it at the same time every day. It will be easier to remember if you take the medication at the same time you do something else every day, such as brushing your teeth in the morning or going to bed at night. Guanethidine usually must be taken for two to seven days before it is fully effective.

Safe dosages of guanethidine for pregnant women and the unborn child have not been established. Therefore, women who are pregnant or think they may be should tell their doctors. Nursing mothers should ask their doctors about continuing to nurse if they are to take guanethidine.

If you forget to take a dose, take it as soon as you remember. However, if you remember a missed dose at the time you are scheduled to take another, take only one dose. *Do not take a double dose to make up for the missed one.*

Do not stop taking this medication without consulting your doctor. Make sure you have enough guanethidine on hand so you can take it exactly as prescribed. Check your supply before holidays and vacations, when it may be difficult to refill your prescription.

Keep this medication in the container it came in, and store it out of the reach of children. Do not allow anyone else to take it.

Hydralazine
(hye dral' a zeen)

Brand names: Apresoline, Dralzine

Hydralazine acts directly on the muscles in the walls of the blood vessels to help lower blood pressure. As these muscles relax, the blood vessels expand and the blood flows more smoothly through the body. To achieve best blood-pressure control, hydralazine usually is prescribed with a diuretic—a water pill—and/or with another drug that lowers blood pressure. (See the section on **diuretics**, page 9, for more information.)

UNDESIRED EFFECTS
Headache, dizziness and rapid heartbeat are the most common side effects during the first few weeks of therapy with hydralazine. If these side effects continue longer than two weeks or are troublesome, contact your doctor. Heart pain (angina) may occur occasionally.

Allergic reactions such as loss of appetite, nausea, vomiting and diarrhea can occur when you take hydralazine. Let your doctor know if you experience these reactions. Mood changes, nervousness or depression should also be reported to your doctor.

In some patients who take hydralazine for long periods of time, the drug can cause a condition that resembles rheumatoid arthritis. The symptoms are fever, chest pain, joint pain, general feeling of discomfort or weakness, numbness or tingling of the fingers or toes, skin rash or itching, swelling of the feet and lower legs and swelling of the lymph glands. This condition requires medical treatment. Contact your doctor if you experience these symptoms.

Hydralazine rarely causes blood problems. Symptoms are chills, fever, sore throat, difficulty in swallowing and sores in the mouth. Contact your doctor immediately if you experience these symptoms.

PRECAUTIONS

If you have heart artery disease, the heart pain that occasionally occurs as a side effect of hydralazine can be severe. Before you begin to take hydralazine, inform your doctor if you have this condition. He will also need to know if you have kidney disease so that he can select the best treatment to lower your blood pressure.

Because other drugs can affect the way hydralazine acts on your body, tell your doctor if you are taking any other prescription or nonprescription drugs. If you do not know the names of the drugs you are taking or what they were prescribed for, take the labeled containers to your doctor or pharmacist.

It is important that you follow your doctor's instructions concerning a low-salt or low-sodium diet. High salt intake can keep hydralazine from working in your system the way it should.

Keep all your appointments with your doctor so that he can do the tests (such as blood counts, liver function tests and electrocardiograms) needed to check on your reaction to hydralazine.

It is not known whether this drug is safe for a pregnant woman and her unborn child. Therefore, if you are pregnant or plan to be, tell your doctor. If you are nursing a baby, ask your doctor about continuing to nurse before taking hydralazine.

DOSAGE AND STORAGE

Hydralazine tablets usually are taken two to four times a day. Your prescription label tells you how many tablets to take and when to take them. Follow the instructions carefully. Your doctor may start treatment with a small dose and increase it gradually. *It is important to follow this dosage schedule.* If you do not understand it, contact your doctor or pharmacist. Hydralazine should be taken with meals or a snack. It may have to be taken for several weeks before it is fully effective.

If you miss a dose, take the missed dose when you remember it. However, if you do not remember a missed dose until another dose is scheduled, take only one dose. *Do not take a double dose to make up for the missed one.*

Do not stop taking this medication without consulting your doctor. Make sure you have enough medication on hand to allow you to take it exactly as prescribed, particularly when you will be away from home and may not be able to refill your prescription.

Keep hydralazine in the container it came in, and keep it out of the reach of children. Do not allow anyone else to take it.

Methyldopa

(meth ill doe′ pa)

Brand name: Aldomet

Methyldopa acts on the center in the brain that controls the nerves governing the blood vessels. The drug decreases the activity of the nerves, and the blood vessels relax and open. This permits the blood to flow more easily through the body and lowers the blood pressure.

Methyldopa is generally given with a diuretic—a water pill. (See the section on **diuretics**, page 9, for more information.) In more severe cases of high blood pressure, methyldopa may be prescribed with other drugs that lower blood pressure to achieve the desired control.

UNDESIRED EFFECTS

Drowsiness is the most common side effect of methyldopa. This effect, which usually occurs 48 to 72 hours after you begin to take the drug or when dosage is increased, should disappear after a period of time. Do not drive a car, operate dangerous machinery or do jobs that require alertness until you know how this drug will affect you.

Methyldopa frequently causes headache, stuffy nose and dry mouth. You can relieve dry mouth by sucking hard candy, chewing gum or drinking fluids.

Dizziness or lightheadedness may occur when you get out of bed or rise from a chair. Get up slowly and give your body time to adjust to the change in position. Check with your doctor if this problem continues or gets worse.

Less common side effects are diarrhea, nausea or vomiting, numbness or tingling of the hands or feet, skin rash, swelling of the breasts or unusually slow heartbeat. These effects tend to disappear as you continue to take the drug and your body becomes used to it. However, if they continue or are bothersome, tell your doctor.

If you develop a fever for no apparent reason, contact your doctor. This is particularly important during the first few weeks when you are taking methyldopa.

If your feet and lower legs swell, contact your doctor. This may mean that methyldopa is having a bad effect on your heart.

Other effects, which are rare but may require medical attention, are flulike illness, mood or mental changes, severe or continuing diarrhea and stomach cramps, unusual bleeding or bruising, and yellowing of the skin and eyes.

Long-term therapy with methyldopa may cause weight gain and blood problems such as anemia.

PRECAUTIONS

If you have ever had liver disease or jaundice, tell your doctor before beginning to take methyldopa. This drug has caused jaundice and liver disorders, so your doctor will want to check your liver function after you've been taking methyldopa for several months.

Certain prescription drugs, such as those for depression or weight reduction, can decrease the effect of methyldopa on blood pressure. Anticoagulants (blood thinners) and the drugs used to treat Parkinson's disease can increase the effect of methyldopa. Before taking methyldopa, inform your doctor of all other prescription or nonprescription drugs you are taking. If you do not know the names of the drugs or what they were prescribed for, take the labeled containers to your doctor or pharmacist.

It is important to follow your doctor's instructions on alcohol consumption, salt or sodium consumption and smoking because these things can keep this medication from working as it should.

Keep all your appointments with your doctor so that he can do the tests (such as blood counts and liver function tests) needed to check your reaction to methyldopa.

If you are pregnant or think you may be, tell your doctor before you start to take methyldopa. If you are nursing a baby, ask your doctor about continuing to nurse if you are to take methyldopa.

DOSAGE AND STORAGE

Methyldopa tablets are usually taken two to four times a day. Your prescription label tells you how much to take and when to take each dose. *Take methyldopa exactly as prescribed.* Follow the instructions carefully and contact your doctor or pharmacist if there is any part you do not understand. Methyldopa usually begins to work six to 12 hours after it is taken, but you will need to take it for one to four full days before you begin to receive its full benefit.

If you forget to take a dose, take it as soon as you remember. Take the remaining doses for that day at regularly spaced intervals.

Do not stop taking this medication without consulting your doctor. If you do, your blood pressure will return to a high level within two days. Make sure you have enough medication on hand to allow you to take it exactly as prescribed. Check your supply before going away from home if it may be difficult to refill your prescription.

Keep this medication in the container that it came in, and keep it out of the reach of children. Do not allow anyone else to take it.

Propranolol
(pro pran' oh lole)

Brand name: Inderal

Propranolol is most commonly prescribed for three important heart and circulation problems: high blood pressure, "heart pain" (angina pectoris) caused by the heart receiving too little oxygen and irregular heartbeat. Propranolol may be useful in treating people who have a combination of these problems. More recently, propranolol has been used to prevent migraine headaches. Propranolol is one of a group of drugs commonly referred to as "beta blockers."

Propranolol "blocks" a chemical reaction in the nervous system. Propranolol therefore has very widespread effects. It prevents certain stimulating chemicals from reaching the nerves in the heart and blood vessels that control the heart's pumping action and the opening and narrowing of blood vessels. Propranolol relieves heart pain by slowing the speed (rate) of the heart so that it needs less oxygen. It slows the movement of nerve messages (impulses) through the electrical system of the heart, which improves the rhythm (beat) of the heart. Because propranolol relaxes the blood vessels, the blood flows more smoothly through the body, and the blood pressure becomes more normal.

USES
High blood pressure: Propranolol is usually prescribed along with a diuretic—a water pill. (See the section on **diuretics**, page 9, for more information.) Propranolol is also given with other medications that reduce blood pressure, particularly when a combination of two drugs will bring the pressure under control with smaller doses of each drug.

Heart pain (angina pectoris): Most frequently the treatment for heart pain is medication that increases the supply of blood to the heart, thus providing the heart with more oxygen. (See the section on **heart pain**, page 39, for a fuller explanation.) However, a person who has not responded to this treatment or who has a decreased blood supply to the heart (sometimes caused by "fatty deposits" in the vessels) may respond to propranolol because its action is entirely different. Rather than increasing the blood supply—and thus the supply of oxygen—to the heart, propranolol decreases the heart's need for oxygen.

For some people, propranolol may reduce the frequency of heart pain attacks; for others, it may allow them to be more active without experiencing heart pain.

Irregular heartbeat: Although propranolol is rarely the drug of choice for any type of irregular heartbeat, it may be useful, along with digitalis drugs, for people whose irregular heartbeat is not controlled by digitalis drugs alone. (See the sections on **digitalis drugs**, page 6, for more information.)

UNDESIRED EFFECTS
Propranolol has a wide variety of effects on many body organ systems. In addition to its desired effects on the heart and blood vessels, propranolol may have undesired effects on the lungs. It may bother some people with lung problems such as hay fever, asthma, bronchitis or emphysema. If propranolol makes you short of breath or if you experience other breathing difficulties, contact your doctor.

A variety of effects on circulation and heart rate can occur and can be harmful, depending on your medical condition.

Propranolol causes some people to become dizzy, lightheaded or drowsy. Do not drive a car or operate dangerous machinery until you know how this drug will affect you.

If this medication causes nausea, vomiting or diarrhea, contact your doctor. He may want to adjust the dosage you are taking. If it upsets your stomach, take this medication with a full eight-ounce glassful of fluid or a light snack.

Some other side effects of propranolol are cold hands and feet, loss of appetite, loss of hair and tiring easily. With long-term therapy, hallucinations (seeing, hearing or feeling things that are not there), mental confusion, nightmares, vivid dreams and sleeping problems can occur, although these effects are rare. Contact your doctor at once if they occur.

Serious side effects of propranolol are blood problems, such as a reduction in the number of white blood cells, and a decrease in one of the substances that helps clot blood. If you experience weakness, bruise easily or have any unusual bleeding, contact your doctor at once.

PRECAUTIONS

Before taking propranolol, inform your doctor if you have any history of allergy or if you have any lung problems such as emphysema, asthma or bronchitis. Your doctor will also need to know if you have diabetes or thyroid, kidney or liver disease.

When taken with other medications, propranolol may have undesired effects. Before you take propranolol, tell your doctor of all other prescription or nonprescription drugs you are taking, especially those for your heart condition or high blood pressure. He will also need to know whether you are taking medicine for diabetes, depression, ulcers or Parkinson's disease. Other drugs that should not be taken with propranolol are sleeping pills, narcotics, allergy or cold medicines that include antihistamines and medicine used to reduce inflammation, including aspirin. If you do not know what drugs you are taking or what they were prescribed for, take the labeled containers to your doctor or pharmacist.

Your doctor may prescribe a low-salt or low-sodium diet, tell you to stop smoking and restrict your intake of alcohol. It is very important that you follow his instructions so you will get the greatest benefit from propranolol.

Your doctor may ask you to check your pulse every day while you take this medication. He will teach you how to take your pulse and what number of beats per minute to check for. If your pulse is slower than it should be, contact your doctor about taking the drug that day.

Keep all your appointments with your doctor so that he can check your response to propranolol. He may want an exercise test with an electrocardiogram, a blood count or other blood tests.

If you go to the dentist or another doctor, be sure to tell him you are taking propranolol. You may want to carry a medical identification card so that, in case of an accident, those treating you will know you are taking propranolol.

Before you start to take propranolol, be sure to tell your doctor if you are pregnant, think you may be or are nursing a baby.

DOSAGE AND STORAGE

Propranolol is usually taken four times a day—before meals and at bedtime. The tablets should be taken with fluids (water, milk, fruit juice, coffee or tea). Follow carefully the instructions on your prescription label that tell you how much to take and when to take each dose. If you do not understand the instructions or have any questions about them, contact your doctor or pharmacist.

If you forget to take a dose, take it as soon as you remember. Then take the other doses for that day at evenly spaced intervals. *Do not take a double dose to make up for the missed one.*

When your supply of tablets is getting low, contact your doctor or pharmacist about refilling your prescription. *Take this medication exactly as your doctor has instructed. Do not stop taking propranolol unless you get permission from your doctor.* Keep the medication in the container it came in, and keep it out of the reach of children. Do not allow anyone else to take it.

Reserpine
(re ser' peen)

Brand names: Rau-sed, Reserpoid, Sandril, Serpalan, Serpanray, Serpasil and others

Reserpine acts on both the vasomotor center (a collection of nerve cells in the brain that control the blood vessel nerves) and the nerves of the blood vessels. It helps keep blood pressure normal by relaxing the blood vessels to permit the blood to flow more easily through the body.

Reserpine is generally more effective when used with a diuretic—a water pill. (See the section on **diuretics**, page 9, for more information.) Reserpine may also be prescribed with other drugs that lower blood pressure to achieve better blood-pressure control.

Reserpine is also used to treat mental illness, particularly when the person is very excited.

UNDESIRED EFFECTS

Dry mouth, stuffy nose, indigestion, tiredness, lethargy and red eyes are some of the more common undesired effects of reserpine. To relieve dry mouth, suck on hard candies, chew gum or drink fluids.

Reserpine causes some people to become drowsy. Do not drive a car or operate dangerous machinery until you know how this medication will affect you. Avoid the use of alcohol and sleeping pills because they can increase the drowsiness.

After you take reserpine, you may experience dizziness when you stand. If you become dizzy, move slowly from a sitting to a standing position. Contact your doctor if the dizziness is severe or continues over a period of time.

Reserpine can cause nightmares, mood changes, nervousness and shaking. If you experience any of these, contact your doctor. Weight gain, breast enlargement in men, changes in menstrual pattern and decreased sexual drive are other undesired effects of reserpine. Contact your doctor if any of these occur.

Depression is the most serious side effect of reserpine. Stop taking it if you begin to feel "blue," lose your appetite or wake much earlier than usual in the morning. Contact your doctor right away and describe to him how you feel.

If reserpine upsets your stomach or gives you diarrhea and cramps, take it with meals or a snack. Contact your doctor if these effects continue or are bothersome.

Although allergic reactions to reserpine seem to be rare, it may cause asthma attacks in people who suffer from asthma.

PRECAUTIONS

Reserpine has caused cancer in laboratory test animals. However, there is some question whether it has this effect on humans. You probably should not take this drug if you have a family history of cancer. Talk this over with your doctor.

Before taking this medication, inform your doctor if you have a peptic ulcer, colitis, depression, epilepsy or gallstones or if you have had any of these problems in the past. Reserpine can aggravate these conditions or make them recur.

Tell your doctor of any other prescription or nonprescription drugs you are taking, especially anticoagulants (blood thinners), any other heart drugs, medicine for seizures and tranquilizers or drugs for depression. If you do not know what drugs you are taking or what they were prescribed for, take the labeled containers to your doctor or pharmacist.

Do not drink carbonated beverages while you are taking reserpine. Follow carefully your doctor's instructions about a low-salt or low-sodium diet, using alcohol and smoking.

Keep all your appointments with your doctor so he can check on your response to reserpine. He may ask you to have blood tests periodically and may also ask you to have your eyes examined.

Reserpine should not be taken during pregnancy or while you are nursing a baby. Tell your doctor if you are pregnant or think you may be.

DOSAGE AND STORAGE

Reserpine comes in tablet and liquid forms to be taken orally and is usually given once or twice a day. Your doctor will select the form best for you. Carefully follow the instructions on your prescription label that tell you how much to take and when to take each dose. If you do not know how to measure the liquid or have any other questions about your prescription, ask your doctor or pharmacist.

If you are to take this medication once a day, take it at the same time— preferably when you do something else each day, such as brushing your teeth in the morning, eating dinner or going to bed at night.

If you forget a dose, *do not take a missed dose when you remember it.* Omit that dose and take the following dose at the next scheduled time. *It is important that you take this medication regularly on the schedule prescribed by your doctor. Do not stop taking this medication without consulting your doctor.*

Make sure you have enough medication on hand so you can take it exactly as directed. Be sure to check your supply before vacations and holidays, when it may be difficult to refill your prescription.

Keep this medication in the container in which it came, and keep it out of the reach of children. Do not allow anyone else to take it.

Irregular Heartbeat or Arrhythmia (A RiTH' ME A)

An irregular heartbeat can be caused by disease such as infection or high blood pressure, by certain drugs including nicotine and caffeine, or by damage to the heart itself in a heart attack. When the heart loses its normal, rhythmic beat, the efficiency of its pumping action decreases. A variation from the normal rhythm of the heartbeat is called an arrhythmia.

There are three principal types of irregular heartbeats or cardiac arrhythmias: slow beat (less than 55 beats per minute), fast beat (more than 100 beats per minute) and an early beat (often described by those who experience it as a "skipped" beat).

The drugs described here are given orally to prevent or treat primarily fast beats and early beats. Other drugs may be given by injection in a hospital to treat more severe irregular heartbeat problems. The drugs in this section are called antiarrhythmics, and they are prescribed to regulate the rhythm of the heartbeat. Artificial pacemakers are also used to correct very slow heartbeats.

ANTIARRHYTHMICS
Procainamide
(proe kane a' mide)

Brand names: Procamide, Procan, Procapan, Pronestyl

Procainamide relaxes an overactive heart by acting on the heart muscle and nerves, slowing down the heart and allowing it to beat at a normal rate and rhythm. This improves the efficiency of the heart's pumping action.

Procainamide is used to maintain normal heart rate and rhythm after they have been established by other means (such as injection of an antiarrhythmic drug or electric shock therapy) and to prevent recurrence of irregular or fast beats. Procainamide is also used to treat early beats.

UNDESIRED EFFECTS
If you experience chills, fever, joint pain, sore throat, itching, hives or skin rash while you are taking procainamide, contact your doctor. Report symptoms similar to those of arthritis to your doctor, since they may indicate development of a potentially serious condition.

Procainamide can cause nausea, diarrhea, bitter taste, loss of appetite, abdominal pain and weakness or lightheadedness. Usually these effects are only mild discomforts, but you should contact your doctor if they become severe. Giddiness or mental depression may also occur.

If you have ever had an allergic reaction to a local anesthetic such as procaine (Novocain), most commonly used in dental procedures, be sure to inform your doctor before you begin to take procainamide.

PRECAUTIONS

Tell your doctor what other prescription or nonprescription drugs you are taking or have taken over the past month. Be sure to tell him if you have taken digitalis drugs or other heart drugs in the past. If you do not know the names of the drugs you are taking or what they were prescribed for, take the labeled containers to your doctor or pharmacist.

Your doctor should also know if you have ever had kidney or liver disease. Patients with myasthenia gravis cannot take procainamide. Keep in close touch with your doctor and pharmacist while taking procainamide. Your doctor may have you visit his office for an electrocardiogram or various blood tests.

Cigarettes and caffeine-containing beverages may increase the irritability of the heart and interfere with the action of procainamide. Follow your doctor's advice about smoking and dietary restrictions.

It is not known whether this drug is safe for a pregnant woman or her unborn child.

DOSAGE AND STORAGE

Procainamide is usually taken four to six times a day. *It is extremely important to take this medication on the exact schedule prescribed by your doctor, even if you must awaken during the night to take it.* Response to this drug may differ a great deal from person to person, and *your* dosage must be carefully tailored to your needs by your doctor. Procainamide must be taken regularly around the clock to keep the heart beating at a normal rate.

Procainamide comes in tablets and capsules to be taken orally. Your prescription label tells you how much to take at each dose. Carefully follow the instructions on your prescription label and ask your doctor or pharmacist to explain any part you do not understand.

If you forget to take a dose, take the missed dose as soon as you remember it. Take the next dose at the regularly scheduled time. However, if you do not remember a missed dose until you are scheduled to take another, take only one dose. *Do not take a double dose to make up for the missed one.*

Be sure you have enough of this medication on hand at all times to take all your doses as prescribed. Check your supply before holidays, vacations or other times when it may be difficult to get more.

Keep procainamide in the container it came in, and keep it out of the reach of children. Do not let anyone else take it.

Propranolol

Brand name: Inderal
(See complete description under **high blood pressure** on page 30.)

Quinidine
(kwin′ i dine)

Brand names: Cardioquin, Duraquin, Quinaglute, Quinidex, Quinora, SK-Quinidine and others

Quinidine relaxes an overactive heart by working on the heart muscles and nerves, slowing down the heart and allowing it to beat at a normal rate and rhythm. This improves the efficiency of the heart's pumping action.

Quinidine is used to maintain normal heart rate and rhythm after it has been established by other means (such as injection of an antiarrhythmic drug or electric shock) and to prevent recurrence of irregular or fast beats.

Quinidine is extracted from the bark of the cinchona tree in South America. This tree also yields quinine. Quinidine is available in three chemical preparations: quinidine gluconate, quinidine polygalacturonate and quinidine sulfate.

UNDESIRED EFFECTS

Some people are allergic to quinidine, so be sure to tell your doctor if you have ever had a reaction to quinidine or quinine (as in tonic water or some cold remedies available without prescription). Quinidine can cause skin rashes, unusual bleeding or bruising, ringing in the ears or changes in hearing, changes in vision, feeling of excitement or apprehension, delirium, dizziness and severe headaches. If you experience any of these symptoms, contact your doctor.

Quinidine naturally affects the heartbeat, and it may also cause your blood pressure to drop. You may experience dizziness or lightheadedness when you move suddenly from lying or sitting to an upright position.

While taking quinidine you may have loss of appetite, stomach pain, nausea or diarrhea. These side effects usually are only mild discomforts, but you should take the medication with food and then contact your doctor if these undesired effects become severe. Do not take antacids or baking soda for stomach upset unless you check first with your doctor or pharmacist.

PRECAUTIONS

Before you start taking quinidine, tell your doctor about any other prescription or nonprescription drugs you are taking or have taken in the past month. Anticoagulants (blood thinners) and some drugs used to treat seizures act in an undesirable way when taken with quinidine. Cough, cold and allergy medications must also be carefully chosen by patients taking quinidine. Be sure to tell your doctor if you have taken digitalis drugs or other heart drugs in the past. If you do not know the names of the drugs you are taking or what they were prescribed for, take the labeled containers to your doctor or pharmacist.

Keep in close touch with your doctor and pharmacist while taking quinidine.

Your doctor may have you visit his office for an electrocardiogram or for blood tests.

Cigarettes and caffeine-containing beverages may increase the irritability of the heart and interfere with the action of quinidine. Follow your doctor's advice about smoking and dietary restrictions.

A woman who is pregnant or who thinks she may be should inform her doctor before taking quinidine.

DOSAGE AND STORAGE

Quinidine usually is taken three or four times a day. *It is extremely important to take this medication on the exact schedule prescribed by your doctor, even if you must awaken during the night to take it.* Response to the drug may differ a great deal from person to person, and *your* dosage must be carefully tailored to your needs by your doctor. Quinidine must be taken regularly to keep the heart beating at a normal rate. Carefully follow the instructions on your prescription label and ask your doctor or pharmacist to explain any part you do not understand.

Quinidine comes in tablets and capsules to be taken orally. Your prescription label tells you how much to take at each dose. This medication may be taken with meals or a snack to prevent upset stomach and to help avoid the bitter taste.

If you forget a dose, take the missed dose as soon as you remember it. Take the next dose at the regularly scheduled time. However, if you remember a missed dose at the time you are scheduled to take another, take only one dose. *Do not take a double dose to make up for the missed one.*

Be sure you have enough of this medication on hand at all times to take all your doses as prescribed. Be sure to check your supply before holidays or at any other time it may be difficult to get more.

Keep this medication in the light-resistant container it came in. When quinidine is exposed to light, it will darken and have a bitter taste. Keep quinidine out of the reach of children. Do not let anyone else take it.

HEART PAIN OR ANGINA PECTORIS (AN ji' NAH pECk' TORE US)

The term "coronary insufficiency" is used to describe the circumstance in which the heart's need for oxygen is greater than its supply of oxygen. When this occurs, heart pain or angina pectoris results. Angina pectoris occurs especially during exercise, exertion or emotional stress. Any disease that causes a decrease in the flow of blood to the heart can cause it, although the most common cause is thought to be fatty deposits that narrow the blood vessels of the heart. Under these circumstances, unusual exercise or emotion increases the heart's need for oxygen, but the blood is unable to flow freely and quickly to the heart, and an angina attack occurs.

Heart pain is experienced not as pain in other parts of the body but as a crushing or squeezing sensation in the area of the breastbone. Occasionally the pain is felt in the neck, shoulder or upper abdomen, where it is often confused with indigestion. The pain frequently spreads down the left arm.

Treatment for an attack of heart pain is rest and drugs that open the blood vessels to permit more oxygen to reach the heart. These drugs are commonly called vasodilators. Your doctor's major goal is to control the pain with as little change in your normal activities as possible. Your doctor will probably ask you to stop smoking, lose weight, get plenty of rest and avoid those things that will bring on heart pain (exertion, overeating, exposure to cold weather and emotional upset).

VASODILATORS
Dipyridamole
(dye peer id' a mole)

Brand name: Persantine

Dipyridamole is one of a group of vasodilator drugs that opens blood vessels to permit more blood to flow to the heart and thus increase the heart's oxygen supply. Dipyridamole is prescribed for long-term treatment of heart pain caused by insufficient oxygen in the heart. It may reduce the frequency and/or severity of attacks of angina pectoris. It will *not* relieve pain if taken *during* an acute attack. In combination with other drugs, it is also used to prevent clots from forming in the blood vessels.

UNDESIRED EFFECTS
Dipyridamole can cause mild headache, dizziness and flushing. Contact your

doctor if these effects continue for an extended period or if they make you too uncomfortable. Patients with low blood pressure probably should not take this drug. Nausea, diarrhea or stomach irritation may occur. If this medication upsets your stomach, try eating a light snack at the time you take it.

PRECAUTIONS

Before you begin to take this medication, tell your doctor what other prescription or nonprescription drugs you are taking, especially any heart medication or anticoagulant (blood thinner) or aspirin. If you do not know the names of the drugs you are taking or what they were prescribed for, show the labeled containers to your doctor or pharmacist.

You should not take this drug if you have just had a heart attack. Sometimes patients will experience an increase in the frequency and/or severity of attacks of heart pain when they first begin to take dipyridamole. If this happens to you, stop taking the drug and contact your doctor. Do not change the dosage on your own initiative.

Follow your doctor's advice about smoking and about use of alcoholic beverages while you are taking dipyridamole.

It is not known whether this drug is safe for a pregnant woman or her unborn child.

DOSAGE AND STORAGE

Dipyridamole tablets usually are taken three times a day, but dosage can vary depending on your response and medical condition. Your prescription label tells you how often to take dipyridamole and how much to take at each dose. Follow the instructions carefully.

Dipyridamole should be taken on an empty stomach and at least one hour before meals. Take it with a full eight-ounce glass of fluid such as water, coffee, tea, milk or fruit juice. You may take dipyridamole with a light snack if the medication makes you nauseous.

If you forget to take a dose, do not take a missed dose when you remember it. Omit it and take only your regular dose at the next scheduled time. This medication must be taken regularly for as long as several months to be effective. Therefore, be sure to take it according to the schedule prescribed by your doctor and keep in touch with your doctor while taking it.

Keep this medication in the container it came in, and keep it out of the reach of children. Do not allow anyone else to take it.

Isosorbide Dinitrate
(eye soe sor' bide dye nye' trate)

Brand names: Angidil, Dilatrate, IsoBid, Isordil, Isotrate, Sorate, Sorbitrate and others

Isosorbide dinitrate, like nitroglycerin, is one of the nitrate group of vasodilators. It relieves heart pain by increasing the blood supply and the oxygen supply to the heart.

Isosorbide dinitrate is available in various forms: chewable tablets and tablets to be dissolved in the mouth for quick relief of angina attacks when they occur, and regular tablets, extended-release tablets and capsules to be swallowed on a regular schedule for prevention of heart pain. Chewable tablets and tablets to be dissolved in the mouth begin to give relief within three minutes and go on working for 30 minutes to two hours. The tablets or capsules to be swallowed begin to work in 30 to 60 minutes; their effectiveness lasts up to six hours.

UNDESIRED EFFECTS

Isosorbide dinitrate can cause headache, flushing, redness of the skin, dizziness, weakness or fainting. These side effects usually are temporary and disappear by themselves. You may wish to sit down for a few minutes after taking a tablet. If these side effects do not disappear or if they keep you from resuming normal activities, contact your doctor or pharmacist.

Allergic reactions may occur, with severe skin rash and peeling of the skin.

Tablets placed under the tongue or between the cheek and gums to dissolve usually produce a tingling or burning sensation. This means they are being absorbed by the lining of the mouth.

PRECAUTIONS

Be sure to tell your doctor about any other prescription or nonprescription drugs you are taking, especially other drugs for your heart condition or blood pressure, drugs for mental depression and medication to treat cough, colds or allergy.

Follow your doctor's advice about smoking and drinking alcoholic beverages while taking this drug.

Isosorbide dinitrate may cause an increase in internal eye pressure in patients with glaucoma, so be sure to tell your doctor if you have glaucoma; he probably will want to check your eye pressure more frequently.

You may develop "tolerance" to isosorbide dinitrate after you have been taking it for a while. This means that you may no longer get relief from the dose your doctor has prescribed for you. Discuss this with your doctor.

Keep in close touch with your doctor and pharmacist while taking this medication. Your doctor will want you to visit his office for periodic examinations and may order various blood tests.

DOSAGE AND STORAGE

Tablets for quick relief of pain: Isosorbide dinitrate comes in two types of tablets to be taken for quick relief when a pain attack occurs—chewable tablets and tablets to be dissolved under the tongue or between the cheek and gums. Your doctor will select the tablet best for you and tell you how many tablets to take for each attack.

If your doctor has prescribed tablets that dissolve in the mouth, remember: Place them under the tongue or between the cheek and gum and leave them there until completely dissolved. Try not to swallow saliva too often until the tablet has completely dissolved.

If chewable tablets have been prescribed for you, remember: To get their full benefit, you should chew them thoroughly before you swallow them.

When an attack occurs, stop whatever you are doing, sit down and take the tablet exactly as you have been instructed to do. Contact your doctor if the pain has not been relieved after you have taken the number of tablets prescribed for each attack.

Carry isosorbide dinitrate tablets with you at all times. You may learn through experience what activities cause angina pectoris. It is a good idea to take a tablet before any activity or stressful situation you know may provoke pain. Talk this over with your doctor and follow his advice for avoiding pain.

Tablets for prevention of angina attacks: Tablets and extended-release tablets or capsules are used to prevent attacks of heart pain. They do not relieve the pain of an angina attack once it occurs.

Isosorbide dinitrate tablets usually are taken four times a day. Your prescription label tells you how often to take them and how much to take at each dose. Follow the instructions carefully and ask your doctor or pharmacist to explain any part you do not understand.

Contact your doctor if you continue to experience angina attacks in spite of the fact that you are taking this medication to prevent them. If you forget to take a dose, take the missed dose as soon as you remember it. Take the remaining doses for that day at regularly spaced intervals. However, if you remember a missed dose at the time you are scheduled to take the next one, take only one dose. *Do not take a double dose to make up for the missed one.*

Keep isosorbide dinitrate tablets in the container they came in and away from excessive heat. Keep this medication out of the reach of children and do not allow anyone else to take it.

Nitroglycerin
(nye troe gli′ ser in)

Brand names: Angibid, Cardabid, Nitro-Bid, Nitroglyn, Nitrol, Nitrong, Nitrospan, Nitrostat, Trates and others

Nitroglycerin is a vasodilator used to treat or to reduce the frequency or severity of attacks of angina pectoris. Nitroglycerin is available in three forms: tablets to be dissolved in the mouth at the time of an angina attack for quick relief; slow-release tablets to be swallowed on a regular schedule for prevention of angina attacks; and an ointment applied to the skin to prevent heart pain.

Nitroglycerin relieves heart pain by relaxing the muscles of the blood vessels in the heart, thus allowing more blood and the oxygen it carries to reach the heart. Tablets dissolved in the mouth begin to give relief within two minutes and go on working for up to 30 minutes. The tablets to be swallowed and the ointment begin to work in about 30 minutes.

UNDESIRED EFFECTS
Nitroglycerin can cause headache, flushing, redness of the skin, increased heart rate, faster pulse, throbbing in the head, dizziness, weakness or fainting. These side effects usually are temporary and disappear by themselves. You may

wish to sit down for a few minutes after taking a tablet. If these effects do not disappear or if they keep you from resuming normal activities, contact your doctor or pharmacist.

Severe skin rash and peeling of the skin are indications of an allergic reaction. Nitroglycerin tablets placed under the tongue or between the cheek and gums usually produce a tingling or burning sensation. This means they are being absorbed as they should.

PRECAUTIONS

Before you start taking nitroglycerin, tell your doctor about any other prescription or nonprescription drugs you are taking, especially other drugs for your heart condition or blood pressure and medications for colds or allergy. Nitroglycerin may cause an increase in internal eye pressure in patients with glaucoma, so be sure to tell your doctor if you have glaucoma; he probably will want to check your eye pressure more frequently.

Do not consume alcohol or smoke if you are taking nitroglycerin. Try to avoid long exposure to cold temperatures, since the effectiveness of nitroglycerin is reduced in cold environments.

You may develop "tolerance" to nitroglycerin after you have been taking it for a while. This means that you may no longer get relief from the dose your doctor has prescribed for you. Discuss this with your doctor.

Keep in close touch with your doctor and pharmacist while taking this medication. Your doctor will want you to visit his office for periodic examinations and may order various blood tests.

DOSAGE AND STORAGE

Tablets to be dissolved in the mouth. Place these small tablets under the tongue or between the cheek and gum and leave them there until they dissolve completely. They should not be swallowed. The medication is absorbed by the lining of the mouth to relieve the pain quickly.

When an attack occurs, stop whatever you are doing and place a tablet under your tongue or between your cheek and gum. Try not to swallow saliva too often until the tablet has completely dissolved. Your doctor will tell you how many tablets to take for each attack.

Carry nitroglycerin tablets with you at all times. Be sure your supply is fresh. Throw away tablets that are more than three months old or that do not cause a tingling or burning sensation in your mouth; these tablets are not fresh. Contact your doctor or pharmacist about a fresh supply. Do not put cotton or other material inside the container for the tablets or carry the tablets loose in your pocket or purse. Nitroglycerin tablets lose their strength after they have been exposed to air.

Contact your doctor if the heart pain has not been relieved after you have taken the number of tablets prescribed for each attack. You may learn through experience what activities cause heart pain. Take a nitroglycerin tablet before any activity or stressful situation you know may provoke heart pain. Talk this over with your doctor and follow his advice for avoiding pain.

Slow-release medication: Swallow these tablets and capsules. Usually you take them two or three times a day. Your prescription label tells you how often to take them and how much to take at each dose. Follow the instructions carefully and ask your doctor or pharmacist about any part of them you do not understand.

Contact your doctor if you continue to experience angina attacks despite your taking nitroglycerin to prevent them. If you forget to take a dose, take the missed dose as soon as you remember it. However, if you do not remember it until you are scheduled to take another dose, take only that dose. *Do not take a double dose to make up for a missed dose.*

Ointment: Use this form especially for angina occurring at night. Carefully follow your doctor's instructions for application of the ointment and any other special instructions he may offer. Ask him to explain anything you do not fully understand.

Keep nitroglycerin tablets and capsules in a cool, dark place. Do not expose them to air, heat or light for too long. *Keep this medication in the container it came in.* Nitroglycerin tablets must be kept in glass containers with tightly fitting metal caps. Keep the bottle closed tightly and do not put any other medicines in it. Keep nitroglycerin out of the reach of children and do not allow anyone else to take it.

Pentaerythritol Tetranitrate
(pen tah eh rith′ ri tall tet rah nye′ trate)

Brand names: Duotrate, Pentritol, Peritrate, Vasolate and others

Like other nitrates, pentaerythritol tetranitrate increases the blood supply to the heart and brings the oxygen supply in balance with the heart's oxygen needs. However, it is not used for quick relief of heart pain when an attack occurs. It is prescribed for long-term prevention of angina attacks and may reduce both the frequency and the severity of pain.

Pentaerythritol tetranitrate begins to work 20 to 60 minutes after it is taken and goes on working for four to five hours.

UNDESIRED EFFECTS

Pentaerythritol tetranitrate can cause headache, flushing, redness of the skin, dizziness, weakness or fainting. These side effects are usually temporary and disappear by themselves. You may wish to sit down for a few minutes if you experience them. If these effects do not disappear or if they keep you from performing your normal activities, contact your doctor or pharmacist.

If you develop a skin rash you may be allergic to this drug. Contact your doctor to find out whether you should continue to take pentaerythritol tetranitrate.

PRECAUTIONS

Inform your doctor of any other prescription or nonprescription drugs you are taking, especially other drugs to treat your heart condition or blood pressure, drugs to treat depression and drugs to treat colds, allergies or cough. If you do not know the names of the drugs or what they were prescribed for, take the labeled containers to your doctor or pharmacist. While taking pentaerythritol tetranitrate, do not consume alcoholic beverages. Alcohol may increase the undesired effects of this drug, and cold environments may reduce its effectiveness.

Pentaerythritrol tetranitrate may increase internal eye pressure in patients with glaucoma. Be sure to tell your doctor if you have glaucoma so he can check your eye pressure frequently.

You may develop "tolerance" to this drug after you have been taking it for a while. This means you may no longer get relief from the dose your doctor has prescribed for you. Discuss this with your doctor.

Keep in close touch with your doctor and pharmacist while taking this medication. Your doctor will want you to visit his office for periodic examinations and may order various blood tests.

DOSAGE AND STORAGE

Pentaerythritol tetranitrate comes in tablets and in extended-release capsules and tablets. The tablets are usually taken four times a day—30 to 60 minutes before meals, or an hour after eating, and at bedtime. The extended-release tablets or capsules usually are taken twice a day.

Your doctor will select the form best for you and indicate on your prescription label how often it should be taken and how much to take at each dose. Follow these instructions carefully and ask your doctor or pharmacist to explain any part you do not understand.

Contact your doctor if you continue to experience angina attacks in spite of taking this medication to prevent them. If you forget to take a dose, take the missed dose as soon as you remember it. Take the remaining doses for that day at regularly spaced intervals. However, if you remember a missed dose at the time you are scheduled to take the next one, take only one dose. *Do not take a double dose to make up for the missed one.*

Keep pentaerythritol tetranitrate in a tightly closed container away from excessive heat. Keep this medication out of the reach of children and do not allow anyone else to take it.

Propranolol

Brand name: Inderal
(See complete description under **high blood pressure**, on page 30.)

Blood Clots

Blood clots can form in the veins of the legs, heart, lungs or brain as a result of inflammation of the veins, a heart attack or poor circulation when the heart is not pumping blood efficiently. Blood clots can be life-threatening. Even those that form in the legs carry the risk that part of the clot may break off and be carried by the bloodstream to a vital organ like the lungs. Blood clots can also cause a heart attack or stroke.

Because they are so serious, blood clots are treated with blood thinners or anticoagulants, drugs that slow up the clotting process. The goal of treatment is to prevent existing clots from getting larger and to prevent the formation of new clots without causing unwanted bleeding inside the body. This delicate balance can be achieved only through frequent blood tests that check the time required for the blood to clot.

Even patients who take anticoagulants as prescribed by their doctors can have serious bleeding. If you are taking anticoagulants or blood thinners, call your doctor immediately if any of these signs of bleeding occur:

- unusual nosebleed or bloody gums after brushing your teeth
- prolonged bleeding from cuts, a heavy menstrual period or blood oozing from a clot
- vomiting or spitting blood that looks either red or brown and resembles coffee grounds
- sudden appearance of bruises or black and blue marks on the skin
- black or bloody bowel movements or red or dark brown urine
- new or unexpected pain such as headaches, stomach pain or backaches

ANTICOAGULANTS

Warfarin
(war' far in)

Brand names: Athrombin-K, Coumadin, Panwarfin

Warfarin helps to prevent blood clots from forming or from getting larger. It is used to treat conditions in which a blood clot may occur or has occurred. These conditions include pulmonary embolism (a blood clot in the lung) and thrombophlebitis (a clot in a blood vessel, usually in the leg).

For people who have an artificial heart valve, warfarin sometimes is used to minimize the chance of clot formation. When the drug heparin has been used to achieve rapid anticoagulation, warfarin frequently is the oral drug taken to maintain this effect. *It is very important to take warfarin exactly on schedule in the precise amount your doctor has prescribed.*

UNDESIRED EFFECTS

Bleeding is the most common undesired effect of warfarin. Contact your doctor at the first sign of any bleeding such as bruising or black and blue marks, blood in the urine (red or dark brown urine) or nosebleed. Also let your doctor know if you develop any unusual pains in the lower back or the abdomen or prolonged headache. *In the event of an accidental overdose, contact your doctor, poison control center or nearest hospital emergency room immediately.*

Bothersome side effects of warfarin may include rash, hives, loss of hair, fever, nausea, vomiting and diarrhea. Any illness that causes vomiting, diarrhea or fever can change the effect of warfarin. If any of these problems last for more than a few days, contact your doctor.

PRECAUTIONS

As long as you are taking warfarin, periodic laboratory tests such as a prothrombin time (a test that measures the time it takes your blood to clot) must be done to check your response to the drug so that the dose can be adjusted if necessary. *Be sure to keep all appointments with your doctor and at the laboratory.*

Prothrombin time tests are repeated more frequently—perhaps daily—when warfarin therapy is first started. Once the proper drug dosage is established and you take your medication properly, the tests can be done less frequently. Failure to keep appointments for these tests could result in improper control of your anticoagulant therapy.

A large number of drugs increase or decrease the anticoagulant effects of warfarin. If you are taking warfarin, do not take aspirin. Inform your doctor of all drugs you are taking—both prescription and nonprescription drugs. If you do not know the names of the drugs or what they were prescribed for, take the labeled containers to your doctor or pharmacist. Among the drugs that are known to alter the effect of warfarin are aspirin, drugs for treatment of arthritis and muscle pains, phenobarbital, antibiotics, clofibrate, disulfiram, phenylbutazone, phenytoin and thyroid hormones.

Do not stop taking any of the medications you are currently taking unless directed to do so by your doctor. Do not take any new drugs unless you have your doctor's permission.

It is important that all the doctors and dentists taking care of you know that you are taking warfarin so they can avoid prescribing medications that would interfere with warfarin's effect.

Be sure your doctor knows about any other medical conditions you have, especially those involving bleeding (ulcers or long or heavy menstrual periods), diabetes, kidney or liver disease or high blood pressure.

Vitamin K can decrease the therapeutic effect of warfarin. Therefore, you should ask your doctor about eating foods that contain vitamin K, including fish, asparagus, bacon, liver, broccoli, cabbage, cauliflower, kale, lettuce, spinach, turnip greens, watercress and onions. Once your doctor has determined the proper dosage of warfarin for you, do not make unusual changes in your diet.

Women who become pregnant while taking warfarin should promptly notify their doctors of their pregnancy. Warfarin should never be taken during pregnancy because the drug passes to the fetus and may cause fatal bleeding in the fetus. Warfarin also passes in milk to the child, so women receiving warfarin should not breast feed their infants.

Avoid any activities that have a high risk of injury. You may want to carry a card or wear a bracelet indicating that you are taking warfarin, so those treating you will know this in the event of an accident.

Avoid excessive consumption of alcoholic beverages while taking warfarin. Ask your doctor how much, if any, alcohol you may consume.

DOSAGE AND STORAGE

Warfarin tablets usually are taken once every 24 hours. Your doctor has determined how often you should take this medication. Carefully follow the instructions on your prescription label, and ask your doctor or pharmacist to explain anything you do not understand. *You must control the amount of warfarin you take.* Your doctor may change the dosage often to find the right amount for you. If you take too much, you may start bleeding. If you take too little, you may get more blood clots.

Do not change your daily dose unless advised to do so by your doctor. To avoid missing any doses, plan to take this medication at the same time every day. Record your doses on a calendar with a mark after you have taken the dose. *You must continue taking warfarin for as long as your doctor tells you to take it.* If you miss a dose, take it as soon as possible. If you do not remember until the next day, do not take two doses. Take only the one scheduled. *Never take a double dose of warfarin.* If you miss doses for two or more days, call your doctor.

Keep warfarin in the container it came in, and keep it out of the reach of children. Do not allow anyone else to take it.

Other Anticoagulants

The most commonly prescribed anticoagulant drug is **warfarin** (described in detail on page 46).

The uses, undesirable effects, precautions and dosage and storage instructions for the following anticoagulants taken orally are generally the same as for warfarin.

Anisindione (brand name, Miradon)
Dicumarol
Phenindione (brand name, Hedulin)
Phenprocoumon (brand name, Liquamar)

High Blood Cholesterol

Cholesterol and triglycerides are fatty acids found in all body tissues, including the blood. People with high levels of fats in their blood have a greater risk of heart disease than do people with lower levels. It is believed that when large amounts of these fatty substances are in the blood, they can harden and build up along the walls of the blood vessels coming from the heart. This buildup is called atherosclerosis. Atherosclerosis decreases the flow of blood, causing heart disease, angina (heart pain), heart attack or stroke.

It has not been established whether lowering the level of cholesterol and triglycerides by means of drugs is helpful in preventing heart disease, angina, heart attack or stroke. However, many doctors hope that bringing blood cholesterol and triglyceride levels to normal and keeping them there can prevent or slow up this clogging process that results in atherosclerosis.

There are generally three causes of too much cholesterol and triglycerides in the blood: diet (eating too many foods high in cholesterol, eating too many fatty foods and drinking too much alcohol), various diseases and heredity.

The first step in therapy is treatment of the underlying disease: exercise and a diet restricting the intake of fat, cholesterol and alcohol. If these means do not have the desired effect, appropriate drugs may be given along with the diet and exercise.

If your doctor has suggested a certain diet or exercise program, follow these plans carefully, even while taking a drug or drugs to lower the level of fat in the blood. You will also have regular blood tests to find out if the drugs, diet and exercise are effective. In addition, you may have tests to determine if the drugs are causing any harmful effects.

Drugs used to lower the levels of fatty acids—cholesterol and triglycerides— are called antilipemics.

ANTILIPEMICS
Cholestyramine
(koe less′ tir a meen)

Brand name: Questran

Cholestyramine is used along with diet therapy to reduce the amount of cholesterol in the blood. Cholestyramine is also prescribed to relieve the itching caused by certain kinds of jaundice.

UNDESIRED EFFECTS
Cholestyramine can cause changes in the appearance of stools or a particularly

unpleasant odor from them. This side effect is harmless and should not worry you.

Other undesired effects are constipation, nausea and bloating. If these occur, contact your doctor. Also contact your doctor if you experience any unusual bleeding, such as bleeding from the gums or rectum, or frequent blushing.

PRECAUTIONS

Cholestyramine may affect the way your body responds to certain other drugs, including anticoagulants (blood thinners). Before you begin to take cholestyramine, tell your doctor what other prescription or nonprescription drugs you are taking. If you don't know the names of the drugs or what they were prescribed for, take the labeled containers to your doctor or pharmacist.

Cholestyramine often interferes with the absorption of other drugs such as digitalis, steroids and those for thyroid conditions. Other drugs should be taken one hour before or several hours after cholestyramine is taken.

Your doctor may want you to have laboratory tests to determine how you are responding to cholestyramine. *Be sure to keep your appointments for these tests* because they give your doctor important information about the effectiveness of the drug.

It is not known whether this drug is safe for a pregnant woman or her unborn child.

DOSAGE AND STORAGE

Cholestyramine is available as a dry powder and is usually taken before meals and at bedtime. Your prescription label tells you when to take this medication and how much to take at each dose. Follow these instructions carefully. Contact your doctor or pharmacist if you have any question about the dosage.

Cholestyramine powder must be mixed with fluids or food. *Do not take the powder alone*. To use the powder, follow these steps:

1. Spread the powder on the surface of a glass of water, milk, fruit juice or soup.

2. Let the powder stand for one minute, then stir it into the beverage and drink it.

3. Put more of the beverage in the glass and drink the beverage to be sure you are consuming all the powder.

The powder also may be mixed with applesauce, crushed pineapple or pureed fruit. The powder should be added to the liquid or food just before you consume it.

If you forget to take a dose, take it as soon as you remember. Take the remaining doses for that day at evenly spaced intervals. However, if you remember a missed dose at the time you are scheduled to take another dose, omit the missed dose and take only the scheduled one. *Do not take a double dose.*

Cholestyramine should be kept in the container it came in, tightly closed and away from moisture. Keep it out of the reach of children and do not allow anyone else to take it.

Clofibrate

(koe fye′ brate)

Brand name: Atromid-S

Clofibrate is used to reduce the amount of fatty substances—cholesterol and triglycerides—in the blood. Clofibrate usually is not prescribed until after it has been determined that diet and exercise alone will not reduce the amount of fatty substances in the blood to the desired levels. A high level of fats in the blood increases the risk of heart disease; use of clofibrate, along with diet and exercise, is intended to reduce this risk. Clofibrate should be used only by people who have not responded sufficiently to diet, exercise or other measures prescribed by their doctors.

UNDESIRED EFFECTS

Clofibrate can cause nausea, vomiting, diarrhea, bloating, weight gain, sore or aching muscles or muscle cramps. Other side effects may include skin reactions (such as itching or rash); loss of hair and dry, brittle hair; headache; dizziness; increased appetite and weight gain; decreased sexual desire; painful or difficult urination; liver problems; anemia; and a decrease of white blood cells. If you experience any of these side effects or get flulike symptoms, contact your doctor.

PRECAUTIONS

Clofibrate may increase the risk of having gallbladder trouble or of getting tumors. The risks have been described in this way:

Two very large studies indicated that taking clofibrate for several years presents important risks. These studies showed a doubling of the risk of getting gallstones or an inflamed gallbladder. For people taking clofibrate for five years, about one patient in 100 may require gallbladder surgery.

One of the studies also suggested that people who take clofibrate have an increased risk of getting cancer. For people taking clofibrate for five years, this study suggested that an additional one person out of 400 would be expected to get cancer during the five-year period; this is about a 30 percent increase above the average cancer rate for the general population. Mice and rats given clofibrate at five to eight times the human dose showed an increased number of liver tumors, some of which were cancerous.

Several other problems relating to the heart and circulation of blood were noted in the other study. These include heart arrhythmia (abnormal heartbeat), blood clotting, angina (chest or heart pain) and blood circulation problems (noticed by pain in the legs).

Because of these risks and the uncertain benefits of this drug (and others used to treat high blood levels of cholesterol and triglycerides), relatively few patients should take clofibrate continuously.

Clofibrate may affect the way your body responds to certain other drugs, particularly anticoagulants (blood thinners). Before you begin to take clofibrate, tell your doctor what other prescription or nonprescription drugs you are taking.

He may have to adjust your dosage of other drugs while you are taking clofibrate. If you don't know the names of the drugs or what they were prescribed for, take the labeled containers to your doctor or pharmacist.

If you have previously had a heart attack, jaundice or liver or kidney disease, inform your doctor before you begin to take clofibrate.

If you have diabetes and you can control it by diet or drugs, your cholesterol and triglyceride levels may also be controlled by them. Therefore, you may not need to take clofibrate to reduce the amount of fatty substances in your blood. If you have a stomach or intestinal ulcer, taking clofibrate may irritate the ulcer.

Laboratory tests are necessary while you are taking clofibrate so that your doctor can determine how your body is responding to it. *Be sure to keep appointments for these tests,* which give your doctor important information.

You should not take clofibrate if you are pregnant or nursing a child. Women capable of becoming pregnant should practice birth control while taking clofibrate. Women who plan to become pregnant should stop taking clofibrate several months before trying to become pregnant.

DOSAGE AND STORAGE

Usually clofibrate capsules are taken two to four times a day. Your prescription label tells you how often to take this medication and how much to take at each dose. Follow the instructions carefully and ask your doctor or pharmacist to explain any part you do not understand.

Take clofibrate between meals without food. *Do not stop taking this medication until your doctor specifically tells you to do so.* Your doctor may decide to stop your clofibrate therapy after a few months if the cholesterol and triglyceride levels in your blood have not decreased. To make sure your doctor can tell how well clofibrate is working, it is important to take it exactly as prescribed.

If you forget to take a dose, take the missed dose as soon as you remember it. If you remember a missed dose at the time you are scheduled to take the next one, take only the regularly scheduled dose and take the remaining doses for that day at evenly. spaced intervals. *Do not take a double dose.*

Keep clofibrate in the container it came in and keep it out of the reach of children. Do not allow anyone else to take it.

Niacin
(nye' a sin)

Brand names: Diacin, Nicotinic Acid, Nicobid, Nicolar and others.

Niacin, also known as nicotinic acid, is one of the B vitamins (B_3). In large doses, niacin reduces the amount of cholesterol and triglycerides in the blood. When given in large doses, niacin also dilates or widens the blood vessels to improve circulation.

Niacin is prescribed for three different conditions. It is used to prevent buildup of fatty deposits inside the blood vessels and, with other vasodilator drugs, to treat conditions caused by poor circulation. It is also used to prevent and treat pellagra (niacin deficiency disease), which can result from an inadequate diet, chronic stomach and intestinal disease or alcoholism.

UNDESIRED EFFECTS

Niacin can cause flushing, itching and a sensation of warmth or burning of the skin (especially the face, neck or ears), headache, nausea, vomiting or diarrhea. These effects usually go away as you continue to take the medicine; but if they continue to bother you, contact your doctor.

Niacin may make you dizzy, especially when moving suddenly from a lying to a sitting position or from a sitting to a standing position. Avoid sudden changes in posture.

PRECAUTIONS

Niacin may affect the way your body responds to certain other drugs, including digitalis drugs, and medications prescribed for high blood pressure, irregular heartbeat or diabetes. Be sure to tell your doctor what other prescription or nonprescription drugs you are taking before you begin to take niacin. If you don't know the names of the drugs or what they were prescribed for, take the labeled containers to your doctor or pharmacist.

Before you begin to take niacin, tell your doctor if you have gallbladder disease or a history of jaundice or liver disease, gout, peptic ulcer or allergy.

Your doctor may want you to have laboratory tests to determine how you are responding to this medication. *Be sure to keep your appointments for these tests* because they give your doctor important information about the effectiveness of the drug.

DOSAGE AND STORAGE

Niacin tablets usually are taken two to four times a day. Take them with cold water, not hot liquids. Your prescription label tells you how often to take niacin and how much to take at each dose. Follow the instructions and contact your doctor or pharmacist if there is any part of them you do not understand.

This drug should be taken with meals or immediately after eating. If you forget to take a dose, take the missed dose as soon as you remember it. Take the remaining doses for that day at evenly spaced intervals. However, if you remember a missed dose at the time you are scheduled to take another dose, omit the missed dose and take only the scheduled one. *Do not take a double dose.*

This medication should be kept in the container it came in, tightly closed and away from moisture. Keep it out of the reach of children and do not allow anyone else to take it.

Miscellaneous Drugs Used in Treating Heart Diseases and Diseases of the Circulatory System

ELECTROLYTE REPLACEMENT

Potassium Supplements

Brand names: K-Lor, K-Lyte, K-Pote, Kaochlor, Kaon, K-tab, KayCiel, Kaylixir, Klotrix, Klorvess, Potasalan, Slow-K, Tri-K, Trikates and others.

A small amount of potassium in the blood is essential for proper function of many parts of the body, including the heart, kidneys, muscles, nerves and digestive system. Usually the food you eat will supply all the potassium you need. However, certain diseases and certain prescription drugs (diuretics or water pills, digitalis, or steroids or cortisone-type drugs, for example) can remove potassium from the body, and it must be replaced. If you are taking a diuretic (water pill) for high blood pressure, for example, your doctor has probably told you to eat more potassium-rich foods or has prescribed a potassium supplement. (See the section on **diuretics**, page 9, for more complete information.)

Potassium supplements are used to prevent and treat potassium loss from the body and the weakness and tiredness that potassium deficiency causes. Several different potassium salts including acetate, bicarbonate, chloride, citrate and gluconate are used alone or in combination as oral medication.

UNDESIRED EFFECTS

Upset stomach is the major undesired effect of potassium supplements. To avoid or diminish this effect, take the medication after eating a meal or snack, or take it with a full glass of water. Contact your doctor if stomach upsets continue to occur.

Too much potassium also can cause problems. *Do not take any more potassium than your doctor tells you to*. While you are taking potassium, keep in touch with your doctor. He will want to check the way you are responding to it. If you are using a salt substitute because you are on a low-salt or no-salt diet, be sure to tell your doctor about the salt substitute. Many salt substitutes contain potassium. If you are taking a salt substitute, it could affect the dosage of potassium supplement you will need.

PRECAUTIONS

Some tablet forms of potassium that are swallowed have produced ulceration and obstruction in the small intestine or stomach. If you develop abdominal or stomach pain, persistent indigestion, vomiting or intestinal bleeding while taking potassium in a tablet, or if you have chronic constipation, you probably should not take potassium in tablet form.

If you are taking another medication along with the potassium supplement and you stop taking the other medication or have your prescription changed to another drug, ask your doctor whether you should continue to take the potassium supplement. Do not take the potassium supplement if you are dehydrated or have muscle cramps from too much exposure to the sun. Contact your doctor. Do not take it if you are taking the drug spironolactone or triamterene. Contact your doctor about these combinations. Be sure your doctor knows about *all* other drugs you are taking, especially steroids or any heart medications. Give your doctor a complete medical history before you begin to take this drug.

DOSAGE AND STORAGE

Potassium supplements come in four forms—powder, liquid, tablets to be dissolved in water before ingestion, and tablets to be swallowed. Instructions for preparing a dose and for taking the drug must be followed closely. The powder and the liquid should be added to water, milk, coffee, tea, soft drinks or fruit juice and mixed well (the powder fully dissolved) just before you take them. Measure each dose carefully to be sure you have the same amount each time you take a dose. *Take potassium with or after food or a meal to avoid stomach irritation.*

The tablets to be dissolved in water should be thoroughly dissolved and mixed well just before you take them. *The tablets to be swallowed must be swallowed, not chewed.* Take them with a full glass of water and with food or after meals.

Your doctor will choose the form best for you, and your prescription label tells you when to take the potassium supplement and how much to take at each dose. Follow the instructions carefully and ask your doctor or pharmacist about any part of them you do not understand.

If you forget to take a dose, take it as soon as you remember. Be sure you have enough of this medication on hand at all times to permit you to take all the doses that have been prescribed for you. Check your supply before holidays or when you plan to be away from home and at any other time it may be difficult to get more.

Keep the potassium supplement in the container it came in, and keep it out of the reach of children. Do not allow anyone else to take it.

Generally, potassium supplements can be used safely during pregnancy as long as dosage is carefully controlled.

Your doctor will want to do certain laboratory tests to help adjust your dosage and to keep your side effects to a minimum.

POOR CIRCULATION
Isoxsuprine
(eye sox′ syoo preen)

Brand name: Vasodilan

Isoxsuprine is a vasodilator drug that relaxes the muscles in the walls of the blood vessels, causing them to widen or expand so that more blood flows more smoothly through them. It is used to improve blood circulation in the brain and, in combination with other types of therapy, to treat diseases of the blood vessels in the arms, legs, hands and feet. Improved circulation results in an increase in the supply of oxygen to body tissues and relieves the symptoms of poor circulation.

UNDESIRED EFFECTS

If you have high blood pressure or severe impairment of circulation to the brain or heart (angina), you may not benefit from this drug, and those conditions may worsen.

Isoxsuprine can cause rapid heart rate or palpitation, flushing, lightheadedness or tiredness. If you experience these effects and if they bother you, contact your doctor. Be sure to tell him if you have ever had an allergic reaction to isoxsuprine.

Contact your doctor if you have nausea, vomiting or abdominal cramps while you are taking isoxsuprine. If you develop a skin rash, contact your doctor to find out whether you should continue to take isoxsuprine.

Isoxsuprine also can cause you to be dizzy when you move. To avoid this effect, change position slowly. Contact your doctor if dizziness continues.

PRECAUTIONS

If you smoke, ask your physician if you may continue to smoke. Nicotine can make isoxsuprine less effective in dilating blood vessels and improving circulation.

You should also avoid exposure to cold because a cold environment or handling cold objects may make this drug less effective.

DOSAGE AND STORAGE

Isoxsuprine tablets usually are taken three or four times a day, preferably with or just following meals to reduce stomach irritation. Your prescription label tells you how often to take isoxsuprine and how much to take at each dose. Dosage is carefully individualized for you. Follow the instructions carefully. If you do not understand any part of them, contact your doctor or pharmacist for an explanation.

Do not take more of this drug than your doctor has prescribed. If you forget a dose, omit that dose completely and take the next dose at the regularly scheduled time. *Do not take a double dose to make up for the one missed.*

Keep isoxsuprine in the container it came in. Keep it out of the reach of children. Do not let anyone else take it.

Papaverine
(pa pav' er een)

Brand names: Cerebid, Cerespan, Pavabid, Vasocap, Vasospan and others.

Papaverine is one of the group of antispasmodic drugs, which means that it improves blood circulation by relieving spasm in the small blood vessels and thereby increasing the diameter of the blood vessel. Papaverine is used to treat people with problems caused by a poor supply of blood to the brain and other parts of the body, especially the extremities. Improved circulation results in an increase in the supply of oxygen to body tissues and relieves the symptoms of poor circulation. Papaverine is also useful in treating heart conditions in which the decreased blood supply causes irregular heartbeats.

Papaverine is obtained from opium, which is also the source for morphine. However, papaverine is very different from morphine in its effects.

UNDESIRED EFFECTS

Papaverine can cause flushing of the face, sweating, irregular pulse, dryness of the mouth or throat, itching, rash, dizziness, headache, stomach irritation, nausea, constipation or loss of appetite. If you experience these effects or if you have disturbances in vision or yellowing of the skin or eyes, contact your doctor.

Papaverine makes some people drowsy or dizzy when they move. Do not drive a car or operate dangerous machinery until you know how papaverine will affect you.

PRECAUTIONS

Papaverine can affect the results of some blood tests. If your doctor prescribes blood tests for you, remind him that you are taking papaverine. You probably will be asked to have laboratory tests to help your doctor monitor how the drug is affecting you. *Be sure to keep all appointments* with your doctor and the laboratory.

If you have severe impairment of circulation to the brain or heart (angina), you may not benefit from this drug and these conditions may worsen.

Before you begin to take papaverine, tell your doctor if you have angina, heart disease, Parkinson's disease or glaucoma or if you have ever had a stroke or an allergic reaction to papaverine. Be sure to tell him what other prescription or nonprescription drugs you are taking. If you do not know the names of the drugs or what they were prescribed for, take the labeled containers to your doctor or pharmacist.

Nicotine can reduce the effectiveness of papaverine, so if you are a smoker, ask your doctor if you may continue to smoke. Papaverine may cause excessive sweating in hot environments; cold environments or exposure to cold may make the drug less effective.

DOSAGE AND STORAGE
Papaverine comes in tablets and capsules and in extended-release tablets and capsules. The regular tablets or capsules usually are taken from three to five times a day, with or immediately following meals or other food to reduce stomach irritation. Extended-release tablets or capsules are usually taken twice a day. Your doctor will select the dosage form he considers best for you. Your prescription label tells you how often to take papaverine and how much to take at each dose. Follow these instructions carefully and contact your doctor or pharmacist if you do not understand any part of it.

If you forget to take a dose, take the missed dose as soon as you remember it; take the remaining doses for that day at evenly spaced intervals. If you do not remember the dose until it is time for you to take another, omit the missed dose completely and take only the scheduled dose. *Do not take a double dose to make up for the missed one.*

Keep papaverine in the container it came in, and keep it out of the reach of children. Do not allow anyone else to take it.

SENILITY
Ergoloid Mesylate
(er' goe lloyd mess' ill ate)

Brand names: Cicanol, Hydergine, Trigot

Ergoloid mesylate is used to treat the problems of "senility" in the elderly, such as dizziness, mental confusion or depression, unsociability and lack of interest in self-care when these problems are thought to be caused by a poor supply of blood to the brain. However, there is no convincing evidence that this drug improves the flow of blood within the brain nor, for that matter, that all these problems are related to impaired flow of blood to the brain! Many health professionals believe that better nutrition and making the elderly feel useful and needed are the best ways to make them more mentally alert. The true causes of the symptoms of "senility" are not really known, and behavioral changes in the elderly are unpredictable. It is difficult, therefore, to measure the effectiveness of drugs intended to treat "senility."

UNDESIRED EFFECTS
When ergoloid mesylate is prescribed as tablets to be placed under the tongue and dissolved, it can cause irritation under the tongue. Skin rash, runny or stuffy nose, lightheadedness, loss of appetite, nausea and vomiting occur rarely. Contact your doctor if they do. Some patients may experience a sudden and severe drop in blood pressure as well as sluggishness, apathy and withdrawal.

An overdose of ergoloid mesylate will cause a severe drop in blood pressure, collapse and possibly coma.

PRECAUTIONS
Before an elderly person takes ergoloid mesylate, he should have a thorough examination to make sure another disease is not causing the problems of "senility." Ergoloid mesylate should not be taken by patients with very low blood pressure. Your doctor should be told of any other medications you are taking, especially drugs to treat a heart condition or high blood pressure.

DOSAGE AND STORAGE
Ergoloid mesylate comes in tablets to be swallowed or in tablets to be placed under the tongue and dissolved. Tablets to be dissolved under the tongue have to be kept there for three to six minutes, and the saliva should be retained in the mouth as long as possible before swallowing; these tablets should *not* be chewed or swallowed whole. Since many elderly patients have difficulty remembering this routine, the tablets to be dissolved under the tongue are not prescribed very frequently for them.

Ergoloid mesylate usually is taken three times a day. Your prescription tells you how much to take and how often to take it. Follow these instructions carefully. Ask your doctor or pharmacist if you do not understand any part of the directions.

Usually three or four weeks of continuous therapy are needed before improvement of the "senility" problem.

Keep ergoloid mesylate in the container it came in, tightly closed and away from heat and moisture. Keep it out of the reach of children. Do not allow anyone else to take it.

INFECTIONS

INFECTIONS

Anti-infectives

The drugs used to help the body combat infections are called, simply, anti-infectives. Infections may be caused by a wide variety of organisms, including bacteria, protozoa, fungi, rickettsiae, spirochetes and viruses. Each anti-infective drug is effective against certain organisms. A few have a broad spectrum of activity, fighting infections caused by a number of different organisms. In addition to being effective only against particular organisms, anti-infectives also must be present in body tissues and fluids in high enough concentration to "overcome" the infection. Some anti-infectives are absorbed into the bloodstream from the stomach or intestines and go throughout the body. Thus these "systemic" anti-infectives (primarily antibiotics) are used to treat "systemic" infections such as pneumonia, flu or other respiratory infections, sore throat, skin infections, ear or sinus infections and venereal infections in a variety of sites in the body. Other anti-infectives reach sufficient concentrations only in certain parts of the body—in the urine, for example. Still others are most effective applied directly to the site of the infection, such as the eye or the skin. These are called "topical" or "local" anti-infectives.

"Antibiotic" is a term used to designate a metabolic product of one organism that is detrimental to the life activities of other organisms. Antibiotics are anti-infectives, generally of biologic origin. They are derived from bacteria, molds, fungi or other living substances. Some synthetic and semi-synthetically produced substances that were originally obtained from microorganisms are also called antibiotics.

Antibiotics can be classified according to their spectrum of activity against the various classes of microorganisms—gram-positive and gram-negative bacteria, rickettsiae, viruses, spirochetes, fungi and protozoa. Those antibiotics that have been effective outside a living body against one or more strains in several classes of organisms are referred to as broad-spectrum antibiotics; those effective against only one or two classes are called narrow-spectrum antibiotics.

When your doctor selects an anti-infective for you, he must take into account the probable infecting organism and the location of the infection in your body. He may do "culture and sensitivity" laboratory tests to determine the causative organism and the best drug to use to treat the infection. In other instances, the organism causing the infection may be obvious (for example, nail infections usually are caused by fungi), or he may know of a community or family "epidemic" of infection caused by a particular organism. In other situations, he may prescribe a broad-spectrum antibiotic because it is effective against a wide range of organisms.

Many anti-infectives, including antibiotics, actually do not destroy the infecting organism. The anti-infectives only slow down or interrupt growth and reproduction of the organism. The patient's body then takes over the fight, and the body's natural defense mechanisms actually "cure" the infection. Thus, when you have a prescription for an anti-infective, it is important that you *take all the medication prescribed.* Since the drug only controls growth and slows down the infection, you must continue to take the medication long enough to give your body a fair chance to overcome the infecting organism. If you stop taking the drug after a few days because you feel better, the infection will flare up again before your body has completed the fight.

There are no anti-infectives effective against the virus that causes the common cold. Antibiotics may be useful in treating other infections, primarily caused by bacteria, that may follow a bad cold. In general, however, a cold should *not* be treated with antibiotics. Treat a cold's symptoms as they occur. (See the section on **allergies and coughs and colds**, page 00.)

Many organisms can become resistant to the anti-infective's used to combat them; the drugs then no longer effectively prevent their growth. Thus, if you are taking one anti-infective and it doesn't seem to be working, your doctor may prescribe a different drug.

If you have medication remaining when your prescription is changed, do not save it for future use or let anyone else take it. Ask your pharmacist how to dispose of it.

When taken orally, anti-infectives generally are absorbed from the stomach and intestines. Solid food and, in some cases, milk and some drugs such as antacids interfere with the absorption of the anti-infective drugs. On the other hand, the absorption of some anti-infectives is not affected by the presence of solid food, milk or other drugs in the stomach. Check with your doctor or pharmacist if you can take the anti-infective drug with meals. If you are told to take it on an "empty stomach" (to be certain that enough of the drug is absorbed to control infection effectively), take the drug one hour before or two hours after a meal or snack. Some anti-infectives may cause nausea or vomiting if taken on an "empty stomach" but can be taken with a light snack to avoid stomach upsets.

Since a number of anti-infectives effectively inhibit the growth of many different organisms, these anti-infectives can stop the growth of bacteria that normally live in the gastrointestinal or urinary tract. These natural bacteria are needed to maintain certain body functions (for example, the breakdown of waste products), and anti-infectives may destroy them. When this bacterial growth stops, other bacteria, fungi and other organisms that are resistant to and not destroyed by the anti-infectives may flourish. Symptoms may include severe diarrhea, nausea and vomiting, a feeling of abdominal fullness, abdominal pain and weakness. The lining of the mouth and the tongue and gums may be covered with white patches that leave reddened surfaces when removed. The vaginal or rectal area may be affected in the same way. *If these symptoms of "super-infection" or overgrowth of nonsusceptible organisms occur, you should stop taking the anti-infective drug and contact your doctor.*

Antibiotic drugs are easily divided into groups (sometimes called "families") that are similar in chemical structure and use in treating infections. Thus, the first part of this chapter discusses several groups of antibiotics—cephalosporins, erythromycins, penicillins and tetracyclines. The drugs in each group have similar base chemical structures. These drugs are used to treat many different kinds of infections. Discussion of these groups of antibiotics in the text is followed by descriptions of some other antibiotics that do not fit neatly into any large family on the basis of their chemistry and uses.

The next groups of anti-infectives are discussed in relationship to the kinds of infections against which they are most commonly used. These include drugs used primarily to treat tuberculosis, urinary tract infections, vaginal infections and eye infections.

Many of the antibiotics discussed in the earlier part of the chapter are also used to treat infections in the urinary tract, vagina or in eyes.

To find the information on the drug you are interested in, use the Index at the back of the book.

CEPHALOSPORINS
Cefaclor
(sef′ a klor)

Brand name: Ceclor

Cefaclor is a cephalosporin antibiotic that is similar to the penicillins in the way it eliminates bacteria. It is used to treat certain types of infections in the throat, ears, skin and urinary tract.

Cefaclor can be used in infections caused by bacteria that produce penicillinase (a substance that makes some penicillins ineffective). However, penicillins are generally preferred to cefaclor in the treatment of "strep" infections and in the prevention of rheumatic fever.

UNDESIRED EFFECTS
Tell your doctor if you have ever had an allergic reaction to any of the cephalosporins or to any form of penicillin.

Allergic reactions, though rare, have occurred with cefaclor. They range from mild rash to serious and sometimes fatal reactions. A serious reaction is more likely to occur in a person with other allergies.

If you get a rash, hives or itching or have difficulty breathing, call your doctor or a hospital. You may need emergency treatment.

The most common side effects of cefaclor are diarrhea, nausea and vomiting. These effects usually are mild and tend to disappear as you continue to take cefaclor and your body adjusts to it. If these effects are severe or last more than two days, contact your doctor.

Cefaclor also can upset your stomach or give you stomach cramps. Usually these reactions can be relieved by taking cefaclor with crackers or a light snack. Contact your doctor if these problems continue.

Some allergic reactions, such as rash and itching all over your body, joint pains, fever or swollen glands, develop only after several days of therapy. Contact your doctor if you experience any of these effects.

In people who are sensitive to this drug, cefaclor can cause blood problems, such as bone marrow depression or a decrease in one of the blood clotting factors. Contact your doctor if you notice any unusual bleeding or easy bruising, get painful sores in your mouth or throat, or develop chills and fever.

Long-term therapy with cefaclor may result in an overgrowth of other organisms in the body. Some symptoms of this condition are itching of the anus, sore mouth or tongue and vaginal infection. If you experience these symptoms, stop taking cefaclor and contact your doctor.

PRECAUTIONS

Before you start taking cefaclor, be sure to tell your doctor or pharmacist if you have ever had an allergic reaction to any cephalosporin or any form of penicillin. Your doctor should be told if you have kidney disease or a history of allergy.

Some other medications, particularly gout medicines, should not be taken with cefaclor. Tell your doctor what other prescription or nonprescription drugs you are taking. If you do not know what drugs you are taking or what they were prescribed for, bring them in their labeled containers to your doctor or pharmacist.

Even if you feel better in a few days after taking cefaclor, take *all* of the medication prescribed for you by your doctor. Bacterial infections take from several days to weeks to be cured completely. If you stop taking the cefaclor, those bacteria still alive can multiply and cause a recurrence of the infection. However, if your symptoms do not improve within a few days or if they become worse, contact your doctor. He may want to change your medication.

Be sure to tell your doctor if you are pregnant or are nursing an infant. Though problems with this medication have not been reported in the literature, your doctor will to consider whether the benefit to you is worth the possible risk to your baby.

Diabetics should be aware that cefaclor can cause false results in some tests for urine sugar. Do not change your diet or the dosage of your diabetes medicine unless you check with your doctor.

Cefaclor also can cause a temporary change in the results of liver function tests. If you have these tests done, be sure the person responsible for reporting the results knows you have been taking cefaclor.

DOSAGE AND STORAGE

Your doctor will determine how often you should take cefaclor. Follow the instructions on your prescription label and ask your doctor or pharmacist to explain any part you do not understand.

Doses of cefaclor should be taken as far apart as possible during the day. If your doctor tells you to take it four times a day, take a dose every six hours. If you give cefaclor to a child, make sure he or she receives it around the clock, even if you have to wake the child for doses.

Cefaclor is best taken on an "empty stomach," one hour before meals or two hours after eating. However, if cefaclor upsets your stomach, it can be taken with meals or a light snack.

Cefaclor comes in capsules, tablets, liquid form and pediatric drops. The tablets and capsules should be taken with a full eight-ounce glass of water.

The container of liquid or pediatric drops (to be taken orally) should be shaken thoroughly to mix the medication evenly before each dose is poured. Measure the prescribed number of drops with the bottle dropper. If there is no dropper with the bottle of liquid, use a specially marked measuring spoon to be sure the dose is accurate. Contact your pharmacist if you have any questions about measuring the liquid.

If you forget to take a dose, take it as soon as you remember. Take any remaining doses for that day at evenly spaced intervals. If you still have symptoms of the infection after you have taken all the medicine, contact your doctor.

When your doctor tells you to stop taking cefaclor, throw away any unused portion of it. Cefaclor may lose it effectiveness after a period of time and should not be saved to treat another infection. Because this medication was prescribed for your particular condition, do not allow anyone else to take your cefaclor.

Keep this medication in the container it came in. Keep liquid cefaclor in the refrigerator but do not freeze it. On the container, you will find an expiration date. Do not take the medication after that date. Throw it away and, if you need more, get a new supply. If you are not sure of the expiration date or have any questions about a refill, contact your pharmacist.

Keep this medication out of the reach of children.

Cephaloglycin
(sef a loe glye' sin)

Brand name: Kafocin

Cephaloglycin is a cephalosporin antibiotic that is used to treat urinary tract infections only. However, some doctors prefer other cephalosporins (such as cephalexin and cephadrine) for these infections because more of these drugs get into the blood to fight infection and they cause fewer stomach and bowel problems.

UNDESIRED EFFECTS
Tell your doctor if you have ever had an allergic reaction to any of the cephalosporins or to any form of penicillin.

Allergic reactions, though rare, have occurred with cephaloglycin. They range from mild rash to serious and sometimes fatal reactions. A serious reaction is more likely to occur in a person with other allergies or a previous reaction to penicillins or cephalosporins.

If you get a rash, hives or itching or have difficulty breathing, call your doctor or a hospital. You may need emergency treatment.

Cephaloglycin can cause serious stomach and intestinal problems that require medical treatment. If you notice bloody or black, tarry stools, or suffer severe stomach cramps, pain or bloating, or have severe diarrhea, you may have an inflammation of the intestines or be bleeding internally. Stop taking cephaloglycin and check with your doctor at once.

Mild diarrhea, nausea or vomiting may occur when you start to take cephaloglycin. These effects tend to disappear as you continue to take cephaloglycin and as your body adjusts to it. Contact your doctor if these effects are severe or last more than two days.

If this medication upsets your stomach or gives you mild stomach cramps, take it with crackers or a light snack. Contact your doctor if these problems continue.

Some allergic reactions, such as rash and itching all over your body, joint pains, fever or swollen glands, develop only after several days of therapy. Contact your doctor if you have any of these effects.

In people who are sensitive to this drug, cephaloglycin can cause blood problems, such as bone marrow depression or a decrease in one of the blood clotting factors. Contact your doctor if you notice any unusual bleeding or easy bruising, get painful sores in the mouth or throat, or develop chills and fever.

Long-term therapy with cephaloglycin may result in an overgrowth of other organisms in the body. If you experience itching of the anus, sore mouth or tongue or vaginal infection, stop taking the medication and contact your doctor.

PRECAUTIONS

Before you start taking cephaloglycin, be sure to tell your doctor or pharmacist if you have ever had an allergic reaction to any cephalosporin or to any form of penicillin. Your doctor should be told if you have kidney disease or a history of any kind of allergy.

Some other medications, particularly probenecid (gout medicine), should not be taken with cephaloglycin because they can increase the undesired effects. Tell your doctor or pharmacist what other prescription or nonprescription drugs you are taking. If you do not know the names of the drugs or what they were prescribed for, bring them in their labeled containers to your doctor or pharmacist. Contact your doctor or pharmacist before starting to take any other medications while you are taking cephaloglycin.

Even if you feel better in a few days, take *all* of the medicine your doctor has prescribed. Bacterial infections take several days to weeks to be cured completely. If you stop taking cephaloglycin, the bacteria still alive can multiply and cause a recurrence of the infection. However, if your symptoms do not improve within a few days or if they become worse, contact your doctor. He may want to change your medication.

Be sure to tell your doctor if you are pregnant or nursing an infant. Though problems with this medication have not been reported in the literature, your doctor will need to consider whether the benefit to you is worth the possible risk to your baby.

Diabetics should be aware that cephaloglycin can cause false results in some tests for sugar in the urine. Do not change your diet or the dosage of your diabetes medicine unless you check with your doctor.

Cephaloglycin also can cause temporary changes in the results of liver function tests. If you have these tests done, be sure the person responsible for reporting the results knows you have been taking cephaloglycin.

Cephaloglycin should not be given to infants under one year of age.

DOSAGE AND STORAGE

Your doctor will determine how often you should take cephaloglycin. Follow the instructions on your prescription label and ask your doctor or pharmacist to explain any part you do not understand.

Doses of cephaloglycin should be taken as far apart as possible during the day. If your doctor tells you to take it four times a day, take a dose every six hours. If you give cephaloglycin to a child, make sure he or she receives it around the clock, even if you must wake the child for doses.

Cephaloglycin comes in capsules that should be taken with a full eight-ounce glass of water. It is best taken on an "empty stomach," one hour before meals, or two hours after eating. However, if this medication upsets your stomach, it can be taken with meals or a light snack.

If you forget to take a dose, take it as soon as you remember. Take the remaining doses for that day at evenly spaced intervals. If you still have symptoms of the infection after you have taken all the medicine, contact your doctor.

When your doctor tells you to stop taking cephaloglycin, throw away any unused portion of it. Cephaloglycin may lose its effectiveness after a period of time and should not be saved to treat another infection. Because this medication was prescribed for your condition, do not allow anyone else to take it.

Keep this medication in the container it came in, tightly closed, away from excessive heat and out of the reach of children.

Cephalexin
(sef a lex′ in)

Brand name: Keflex

Cephalexin is a cephalosporin antibiotic that is similar to the penicillins in the way it eliminates bacteria. It is used to treat certain types of infections in the throat, ears, skin and urinary tract.

Cephalexin can be used against infections caused by bacteria that produce penicillinase (a substance that makes some penicillins ineffective). However, penicillins are generally preferred to cephalexin in the treatment of "strep" infections and in the prevention of rheumatic fever.

UNDESIRED EFFECTS

Tell your doctor if you have ever had an allergic reaction to any of the cephalosporins or to any form of penicillin.

Allergic reactions, though rare, have occurred with cephalexin. They range from mild rash to serious and sometimes fatal reactions. A serious reaction is more likely to occur in a person with other allergies.

If you get a rash, hives or itching or have difficulty breathing, call your doctor or a hospital. You may need emergency treatment.

The most common side effects of cephalexin are diarrhea, nausea and vomiting. These effects usually are mild and tend to disappear as you continue to take cephalexin and as your body adjusts to it. If these effects are severe or last more than two days, contact your doctor.

Cephalexin can also upset your stomach or give you stomach cramps. Usually these reactions can be relieved by taking the medication with crackers or a light snack. Contact your doctor if these problems continue.

Some allergic reactions, such as rash and itching all over your body, joint pains, fever or swollen glands, develop only after several days of therapy. Contact your doctor if you have any of these effects.

In people who are sensitive to this drug, cephalexin can cause blood problems, such as bone marrow depression or a decrease in one of the blood clotting factors. Contact your doctor if you notice any unusual bleeding or easy bruising, get painful sores in the mouth or throat, or develop chills and fever.

Long-term therapy with cephalexin may result in an overgrowth of other organisms in the body. Some symptoms of this condition are itching of the anus, sore mouth or tongue and vaginal infection. Stop taking cephalexin and contact your doctor.

PRECAUTIONS

Before you start taking cephalexin, be sure to tell your doctor or pharmacist if you have ever had an allergic reaction to any cephalosporin or to any form of penicillin. Your doctor should be told if you have kidney disease or a history of allergy.

Some other medications, particularly gout medicines, should not be taken with cephalexin. Tell your doctor what other prescription or nonprescription drugs you are taking. If you do not know what drugs you are taking or what they are prescribed for, bring them in their labeled containers to your doctor or pharmacist.

Even if you feel better in a few days, take *all* of the medication prescribed for you by your doctor. Bacterial infections take several days to weeks to be cured completely. If you stop taking cephalexin, the bacteria still alive can multiply and cause a recurrence of the infection. However, if your symptoms do not improve within a few days or if they become worse, contact your doctor. He may want to change your medication.

Be sure to tell your doctor if you are pregnant or are nursing an infant. Though problems with this medication have not been reported in the literature, your doctor will need to consider whether the benefit to you is worth the possible risk to your baby.

Diabetics should be aware that cephalexin can cause false results in some tests for urine sugar. Do not change your diet or the dosage of your diabetes medicine until you check with your doctor.

Cephalexin can also cause a temporary change in the results of liver function tests. If you have these tests done, be sure the person responsible for reporting the results knows you have been taking cephalexin.

DOSAGE AND STORAGE

Your doctor will determine how often you should take cephalexin. Follow the instructions on your prescription label and ask your doctor or pharmacist to explain any part you do not understand.

Doses of cephalexin should be taken as far apart as possible during the day. If your doctor tells you to take it four times a day, take a dose every six hours. If you give cephalexin to a child, make sure he or she receives it around the clock, even if you have to wake the child for doses.

Cephalexin is best taken on an "empty stomach," one hour before meals or two hours after eating. However, if this medication upsets your stomach, it can be taken with meals or a light snack.

Cephalexin comes in capsules, tablets, liquid form and pediatric drops. The tablets and capsules should be taken with a full eight-ounce glass of water.

The liquid and pediatric drops should be shaken thoroughly to mix the medication evenly before each dose is poured. Measure the prescribed number of drops with the bottle dropper. If there is no dropper with the bottle of liquid, use a specifically marked measuring spoon to be sure the dose is accurate. Contact your pharmacist if you have any questions about measuring the liquid.

If you forget to take a dose, take it as soon as you remember. Take any remaining doses for that day at evenly spaced intervals. If you still have symptoms of the infection after you have taken all the medicine, contact your doctor.

When your doctor tells you to stop taking cephalexin, throw away any unused portion of it. Cephalexin may lose its effectiveness after a period of time and should not be saved to treat another infection. Because this medication was prescribed for your particular condition, do not allow anyone else to take it.

Keep cephalexin in the container it came in. Keep liquid cephalexin in the refrigerator but do not freeze it. On the container, you will find an expiration date. Do not take the medication after that date. Throw it away and, if you need more, get a new supply. If you are not sure of the expiration date or have any questions about a refill, contact your pharmacist.

Keep this medication out of the reach of children.

ERYTHROMYCINS

Erythromycins

(eh rith roe mye' sins)

Brand names: Erythromycin—E-Mycin, Ilotycin, Kesso-mycin, RP-Mycin Robimycin; Erythromycin Ethylsuccinate—EES, E-Mycin E, Pediamycin, Wyamycin; Erythromycin Stearate—Bristamycin, Erypar, Erythrocin, Ethril, Pfizer-E, SK-Erythromycin, Wyamycin S

The erythromycins are available in a number of chemical forms, including erythromycin, the ethylsuccinate ester and the stearate ester. Erythromycin and erythromycin ethylsuccinate and stearate are described here, and the term erythromycins used here refers to all three chemical forms. Another erythromycin, erythromycin estolate, shares the uses of the erythromycins discussed here, but it produces liver problems more frequently than the other erythromycins. (See **erythromycin estolate**, page 74.)

The erythromycins are systemic antibiotics used to treat a wide variety of infections, including throat, ear and skin infections, pneumonia and diphtheria. They are considered good drugs to treat "strep" infections in people who have a history of rheumatic fever or rheumatic heart disease and who may be sensitive or allergic to penicillins.

The erythromycins are the preferred drugs to eliminate diphtheria-causing bacteria from people who show no signs of the disease but are infecting others. There appears to be some evidence that erythromycins are effective against Legionnaires' disease.

UNDESIRED EFFECTS

Serious side effects are rare.

Allergic reactions, ranging from mild rash and hives to a serious or sometimes fatal reaction, are rare. No one who has ever had an allergic reaction to any of the erythromycins should take these medications again.

When you start taking an erythromycin, you may have nausea, diarrhea or vomiting. These effects tend to go away as you continue to take it and as your body adjusts to the medicine. Contact your doctor if these problems get worse or last more than two days.

If an erythromycin upsets your stomach, take the medicine with crackers or a light snack. Contact your doctor if you continue to have stomach upsets.

When you take any of the erythromycins for a long period of time, bacteria it does not eliminate may multiply too rapidly. Some symptoms of this overgrowth are itching of the rectal and genital areas, sore mouth or tongue and vaginal infection. If you have any of these effects, contact your doctor.

Erythromycins rarely cause inflammation of the liver.

PRECAUTIONS

Before you start taking an erythromycin, be sure to tell your doctor if you have liver disease, if you have ever had an allergic reaction to any one of the erythromycins or if you have a history of drug allergy.

Certain other medications (such as those used to treat asthma attacks) and certain other antibiotics, including penicillins, can effect the way your body responds to the erythromycins. Tell your doctor what other prescription or nonprescription drugs you are taking. If you do not know the names of the drugs or what they are prescribed for, bring them in their labeled containers to your doctor or pharmacist.

Food and beverages that contain acids may also effect the way you respond to these medicines. Do not take these medicines with or immediately after drinking fruit juice or carbonated beverages.

Even if you feel better in a few days after taking an erythromycin, take *all* of the medicine your doctor has prescribed. This is particularly important if you have a "strep" infection. Serious heart problems can result later if the infection is not completely cured. Bacterial infections take several days to weeks to be cured completely. However, if your symptoms do not improve in a few days or get worse, contact your doctor. He may want to change your medication.

Although no problems have been reported in the literature when erythromycins have been given to pregnant women or nursing mothers, tell your doctor if you are pregnant or nursing your baby. This information will help him select the treatment best for you and your baby.

DOSAGE AND STORAGE

Your doctor will determine how much erythromycin you should take and how often you should take it. Carefully follow the instructions on your prescription label and ask your doctor or pharmacist to explain any part you do not understand.

Doses of the erythromycins should be taken as far apart as possible during the day. If your doctor instructs you to take this medication four times a day, take a dose every six hours. If you give one of the erythromycins to a child, be sure he or she receives it around the clock, even if you have to wake the child for doses.

The erythromycins come in tablets that should be taken with a full eight-ounce glass of water. Some tablets are to be chewed or crushed before they are swallowed, and your prescription label will include that direction. Erythromycins are best taken on an "empty stomach," one hour before meals or two hours after eating. However, some brands of coated tablets can be taken without regard to meals. The containers of liquid should be shaken well before each use to mix the medication evenly in each dose. The liquid should be measured in a specially marked dropper or measuring spoon to make certain of an accurate dose. (The drops for children are to be taken orally even though they are in a dropper bottle.)

If you forget a dose, take it as soon as you remember it. However, if it is almost time for the next dose, you may either double the next dose or space the missed dose and the next dose one to two hours apart. Then go back to your regular dosing schedule.

If you still have symptoms of the infection when you have taken all the medicine prescribed, contact your doctor. When he tells you to stop taking an erythromycin, throw away any unused part of it. This medication may lose its effectiveness over a period of time and should not be saved to treat another infection. Because an erythromycin was prescribed for your particular condition, do not allow anyone else to take it.

Keep this medication in the container it came in and store the tablets at room temperature. The liquid preparations should be kept in the refrigerator but not frozen. Check these containers for an expiration date. Do not take this medication after the expiration date. Throw away the medication and, if you need more, get a new supply. Contact your pharmacist if you are not sure of the expiration date or need information about a refill.

Keep this and all medication out of the reach of children.

Erythromycin Estolate
(eh rith roe mye' sin ess'toe late)

Brand name: Ilosone

Erythromycin estolate is a systemic antibiotic used to treat a wide variety of infections, including throat, ear and skin infections, pneumonia and diphtheria. It is considered a good drug to treat "strep" infections in people who are sensitive to penicillin.

The erythromycins are the preferred drugs to eliminate diphtheria-causing bacteria from people who show no signs of disease but are infecting others. There appears to be some evidence that erythromycin estolate is effective against Legionnaires' disease.

While the uses of this drug are identical to those of the other erythromycins, it produces liver problems more frequently than the other erythromycins.

UNDESIRED EFFECTS
The most serious side effect of erythromycin estolate is inflammation of the liver. Some symptoms of this problem are severe stomach pain, unusual weakness or tiredness, yellowing of the eyes or skin (jaundice), dark or amber urine and pale stools. If you have any of these symptoms, stop taking the medication and contact your doctor. Liver problems occur more frequently in adults than in children.

Allergic reactions, ranging from mild rash and hives to a serious and sometimes fatal reaction, are rare. No one who has ever had an allergic reaction to any of the erythromycins should take erythromycin estolate.

When you start taking erythromycin estolate, you may have nausea, diarrhea or vomiting. As you continue to take it and your body adjusts to it, these effects tend to lessen or disappear. Contact your doctor if they get worse or last more than two days.

If erythromycin estolate upsets your stomach, take the medicine with crackers or a light snack. Contact your doctor if you continue to have stomach upsets.

During long-term therapy with erythromycin estolate, bacteria that are resistant to it may multiply too rapidly. Itching of the rectal and genital areas, sore mouth or tongue, and vaginal infection can be caused by this overgrowth. If you experience any of these effects, contact your doctor.

PRECAUTIONS
Erythromycin estolate should not be taken by people with liver disease. Tell your doctor if you have or have ever had liver disease or jaundice. He will also need to know if you have ever had an allergic reaction to any erythromycin or have previously had any problems with erythromycin estolate.

Certain other medications, such as those used to treat asthma attacks and certain other antibiotics, including penicillins, can affect the way your body responds to erythromycin estolate. Tell your doctor what other prescription or nonprescription drugs you are taking. If you do not know the names of the drugs or what they were prescribed for, bring them in their labeled containers to your doctor or pharmacist.

Food and beverages that contain acids may also affect your response to this medication. Do not take erythromycin estolate with or immediately after drinking fruit juice or carbonated beverages.

Take *all* the medicine your doctor has prescribed, even if you feel better a few days after taking erythromycin estolate. This is particularly important if you have a "strep" infection. Serious heart problems can result later if the infection is not completely cured. Bacterial infections take several days or weeks to be cured completely. However, if your symptoms do not improve or get worse within a few days after you start taking erythromycin estolate, contact your doctor. He may want to change your medication.

Tell your doctor if you are pregnant or are nursing a baby. Your doctor will select the best treatment for you and your baby. Problems with this drug have not been reported in the literature, but the benefit to you has to be balanced against possible risk to the baby.

While you are taking erythromycin estolate, your doctor may want to test its effect on your liver function. *Keep all appointments for these tests.*

DOSAGE AND STORAGE

Your doctor will determine how much erythromycin estolate you should take and how often you should take it. Follow the instructions on your prescription label carefully and ask your doctor or pharmacist to explain any part you do not understand.

Doses of erythromycin estolate should be taken as far apart as possible during the day, take a dose every six hours. If you give erythromycin estolate to a child, be sure he or she receives it around the clock, even if you have to wake the child for doses.

Erythromycin estolate comes in capsules, tablets to be swallowed, tablets to be chewed and liquid form. Erythromycin in any of these forms can be taken without regard for meals.

Capsules and tablets to be swallowed should be taken with a full eight-ounce glass of water. Chewable tablets should not be swallowed whole but should be chewed completely before they are swallowed. The container of liquid erythromycin estolate should be shaken well before each use to mix the medication evenly in each dose. Measure your dose with a specially marked measuring spoon to ensure an accurate dose.

If you forget to take a dose, take it as soon as you remember. However, if it is almost time for the next dose, you may either double it or space the missed dose and the next dose one to two hours apart. Then go back to your regular dosing schedule.

If you have taken all the medicine prescribed and still have symptoms of the infections, contact your doctor. When he tells you to stop taking erythromycin estolate, do not save it to treat another infection. Throw away any unused portion of it. Erythromycin estolate may lose its effectiveness over a period of time. Do not allow anyone else to take the erythromycin estolate that was prescribed for your particular condition.

Keep this medication in the container it came in. Store liquid erythromycin estolate in the refrigerator. Store the tablets and capsules at room temperature.

Check the bottle of liquid for an expiration date, and do not take it after this date. Throw away the liquid and, if necessary, get a new supply. Contact your pharmacist if you are not sure of the expiration date or have any questions about a refill.

Keep this medication out of the reach of children.

PENICILLINS

Penicillins are antibiotic anti-infective drugs derived originally from a mold called Penicillium. Now, a variety of different penicillins are produced by chemically modifying the basic chemical from this mold. All penicillins contain the same basic chemical structure, but this structure is modified to produce drugs with different antibacterial characteristics that may make one preferable to another in a given situation.

The penicillins may either kill organisms causing infection or merely slow them down to allow the body's defenses to take over. Some penicillins are active only against a few bacteria, while others are effective against a wide variety of bacteria. For example, some bacteria produce a substance called penicillinase, which destroys some penicillins, making them not effective in treating infections caused by those bacteria. Other penicillins, however, are not affected by penicillinase-producing bacteria.

Penicillins are not effective against viruses, fungi, rickettsiae or yeasts.

Penicillins are available in several forms, including tablets, capsules, liquid and injection. Your doctor will choose the form best for you and will give you specific instructions on how to take it.

In order to kill or immobilize bacteria, it is necessary to keep a certain amount of penicillin in your bloodstream at all times. Therefore, you should try to take each dose on schedule.

It is best to take penicillins on an "empty stomach," either one hour before meals or two hours after meals.

It is important to use all of the penicillin your doctor has prescribed even though you will begin to feel better before you finish your prescribed dosage. If you stop taking the penicillin too soon, the bacteria still alive may be able to cause a recurrence of the infection. This is particularly important when treating "strep" infections, because heart problems can develop if the infection is not completely cured.

If your doctor prescribes a liquid form of penicillin, be sure to read all of the labels on the bottle. Liquid penicillins must be stored in the refrigerator (not in the freezer) and needs to be shaken thoroughly each time a dose is poured. Ask your pharmacist for a special spoon so that you can measure the doses accurately.

Your prescription bottle will have an expiration date on it. Do not use liquid penicillin after that date—throw it away and get a fresh supply.

Before you begin to take penicillin, you should tell your doctor if you are taking other medicines and about any chronic health problems you may have. *Inform your doctor if you have ever had an allergic reaction to any penicillin product.*

Penicillins usually begin to clear up infections within a few days. If you do not begin to feel better a few days after your prescribed doses or if your symptoms get worse, contact your doctor.

Amoxicillin

(a mox' i sill in)

Brand names: Amoxil, Larotid, Polymox, Robamox, Sumox, Trimox, Ultimox, Wymox

Amoxicillin is a penicillinlike antibiotic, very similar in chemical structure and activity to ampicillin. It is a broad-spectrum antibiotic, which means it eliminates a number of different bacteria. It is, however, inactivated by penicillinase and cannot be used in infections caused by penicillinase-producing bacteria.

Amoxicillin is used to treat certain types of pneumonia and infections of the ear, urinary tract and skin. Sometimes it is used to treat gonorrhea.

UNDESIRED EFFECTS

Tell your doctor if you have ever had an allergic reaction to any form of penicillin, cephalosporin or amoxicillin.

Allergic reactions are the most common side effects of amoxicillin. Serious and sometimes fatal allergic reactions have occurred, although they are rare, particularly when the medication is taken by mouth. A serious reaction is more likely in a person with other allergies, but it can happen even if you have taken penicillin before with no problems.

Call your doctor or a hospital immediately if you start wheezing or have difficulty breathing immediately after taking amoxicillin or if you develop a rash, itching or hives. You may need emergency treatment.

Amoxicillin can cause nausea and vomiting, irritation of the mouth and tongue and diarrhea. These effects tend to decrease or disappear as you continue to take amoxicillin and as your body adjusts to it. Nausea and vomiting may be relieved if you take amoxicillin with food or a light snack. If diarrhea is severe or lasts for more than two days, contact your doctor.

Other allergic reactions may take longer to develop, such as rash and itching all over the body and in the mouth, fever, joint pain and swollen glands. Contact your doctor if you experience these effects.

In people who are sensitive to amoxicillin, it can cause blood problems such as bone marrow depression or a decrease in the number of blood platelets. If you experience unusual bleeding, easy bruising, painful sores of the mouth and throat or chills and fever, contact your doctor.

PRECAUTIONS

Before you start taking amoxicillin, be sure to tell your doctor or pharmacist if you have ever had an allergic reaction to any form of penicillin, cephalosporin or amoxicillin. Your doctor should be informed if you have or have ever had any kind of allergy, including asthma and hay fever, and if you have kidney disease.

To help your doctor select the best treatment for your problem, you will need to tell him what other medicines you are taking, including medicine for gout and tetracyclines (another type of antibiotic). If you do not know what drugs you are taking or what they were prescribed for, take the labeled containers to your doctor or pharmacist. Contact your doctor or pharmacist before starting to take any other medication, including aspirin, while you are taking amoxicillin.

Take *all* of the medication prescribed for you by your doctor, even if you feel better a few days after your start taking amoxicillin. It takes several days or weeks to cure most infections. If you stop taking amoxicillin before you are cured, the bacteria still alive will begin to multiply and cause a recurrence of the infection. However, if your symptoms do not improve within a few days or if they become worse, contact your doctor. He may wish to change the medication.

It is not known whether amoxicillin is safe for a pregnant woman and her unborn child. However, pregnant women with infections may be given amoxicillin to protect the child from the infection. This medication can pass through the milk to a nursing infant, so your doctor should be told if you are nursing a baby.

DOSAGE AND STORAGE

Your doctor has determined how often you should take amoxicillin. Follow his instructions carefully and ask your doctor or pharmacist to explain anything you do not understand. Doses of this medication should be taken as far apart as possible during the day. If your doctor instructs you to take it three times a day, take a dose every eight hours. If you give amoxicillin to a child who normally sleeps more than eight hours a night, wake the child and give him or her the dose when it is scheduled.

Amoxicillin comes in capsules, in liquid form and in pediatric drops to be taken orally. The container of liquid or pediatric drops should be shaken well before each use to mix the medication. Measure with the bottle dropper the number of drops your doctor has prescribed. If there is no dropper with the bottle of liquid, use the special calibrated measure from your pharmacist to be sure the dose is accurate.

The liquid dose may be added to infant formula, milk, fruit juice, water or ginger ale and then taken immediately.

If you forget to take a dose, take it as soon as you remember, and take the remaining doses for that day at evenly spaced intervals. Take all of this medication exactly as prescribed. If you still have symptoms of the infection after you have taken all the medication, contact your doctor.

After your doctor tells you to stop taking amoxicillin, throw away any unused portion of it. Amoxicillin may lose its effectiveness after a period of time and should not be saved to treat another infection. Because this medication was prescribed for your particular condition, do not allow anyone else to take your amoxicillin.

Keep this medication in the container it came in. Keep liquid amoxicillin in the refrigerator, but do not freeze it. You will find an expiration date on the container. Do not take liquid amoxicillin after that date. Throw it away and, if you need more, get a new supply. If you are not sure of the expiration date or have any questions about a refill of your prescription, contact your pharmacist.

Keep this medication out of the reach of children.

Ampicillin
(am pi sill' in)

Brand names: Amcill, Omnipen, Penbritin, Pensyn, Pfizerpen A, Polycillin, Principen, Totacillin and others

Ampicillin is one of the penicillin family of antibiotics, which has a broad spectrum of activity against bacteria, which means it eliminates a number of different bacteria. It eliminates many of the bacteria that penicillin G eliminates, in addition to several others against which penicillin G is not effective. Ampicillin is, however, inactivated by penicillinase and cannot be used in infections caused by penicillinase-producing bacteria.

Ampicillin is used to treat many kinds of infections caused by bacteria known to be sensitive to it. These infections include pneumonia and bronchitis and infections in the ears, urinary tract and skin. It is sometimes used as a single-dose treatment for gonorrhea.

UNDESIRED EFFECTS
Tell your doctor if you have ever had an allergic reaction to any form of penicillin, cephalosporin or ampicillin.

Allergic reactions are the most common side effects of ampicillin. Serious and sometimes fatal allergic reactions have occurred, although they are rare, particularly when the medication is taken orally. A serious reaction is more likely to occur in a person with other allergies, but it can happen even if you have taken penicillin before with no problems.

Call your doctor or a hospital immediately if you start wheezing or have difficulty breathing right after you take ampicillin or if you develop a rash, itching or hives. You may need emergency treatment.

Ampicillin can cause diarrhea, especially in children. It can also cause nausea, vomiting and irritation of the mouth and tongue. These effects tend to decrease or disappear as you continue to take ampicillin and as your body adjusts to it. If these effects are severe or last more than two days, contact your doctor.

Other allergic reactions may take longer to develop, such as rash and itching all over the body and in the mouth, joint pain, fever and swollen glands. Contact your doctor if you experience these effects.

In people sensitive to ampicillin, it can cause blood problems such as bone marrow depression or a decrease in the number of blood platelets. If you experience unusual bleeding, easy bruising, painful sores of the mouth and throat or chills and fever, contact your doctor.

PRECAUTIONS

Before you start taking ampicillin, be sure to tell your doctor or pharmacist if you have ever had an allergic reaction to any form of penicillin, cephalosporin or ampicillin. Your doctor should be informed if you have kidney disease and if you have now or ever have had any kind of allergy, including asthma and hay fever.

Tell your doctor what other prescription or nonprescription drugs you are taking, particularly medications for gout and the antibiotic tetracycline. If you do not know what drugs you are taking or what they were prescribed for, bring the labeled containers to your doctor or pharmacist. While you are taking ampicillin, do not start to take any other medicines, including aspirin, unless you first check with your doctor or pharmacist.

Take *all* of the medication prescribed for you, even if you feel better after taking it for a few days. Most infections take several days or weeks to cure. If you stop taking ampicillin before you are cured, bacteria still alive can multiply and cause a recurrence of the infection. However, if your symptoms do not improve within a few days after you start taking ampicillin or if they become worse, contact your doctor. He may want to change the medication.

When your doctor prescribes ampicillin for your baby, he will probably want laboratory tests such as blood counts and tests for kidney and liver function to determine what effect this medication is having.

Diabetics should know that ampicillin can cause false results for some urine sugar tests. Check with your doctor before changing your diet or the dosage of your diabetes medicine.

It is not known whether ampicillin is safe for a pregnant woman and her unborn child. However, pregnant women with infections may be given ampicillin to protect the child from the infections. This medication can pass through the milk to a nursing infant; before your doctor decides on treatment for your problem, he should be told if you are breast-feeding a baby.

DOSAGE AND STORAGE

Your doctor will determine how often you should take ampicillin. Carefully follow the instructions on your prescription label. Doses of this medication should be taken as far apart as possible during the day. If your doctor instructs you to take it four times a day, take a dose every six hours. If you give ampicillin to a child, make sure he or she receives it around the clock, even if you must wake the child for doses.

Ampicillin is best taken on an "empty stomach," one hour before meals or two hours after meals, unless your doctor gives you different directions. Ampicillin is available in capsules, chewable tablets and liquid form. Capsules should be taken with a full eight-ounce glass of water. The chewable tablets should not be swallowed whole but should be thoroughly crushed or chewed before they are swallowed.

The container of liquid should be shaken thoroughly before each use to mix the medication evenly. Measure with the bottle dropper the number of drops your doctor has prescribed. If there is not a dropper with the bottle of liquid, use the special calibrated measure from your pharmacist to ensure an accurate dose. These drops are to be taken orally.

If you forget to take a dose, take it as soon as you remember and take the remaining doses for that day at evenly spaced intervals. Take all of this medication exactly as prescribed. If you still have symptoms of the infection after you have taken all the medication, contact your doctor.

After your doctor tells you to stop taking ampicillin, throw away any unused portion of it. Ampicillin may lose its effectiveness after a period of time and should not be saved to treat another infection. Because this medication was prescribed for your particular condition, do not allow anyone else to take it.

Keep this medication in the container it came in. Keep liquid ampicillin in the refrigerator, but do not freeze it. You will find an expiration date on the container. Do not take the liquid after that date. Throw away the liquid and, if you need more, get a new supply. If you are not sure of the expiration date or have any questions about a refill of your prescription, contact your pharmacist.

Keep this medication out of the reach of children.

Carbenicillin
(kar ben i sill' in)

Brand names: Geocillin, Geopen, Pyopen

Carbenicillin is one of the penicillin antibiotics that act against the bacteria that cause problems in the urinary tract. Carbenicillin eliminates bacteria in the urinary tract that are resistant to ampicillin. It is, however, inactivated by penicillinase and cannot be used against infections caused by penicillinase-producing bacteria.

Carbenicillin is used only for infections of the urinary tract and the prostrate gland that are sensitive to this drug.

UNDESIRED EFFECTS
Do not take carbenicillin if you have ever had an allergic reaction to any form of penicillin, cephalosporin or carbenicillin.

Allergic reactions are the most common side effects of carbenicillin. Serious and sometimes fatal allergic reactions have occurred, although they are rare, particularly when the medication is taken orally. A serious reaction is more likely to occur in a person with other allergies, but it can happen even if you have taken penicillin before with no problems.

If you get hives, itching or rash, start wheezing or have difficulty breathing right after you take carbenicillin, call your doctor or a hospital immediately. You may need emergency treatment.

Carbenicillin can cause a bitter or unpleasant taste, diarrhea, nausea or vomiting. These effects tend to decrease or disappear as you continue to take carbenicillin and as your body adjusts to it. Contact your doctor if these effects are severe or last more than two days.

Other allergic reactions may take longer to develop, such as rash and itching all over the body and in the mouth, joint pain, fever or swollen glands. Contact your doctor if you experience these effects.

In people who are sensitive to carbenicillin, it can cause blood problems such as bone marrow depression or a decrease in one of the blood clotting factors. If you experience unusual bleeding, easy bruising, painful sores of the mouth and throat or chills or fever, contact your doctor.

PRECAUTIONS

Before you start taking carbenicillin, be sure to tell your doctor or pharmacist if you have ever had an allergic reaction to any form of penicillin, cephalosporin or carbenicillin. Your doctor also needs to know if you have liver disease and if you have now or have ever had any allergies, including asthma, hay fever, skin rash or hives.

Some other drugs, particularly medications for gout and arthritis and another antibiotic, tetracycline, can increase the effect of carbenicillin and the possibility of allergic reaction. Be sure to tell your doctor what other prescription or nonprescription drugs you are taking. If you do not know what drugs you are taking or what they were prescribed for, take the labeled containers to your doctor or pharmacist. While you are taking carbenicillin, do not start to take any other medicine, including nonprescription medications, unless you have permission from your doctor.

Take *all* of the medication prescribed by your doctor, even if you feel better a few days after you start taking carbenicillin. Most infections take several days or weeks to cure. If you stop taking carbenicillin before your infection is cured, the bacteria still alive can begin to multiply and cause a recurrence of the infection. However, if your symptoms do not improve within a few days after you start taking this medication or if they become worse, contact your doctor. He may want to change your medication.

Carbenicillin can interfere with certain blood tests done to study liver function. Be sure the person who will be evaluating such tests knows you are taking carbenicillin.

Carbenicillin should not be given to children. To date, not enough studies have been done to ensure the safe use of this drug in children.

Tell your doctor if you are nursing a baby. He will need this information because carbenicillin is passed to the baby through breast milk. It is not known whether this drug is safe for a pregnant woman or her unborn child.

DOSAGE AND STORAGE

Carbenicillin usually is taken four times a day in doses six hours apart. Your doctor will determine how often you should take it. Carefully follow his instructions on your prescription label and check with your doctor or pharmacist if there is anything about the instructions you do not understand.

Carbenicillin tablets should be taken on an "empty stomach." Take them one hour before or two hours after meals with a full eight-ounce glass of water.

Take all of this medication exactly as prescribed and do not miss any doses. If you forget to take a dose, take it as soon as you remember. Then take the remaining doses for that day at evenly spaced intervals. If you still have symptoms of the infection after you have taken all the medication, contact your doctor.

After your doctor tells you to stop taking carbenicillin, throw away any unused portion of your prescription. Carbenicillin may lose its effectiveness after a period of time and should not be saved to treat another infection. Because this medication has been prescribed for your particular condition, do not allow anyone else to take your carbenicillin.

Keep this medication in the container it came in. Carbenicillin usually comes with a drying agent in a packet to keep the tablets from breaking down. *Do not swallow the drying agent.* Keep it in the container with the tablets until they are used; then throw away the drying agent.

Keep this medication out of the reach of children.

Cloxacillin
(klox a sill' in)

Brand names: Cloxapen, Tegopen

Cloxacillin is a penicillinase-resistant penicillin. It is used principally to treat infections caused by bacteria that produce penicillinase. These infections include certain types of pneumonia, skin infections and systemic infections.

UNDESIRED EFFECTS
Tell your doctor if you have ever had an allergic reaction to any form of penicillin, cephalosporin or cloxacillin.

Allergic reactions are the most common side effects of cloxacillin. Serious and sometimes fatal allergic reactions have occurred, although they are rare, particularly when the medication is taken orally. A serious reaction is more likely to occur in a person with other allergies, but it can occur even if you have taken penicillin before with no problems.

If you start wheezing or have difficulty breathing right after you take cloxacillin or if you develop a rash, hives or itching, call your doctor or a hospital immediately. You may need emergency treatment.

You may also experience diarrhea, nausea or vomiting after you take cloxacillin. These effects tend to decrease or disappear as you continue to take cloxacillin and as your body adjusts to it. If these effects are severe or last more than two days, contact your doctor.

Other allergic reactions, such as rash and itching all over the body, joint pain, fever and swollen glands, may take longer to develop. If cloxacillin causes any of these effects, contact your doctor.

In people who are sensitive to this drug, cloxacillin can cause blood problems such as bone marrow depression or a decrease in one of the blood clotting factors. If you experience unusual bleeding, easy bruising, painful sores of the mouth and throat or chills and fever, contact your doctor.

PRECAUTIONS

Before you start to take cloxacillin, be sure to tell your doctor or pharmacist if you have ever had an allergic reaction to any form of penicillin, cephalosporin or cloxacillin. Your doctor will also need to know if you have kidney disease and if you now have or have ever had any kind of allergy, including hay fever, asthma, hives or rash.

Some other medications, such as tetracyclines (another antibiotic) and gout medicines, can increase the effect of cloxacillin and the possibility of allergic reaction. Tell your doctor what other prescription or nonprescription drugs you are taking. If you do not know the names of the drugs or what they were prescribed for, bring the labeled containers to your doctor or pharmacist. Do not start to take any other medication, including aspirin, unless you have permission from your doctor.

Even if you feel better a few days after you start taking cloxacillin, continue to take it until you have used *all* that was prescribed. This is particularly important if you have a "strep" infection. Serious heart problems can develop later if the infection is not completely cured.

If your symptoms do not improve within a few days after you start to take cloxacillin or if they become worse, contact your doctor. He may wish to change your medication.

During long-term therapy, your doctor may want laboratory tests such as blood counts and tests for kidney and liver function to determine your response to cloxacillin.

Though the safety of cloxacillin's use during pregnancy has not been established, a pregnant woman with an infection may be given cloxacillin. Your doctor must weigh the benefit against the possible risk. Your doctor should be told if you are nursing a baby, because cloxacillin passes through the milk to the baby.

DOSAGE AND STORAGE

Your doctor has determined how often you should take cloxacillin, and this information is indicated on your prescription label. Carefully follow the instructions and check with your doctor or pharmacist if you do not understand any part of the instructions.

Doses of cloxacillin should be taken as far apart as possible during the day. If your doctor instructs you to take it four times a day, take a dose every six hours. If you give cloxacillin to a child, be sure he or she receives it around the clock, even if you have to wake the child for doses.

Cloxacillin is available in capsules and in liquid form. It is best taken on an "empty stomach," one hour before meals or two hours after eating, unless your doctor gives you different directions.

Capsules should be taken with a full eight-ounce glass of water. The container of liquid cloxacillin should be shaken thoroughly before each use to mix the medication. Measure doses with a specially marked measuring spoon.

If you forget to take a dose, take it as soon as you remember and take the remaining doses for that day at evenly spaced intervals. However, if it is almost time for another dose, you may either double the next dose or space the missed dose and the next dose one or two hours apart. Then go back to your regular dosing schedule.

Take all the cloxacillin exactly as prescribed. If you still have symptoms of the infection after you have taken all the medication, contact your doctor.

After your doctor tells you to stop taking cloxacillin, throw away any unused portion of it. Cloxacillin may lose its effectiveness after a period of time and should not be saved to treat another infection. Because this medication was prescribed for your particular condition, do not allow anyone else to take your cloxacillin.

Keep the cloxacillin in the container it came in. Keep liquid cloxacillin in the refrigerator, but do not freeze it. Check the expiration date on the container and do not take the liquid after that date. Throw away the liquid and, if you need more, get a new supply. If you are not sure of the expiration date or have any questions about a refill of your prescription, contact your pharmacist.

Keep this medication out of the reach of children.

Dicloxacillin
(dye klox a sill' in)

Brand names: Dycill, Dynapen, Pathocil, Veracillin

Dicloxacillin is a penicillinase-resistant penicillin. Dicloxacillin is used principally to treat infections caused by bacteria that produce penicillinase. These infections include certain types of pneumonia, skin infections and systemic infections.

UNDESIRED EFFECTS
Tell your doctor if you have ever had an allergic reaction to any form of penicillin, cephalosporin or dicloxacillin.

Allergic reactions are the most common side effects of dicloxacillin. Serious and sometimes fatal allergic reactions have occurred, although they are rare, particularly when the medication is taken orally. A serious reaction is more likely to occur in a person with other allergies, but it can occur even if you have taken penicillin before with no problems.

Call your doctor or a hospital immediately if you start wheezing or have difficulty breathing right after you take dicloxacillin or if you develop a rash, hives or itching. You may need emergency treatment.

You may also experience diarrhea, nausea or vomiting with dicloxacillin. These effects tend to decrease or disappear as you continue to take dicloxacillin and as your body adjusts to it. If these effects are severe or last more than two days, call your doctor.

Other allergic reactions may take longer to develop. If, after you have been taking dicloxacillin for several days, you get a rash and itching all over your body, joint pain, fever or swollen glands, contact your doctor.

In people who are sensitive to this drug, dicloxacillin can cause blood problems such as bone marrow depression or a decrease in one of the blood clotting factors. If you experience unusual bleeding, easy bruising, painful sores of the mouth and throat or chills and fever, contact your doctor.

PRECAUTIONS

Before you start to take dicloxacillin, be sure to tell your doctor or pharmacist if you have ever had an allergic reaction to any form of penicillin, cephalosporin or dicloxacillin. To select the medicine right for you, your doctor will need to know if you have kidney disease and if you have any history of allergies, including hay fever, asthma, rash or hives.

Some other medications, including tetracyclines and gout medicines, can increase the effect of dicloxacillin and the possibility of allergic reaction; tetracyclines may also decrease the ability of dicloxacillin to kill bacteria rapidly. Tell your doctor what other prescription or nonprescription drugs you are taking. If you do not know the names of the drugs or what they were prescribed for, bring them in their labeled containers to your doctor or pharmacist. Do not start to take any other medication, including aspirin, unless you have permission from your doctor.

Do not stop taking dicloxacillin even if you feel better a few days after taking it. It is important that you take *all* of this medication as prescribed if your infection is to be cured. This is particularly important if you have a "strep" infection. Serious heart problems can develop later if the infection is not completely cured.

If your symptoms do not improve or become worse a few days after you start to take dicloxacillin, contact your doctor. He may want to change your medication.

During long-term therapy, your doctor may want tests, such as blood counts and tests for kidney and liver function, to determine your response to dicloxacillin.

Dicloxacillin passes through the milk to a breast-fed infant, so you should tell your doctor if you are nursing a baby. The safety of dicloxacillin's use during pregnancy has not been established, but it may be necessary to give it to a pregnant woman with an infection to protect the baby from the infection.

DOSAGE AND STORAGE

Your doctor will determine how often you should take dicloxacillin. Carefully follow the instructions on your prescription label and check with your doctor or pharmacist if you do not understand any part of the instructions.

Doses of dicloxacillin should be taken as far apart as possible during the day. If your doctor instructs you to take it four times a day, take a dose every six hours. If you give dicloxacillin to a child, be sure he or she receives it around the clock, even if you have to wake the child for doses.

Dicloxacillin is available in capsules and liquid form. It should be taken on an "empty stomach," one hour before or two hours after meals, unless your doctor gives you different directions.

Dicloxacillin capsules should be taken with a full eight-ounce glass of water. The liquid should be shaken thoroughly before each use to mix the medication. Measure doses with a specially marked measuring spoon.

If you forget to take a dose, take it as soon as you remember and take the remaining doses for that day at evenly spaced intervals. However, if it is almost time for another dose, you may either double the next dose or space the missed dose and the next dose one or two hours apart. Then go back to your regular dosing schedule.

Take all of this medication exactly as prescribed. If you still have symptoms of the infection after you have taken all the dicloxacillin, contact your doctor.

After your doctor tells you to stop taking dicloxacillin, throw away any unused portion of it. Dicloxacillin may lose its effectiveness after a period of time and should not be saved to treat another infection. Because this medication was prescribed for your particular condition, do not allow anyone else to take your dicloxacillin.

Keep this medication in the container it came in. Keep liquid dicloxacillin in the refrigerator, but do not freeze it. Check the expiration date on the container and do not take the liquid after that date. Throw away the liquid and, if you need more, get a new supply. Contact your pharmacist if you are not sure of the expiration date or have questions about a refill.

Keep this medication out of the reach of children.

Hetacillin

(het a sill' in)

Brand name: Versapen

Hetacillin itself is not active against bacteria, but once in the body it is rapidly converted into ampicillin. Like ampicillin, hetacillin is prescribed to treat many kinds of infections caused by bacteria. Hetacillin is used to treat certain types of pneumonia and bronchitis and infections of the ears, urinary tract and skin. It is, however, inactivated by penicillinase and cannot be used against infections caused by penicillinase-producing bacteria.

UNDESIRED EFFECTS

Tell your doctor if you have ever had an allergic reaction to any form of penicillin, cephalosporin, ampicillin or hetacillin.

Allergic reactions are the most common side effects of hetacillin. Serious and sometimes fatal allergic reactions have occurred, although they are rare, particularly when the medication is taken by mouth. A serious reaction is more likely to occur in a person with other allergies, but it can occur even if you have taken penicillin before with no problems.

Call your doctor or a hospital immediately if you start wheezing or have difficulty breathing right after you take hetacillin or if you get a rash, itching or hives. You may need emergency treatment.

Hetacillin can cause diarrhea, especially in children. Other common side effects are nausea, vomiting and irritation of the mouth and tongue. As you continue to take hetacillin and as your body adjusts to it, these effects tend to decrease or disappear. If these effects are severe or last more than two days, contact your doctor.

Other allergic reactions may take longer to develop. If, after you have been taking hetacillin for several days, you get a rash and itching all over your body, joint pain, fever or swollen glands, contact your doctor.

In people who are sensitive to hetacillin or ampicillin, it can cause blood problems such as bone marrow depression or a decrease in one of the blood clotting factors. If you experience unusual bleeding, easy bruising, or painful sores of the mouth and throat or chills and fever after taking hetacillin, contact your doctor.

PRECAUTIONS

Before you start taking hetacillin, be sure to tell your doctor or pharmacist if you have ever had an allergic reaction to any form of penicillin, cephalosporin, ampicillin or hetacillin. Your doctor also needs to know if you have kidney disease and if you have a history of any kind of allergy, including asthma, hay fever, rash or hives.

When taken with hetacillin, medicines for gout can increase the possibility of allergic reaction. Tetracycline can prevent hetacillin from rapidly killing bacteria. Tell your doctor what other prescription or nonprescription drugs you are taking. If you do not know the names of the drugs or what they were prescribed for, bring them in their labeled containers to your doctor or pharmacist. While you are taking hetacillin, do not start to take any other medicines, including aspirin, unless you first check with your doctor or pharmacist.

Take *all* the medication prescribed for you, even if you feel better after taking hetacillin for a few days. This is particularly important if you have a "strep" infection. Serious heart problems can result later if your infection is not completely cured. However, if your symptoms do not improve or become worse within a few days after you start taking hetacillin, contact your doctor. He may want to change your medication.

With long-term therapy in an adult or when a baby is taking hetacillin, your doctor will probably want tests, such as blood counts and tests for kidney and liver function, to determine what effect the hetacillin is having.

Diabetics should know that hetacillin can cause false results in some urine sugar tests. Check with your doctor before changing your diet or the dosage of your diabetes medicine.

It is not known whether hetacillin is safe for a pregnant woman and her unborn child. However, a pregnant woman with an infection may be given hetacillin. Your doctor must weigh the benefit against the possible risk. This medication can pass through the milk to a nursing infant. Your doctor should be told that you are nursing a baby before he decides on treatment for your problem.

DOSAGE AND STORAGE

How often you should take hetacillin has been determined by your doctor and is indicated on your prescription label. Carefully follow his instructions. Doses of this medication should be taken as far apart as possible during the day. If your doctor instructs you to take it four times a day, take a dose every six hours. If you give hetacillin to a child, make sure he or she receives it around the clock, even if you have to wake the child for doses.

Hetacillin should be taken on an "empty stomach," one hour before meals or two hours after eating, unless your doctor gives you different directions. It is available in capsules, liquid form and pediatric drops. Capsules should be taken with a full eight-ounce glass of water.

The container of liquid or pediatric drops to be taken orally should be shaken well before each use to mix the medication evenly. Measure with the bottle dropper the number of drops your doctor has prescribed. If you do not know how to do this, ask your pharmacist to show you how. If there is no dropper with the liquid, use a special calibrated measure to be sure the dose is accurate.

If you forget to take a dose, take it as soon as you remember and take the remaining doses for that day at evenly spaced intervals. Take all the hetacillin exactly as prescribed. If you still have symptoms of the infection after you have taken all the medication, contact your doctor.

When your doctor tells you to stop taking hetacillin, throw away any unused portion of it. Hetacillin may lose its effectiveness after a period of time and should not be saved to treat another infection. Because this medication was prescribed for your particular condition, do not allow anyone else to take your hetacillin.

Keep this medication in the container it came in. Keep liquid hetacillin in the refrigerator but do not freeze it. You will find an expiration date on the container. Do not take the liquid after that date. Throw away the liquid and, if you need more, get a new supply. If you are not sure of the expiration date or have any questions about a refill, contact your pharmacist.

Keep this medication out of the reach of children.

Methicillin
(meth eh sill' in)

Brand names: Azapen, Celbenin, Staphcillin

Methicillin is a penicillinase-resistant penicillin that is given only by injection. Newborn infants, elderly people in poor general health and people recovering from surgery are at great risk of infection while they are in the hospital. In newborns, the infection may not show up until several days or weeks after they are home. Many of these "hospital acquired" infections cannot be cured by penicillin G because they are caused by penicillinase-producing "staph" bacteria. Methicillin is particularly useful in treating moderate to severe infections of this kind.

UNDESIRED EFFECTS

Tell your doctor if you have ever had an allergic reaction to any form of penicillin, cephalosporin or methicillin.

Allergic reactions are the most common side effects of methicillin. Serious and sometimes fatal allergic reactions have occurred, although they are rare. A serious reaction is more likely to occur in a person with other allergies, but it can occur even if you have taken penicillin before with no problems.

Wheezing, difficulty in breathing, rash, itching and hives occurring right after an injection of methicillin are symptoms of an allergic reaction and usually require emergency treatment.

Methicillin can also cause diarrhea, nausea or vomiting. These effects tend to disappear or decrease as the body adjusts to the medication and require medical attention only if they are severe or last more than two days.

Other allergic reactions may take longer to develop. These include a rash and itching all over the body, joint pain, fever and swollen glands. Contact your doctor if these occur.

In people sensitive to this drug, methicillin can cause blood problems such as bone marrow depression or a decrease in one of the blood clotting factors. If you experience unusual bleeding, easy bruising, painful sores of the mouth and throat or chills and fever, contact your doctor.

Kidney failure can occur with methicillin therapy, although this reaction is rare. Symptoms are blood in the urine, passage of large amounts of light-colored urine, swelling of the face and ankles, troubled breathing and unusual tiredness or weakness. If you experience any of these symptoms, contact your doctor. While you are taking methicillin, your doctor will probably want tests of your kidney function.

PRECAUTIONS

Before you start to take methicillin, be sure to tell your doctor if you have ever had an allergic reaction to any form of penicillin, cephalosporin or methicillin. He will also need to know if you have kidney disease and if you have any history of allergies, including hay fever, asthma, hives or rash.

If you receive an injection of methicillin in the doctor's office, stay there for 30 minutes after the injection so you will have medical treatment readily available if you have a serious allergic reaction to the injection.

Some other medications should not be taken with methicillin, such as gout medicine, which can increase the possibility of allergic reaction, and tetracyclines, which can prevent the rapid killing of bacteria. Tell your doctor what other prescription or nonprescription drugs you are taking. Do not start to take any other medication, including nonprescription medications, while you are taking methicillin unless you have your doctor's permission.

Before starting to take methicillin, tell your doctor if you are pregnant or are nursing a baby.

DOSAGE AND STORAGE

Methicillin is always given by injection under the supervision of a doctor.

Nafcillin
(naf sill' in)

Brand names: Nafcil, Unipen

Nafcillin is a penicillinase-resistant penicillin. Nafcillin is used primarily to treat infections caused by penicillinase-producing "staph" bacteria. These infections include certain types of pneumonia, skin infections and systemic infections.

UNDESIRED EFFECTS

Do not take nafcillin if you have ever had an allergic reaction to any form of penicillin, cephalosporin or nafcillin.

Allergic reactions are the most common side effects of nafcillin. Serious and sometimes fatal allergic reactions have occurred, although they are rare, particularly when the medication is take orally. A serious reaction is more likely to occur in a person with other allergies, but it can occur even if you have taken penicillin before with no problems.

If you get hives, itching or rash or if you start wheezing or have difficulty breathing after taking nafcillin, call your doctor or a hospital immediately. You may need emergency treatment.

Diarrhea, nausea or vomiting may occur when you begin to take nafcillin. These effects tend to decrease or disappear as you continue to take nafcillin and as your body adjusts to it. If these effects are severe or last more than two days, contact your doctor.

Other allergic reactions may take longer to develop. If you experience rash and itching all over your body, joint pain, fever or swollen glands while you are taking nafcillin, contact your doctor.

In people who are sensitive to this drug, nafcillin can cause blood problems such as bone marrow depression or a decrease in one of the blood clotting factors. The symptoms of these problems are unusual bleeding, easy bruising, painful sores in the mouth and throat and chills and fever. If you develop any of these symptoms, contact your doctor.

PRECAUTIONS

Before you start to take nafcillin, be sure to tell your doctor or pharmacist if you have ever had an allergic reaction to any form of penicillin, cephalosporin or nafcillin. Your doctor will also need to know if you have kidney disease and if you have a history of any allergies, including hay fever, asthma, hives or rash.

Some other medications, such as gout medicine, can increase the effect of nafcillin and the possibility of allergic reaction. Tell your doctor what other prescription or nonprescription drugs you are taking. If you do not know the names of the drugs or what they were prescribed for, bring them in the labeled containers to your doctor or pharmacist. While you are taking nafcillin, do not start to take any other medication, including nonprescription medications, unless you have permission from your doctor.

Do not stop taking nafcillin, even if you feel better a few days after you start taking it. Take *all* the medication that was prescribed for you. Most infections take several days or weeks to be cured, and if you do not continue to take the medication, some bacteria may remain alive and cause a recurrence of the infection.

If your symptoms do not improve or if they become worse within a few days after you start to take nafcillin, contact your doctor. He may want to change your medication.

During long-term therapy, your doctor may want tests to check on your reaction to nafcillin. These will probably be blood counts and tests of your kidney and liver function.

To help your doctor select the right therapy for you, tell him if you are pregnant or are nursing a baby. Though no major problems with this drug have been reported in the literature, he will want to consider whether the benefit to you is worth the risk to your baby.

DOSAGE AND STORAGE

Your doctor has determined how often you should take nafcillin, and this information is indicated on your prescription label. Carefully follow the instructions and check with your doctor or pharmacist if you do not understand any part of the instructions.

Doses of nafcillin should be taken as far apart as possible during the day. If your doctor instructs you to take nafcillin four times a day, take a dose every six hours. If you give nafcillin to a child, be sure he or she receives it around the clock, even if you must wake the child for doses.

Nafcillin should be taken on an "empty stomach," at least one hour before meals or two hours after eating, unless your doctor gives you different directions.

Nafcillin is available in capsules, tablets and liquid form. Capsules and tablets should be taken with a full eight-ounce glass of water. The container of liquid should be shaken thoroughly before each use to mix the medication. Measure doses with a specially marked measuring spoon.

If you forget to take a dose, take it as soon as you remember and take the remaining doses for that day at evenly spaced intervals. However, if it is almost time for another dose, you may either double the next dose or space the missed dose and the next dose one or two hours apart. Then go back to your regular dosing schedule.

Take all the nafcillin exactly as prescribed. If you still have symptoms of the infection after you have taken all the medication, contact your doctor.

After your doctor tells you to stop taking nafcillin, throw away any unused portion of it. Nafcillin may lose its effectiveness after a period of time and should not be saved to treat another infection. Because this medication was prescribed for your particular condition, do not allow anyone else to take your nafcillin.

Keep this medication in the container it came in. Keep liquid nafcillin in the refrigerator, but do not freeze it. Check the expiration date on the container and, if you need more nafcillin, get a new supply. If you are not sure of the

expiration date or have any questions about a refill, contact your pharmacist.
Keep this medication out of the reach of children.

Oxacillin

(ox a sill' in)

Brand names: Bactocill, Prostaphlin
Oxacillin is a penicillinase-resistant penicillin. Oxacillin is used principally
to treat infections caused by penicillinase-producing "staph" bacteria. Some of
these are certain types of pneumonia, skin infections and systemic infections.

UNDESIRED EFFECTS

*Tell your doctor if you have ever had an allergic reaction to any form of
penicillin, cephalosporin or oxacillin.*

Allergic reactions are the most common side effects of oxacillin. Serious and
sometimes fatal allergic reactions have occurred, although they are rare, particularly when the medication is taken orally. A serious reaction is more likely
to occur in a person with other allergies, but it can occur even if you have taken
penicillin in the past with no problems.

If you get a rash, hives or itching or start wheezing and have difficulty
breathing right after you take oxacillin, call your doctor or a hospital immediately. You may need emergency treatment.

Oxacillin also can cause diarrhea, nausea or vomiting. These effects tend to
decrease or disappear as you continue to take oxacillin and as your body adjusts
to it. Contact your doctor if these effects are severe or last more than two days.

Other allergic reactions may take longer to develop. If you experience a rash
and itching all over your body, joint pain, fever or swollen glands after several
days of therapy, contact your doctor.

In people sensitive to this drug, oxacillin can cause blood problems such as
bone marrow depression or a decrease in one of the blood clotting factors. Some
symptoms of these problems are unusual bleeding, easy bruising, painful sores
of the mouth and throat and chills and fever. Contact your doctor if you experience any of these symptoms.

PRECAUTIONS

Before you start to take oxacillin, be sure to tell your doctor or pharmacist
if you have ever had an allergic reaction to any form of penicillin, cephalosporin
or oxacillin. Your doctor will also need to know if you have kidney disease or
if you have a history of any allergy, including rash, hives, hay fever and asthma.

Certain other medications should not be taken with oxacillin. For example,
gout medicines can increase the effect of oxacillin and the possibility of allergic
reaction, while tetracyclines decrease the ability of oxacillin to kill bacteria
rapidly. Tell your doctor what prescription or nonprescription medications you
are taking. If you do not know the names of the drugs or what they were
prescribed for, bring them in the labeled containers to your doctor or pharmacist.
Do not start to take any other medication, including aspirin, while you are
taking oxacillin unless you have your doctor's permission.

Even if you feel better a few days after you start taking oxacillin, continue to take it, and take *all* that was prescribed for you. This is particularly important if you have a "strep" infection. Serious heart problems can develop later if the infection is not completely cured.

If your symptoms do not improve within a few days after you start to take oxacillin or if they become worse, contact your doctor. He may want to change your medication.

Newborns and infants can develop kidney problems when they are taking large doses of oxacillin. During therapy of this kind, the kidney function of the baby should be carefully checked.

During long-term therapy, your doctor may want tests, such as blood counts and tests for kidney and liver function, to determine your response to oxacillin.

Before starting to take oxacillin, tell your doctor if you are pregnant or are nursing a baby. Though problems in these situations have not been reported in the literature, your doctor will need this information to decide whether the benefit of this drug to you is worth the possible risk to your baby.

DOSAGE AND STORAGE

In serious infections, oxacillin may first be given by injection and then continued with one of the forms to be taken orally, capsules or liquid.

Your doctor will determine how often you should take oxacillin orally. Carefully follow the instructions on your prescription label and check with your doctor or pharmacist if you do not understand any part of the instructions.

Doses of oxacillin should be taken as far apart as possible during the day. If your doctor instructs you to take it four times a day, take a dose every six hours. If you give oxacillin to a child, be sure he or she receives it around the clock, even if you must wake the child for doses.

Oxacillin is best taken on an "empty stomach," one hour before meals or two hours after eating, unless your doctor gives you different directions. Capsules should be taken with a full eight-ounce glass of water. The liquid should be shaken thoroughly before each use to mix the medication. Measure doses with a specially marked measuring spoon.

If you forget to take a dose, take it as soon as you remember it and take the remaining doses for that day at evenly spaced intervals. However, if it is almost time for another dose, you may either double the next dose or space the missed dose and the next dose one or two hours apart. Then go back to your regular dosing schedule.

Take *all* the oxacillin exactly as prescribed. If you still have symptoms of the infection after you have taken all the medication, contact your doctor.

After your doctor tells you to stop taking oxacillin, throw away any unused portion of it. Oxacillin may lose its effectiveness after a period of time and should not be saved to treat another infection. Because this medication was prescribed for your particular condition, do not allow anyone else to take your oxacillin.

Keep this medication in the container it came in. Keep liquid oxacillin in the refrigerator but do not freeze the oxacillin. Check the expiration date on the container and do not take the liquid after that date. Throw away the liquid and, if you need more, get a new supply. If you are not sure of the expiration date or have any questions about a refill, contact your pharmacist.

Keep this medication out of the reach of children.

Penicillin G
(pen i sill′ in)

Brand names: Kesso-Pen, Pentids, Pfizerpen G and others

Penicillin G is the most effective of the penicillins in eliminating bacteria sensitive to penicillin. Penicillin G is, however, inactivated by penicillinase (a substance produced by bacteria) and cannot be used against infections caused by penicillinase-producing bacteria.

Penicillin G often is the preferred drug in treating certain types of pneumonia, scarlet fever and throat and skin infections. Penicillin G is also used to prevent a recurrence of rheumatic fever. The injectable form of penicillin G is used to treat gonorrhea and syphilis.

UNDESIRED EFFECTS
Tell your doctor if you have ever had an allergic reaction to any form of penicillin, cephalosporin or penicillin G.

Allergic reactions are the most common side effects of penicillin G. Serious and sometimes fatal allergic reactions have occurred, although they are rare, particularly when the medication is taken orally. A serious reaction is more likely to happen in a person with other allergies, but it can occur even if you have taken penicillin before with no problems.

If you get a rash, hives or itching or start wheezing and have difficulty breathing right after you take penicillin G, call your doctor or a hospital immediately. You may need emergency treatment.

Penicillin G can cause diarrhea, nausea and vomiting, which tend to decrease or disappear as you continue to take penicillin G and as your body adjusts to it. If these effects are severe or last more than two days, call your doctor. In some people, penicillin G may cause the tongue to darken or discolor. This effect is temporary and will go away when you stop taking the medication.

Other allergic reactions may develop only after several days of therapy. If you experience a rash and itching all over your body, joint pains, fever or swollen glands, contact your doctor.

In people sensitive to this drug, penicillin G can cause blood problems, such as bone marrow depression or a decrease in one of the blood clotting factors. The symptoms of such problems are unusual bleeding, easy bruising, painful sores of the mouth and throat and chills and fever. Contact your doctor if you have any of these symptoms.

PRECAUTIONS
Before you start taking penicillin G, be sure to tell your doctor or pharmacist if you have ever had an allergic reaction to any form of penicillin, cephalosporin

or penicillin G. Your doctor should be told if you have kidney disease or a history of any kind of allergy, including asthma, hay fever, rash or hives.

Some other medications should not be taken with penicillin G because they increase or decrease its effect. Gout medicines can increase the effect of penicillin G and, therefore, the possibility of allergic reaction. Tetracyclines can prevent the rapid killing of bacteria needed for certain infections. Tell your doctor what other prescription or nonprescription drugs you are taking. If you do not know the names of these drugs or what they were prescribed for, bring them in their labeled containers to your doctor or pharmacist. Do not start to take any other medications, including nonprescription medications, without permission from your doctor while you are taking penicillin G.

Take *all* of the medication prescribed for you by your doctor, even if you feel better a few days after you start taking it. This is particularly important if you have a "strep" infection. Serious heart problems can result later if the infection is not completely cured.

To help your doctor select the treatment best for you, tell him if you are pregnant or are nursing a baby. Penicillin G is passed to an unborn child and to a nursing infant through the mother's milk.

If you have diabetes, penicillin G can cause false results in some tests of sugar urine. Do not change your diet or the dosage of your diabetes medicine unless you check first with your doctor.

If you get an injection of penicillin G in the doctor's office, stay there for 30 minutes after the injection so you will be close to medical care if you should have a serious allergic reaction to the injection.

DOSAGE AND STORAGE

Your doctor will determine how often you should take penicillin G. Carefully follow the instructions on your prescription label and ask your doctor or pharmacist to explain any part of the instructions you do not understand. Doses of this medication should be taken as far apart as possible during the day. If your doctor tells you to take it three times a day, take a dose every eight hours. If you give penicillin G to a child, make sure he or she receives it around the clock, even if you must wake the child for doses.

Penicillin G should be taken on an "empty stomach," one hour before meals or two hours after eating. It comes in tablets or in liquid form. The tablets should be taken with a full eight-ounce glass of water. The container of liquid should be shaken thoroughly before each use to mix the medication evenly. Use a specially marked measuring spoon to be sure of an accurate dose.

If you forget to take a dose, take it as soon as you remember. However, if it is almost time for your next dose, you may either double the next dose or space the missed dose and the next dose one to two hours apart. Then go back to your regular dosing schedule. Take all of the penicillin G as prescribed. If you still have symptoms of the infection after you have taken all the medication, contact your doctor.

After your doctor tells you to stop taking penicillin G, throw away any unused portion of it. Penicillin G may lose its effectiveness after a period of time and should not be saved to treat another infection. Because this medication was prescribed for your particular condition, do not allow anyone else to take your penicillin G.

Keep this medication in the container it came in. Keep liquid penicillin G in the refrigerator but do not freeze it. You will find an expiration date on the container. Do not take the medication after that date. Throw it away and, if you need more, get a new supply. If you are not sure of the expiration date or have any questions about a refill, contact your pharmacist.

Keep this medication out of the reach of children.

Penicillin V
(pen i sill' in)

Brand names: Ledercillin-VK, Pen-Vee K, Pfizerpen VK, Robicillin VK, Uticillin VK, V-Cillin K, Veetids and others

Penicillin V is absorbed better than pencillin G, so pencillin V gets into the bloodstream faster than pencillin G to fight the infection. Pencillin V is, however, inactivated by penicillinase (a substance produced by bacteria) and cannot be used against infections caused by penicillinase-producing bacteria.

Penicillin V is used to treat mild to moderate infections of the throat, ears and skin and scarlet fever. Penicillin V is also given to prevent a recurrence of rheumatic fever. Because penicillin V is available in oral form only, it is not used for serious infections that require very rapid elimination of bacteria.

UNDESIRED EFFECTS
Tell your doctor if you have ever had an allergic reaction to any form of penicillin, cephalosporin or penicillin V.

Allergic reactions are the most common side effects of penicillin V. Serious and sometimes fatal allergic reactions have occurred, although they are rare, particularly when the medication is taken orally. A serious reaction is more likely to happen in a person with other allergies, but it can occur even if you have taken penicillin before with no problems.

If you get a rash, hives or itching or start wheezing and have difficulty breathing right after you take penicillin V, call your doctor or a hospital immediately. You may need emergency treatment.

Diarrhea, nausea and vomiting are other undesired effects of penicillin V. Although these effects tend to decrease or disappear as you continue to take penicillin V and as your body adjusts to it, call your doctor if they are severe or last more than two days. In some people, penicillin V may cause the tongue to darken or discolor. This effect is temporary and will go away when you stop taking the medication.

Other allergic reactions, such as rash and itching all over the body, joint pains, fever or swollen glands, may develop only after several days of therapy. If you experience any of these effects, contact your doctor.

In people sensitive to this drug, penicillin V can cause blood problems, such as bone marrow depression or a decrease in one of the blood clotting factors. Symptoms of such problems are unusual bleeding, easy bruising, painful sores of the mouth and throat and chills and fever. Contact your doctor if you have any of these symptoms.

PRECAUTIONS

Before you start taking penicillin V, be sure to tell your doctor or pharmacist if you have ever had an allergic reaction to any form of penicillin, cephalosporin or penicillin V. Your doctor should be told if you have kidney disease or a history of any kind of allergy, including asthma, hay fever, rash or hives.

Some other medications, such as gout medicines and tetracyclines, should not be taken with penicillin V. They can increase the effect of this drug and, therefore, the possibility of allergic reactions, or they can decrease the bacteria-killing effect of penicillin V. Tell your doctor what other prescription or non-prescription drugs you are taking. If you do not know the names of the drugs or what they are prescribed for, bring them in their labeled containers to your doctor or pharmacist. While you are taking penicillin V, do not start to take any other medications, including aspirin, without permission from your doctor.

Even if you feel better a few days after you start taking penicillin V take *all* of the medication prescribed for you by your doctor. This is particularly important if you have a "strep" infection. Serious heart problems can result later if the infection is not completely cured.

Before taking penicillin V, tell your doctor if you are pregnant or are breast-feeding a baby. He needs this information to select the treatment best for you because penicillin V is passed by the mother to her unborn child and to a nursing infant through the mother's milk.

DOSAGE AND STORAGE

Your doctor will determine how often you should take penicillin V. Follow the instructions on your prescription label and ask your doctor or pharmacist to explain any part of the instructions you do not understand.

Doses of this medication should be taken as far apart as possible during the day. If your doctor tells you to take it four times a day, take a dose every six hours. If you give penicillin V to a child, make sure he or she receives it around the clock, even if you have to wake the child for doses.

Penicillin V should be taken on an "empty stomach," one hour before meals or two hours after eating. It comes in capsules, tablets and liquid form. The tablets and capsules should be taken with a full eight-ounce glass of water.

The liquid should be shaken thoroughly before each use to mix the medication evenly. Use a specially marked measuring spoon to be sure of an accurate dose.

If you forget to take a dose, take it as soon as you remember. However, if it is almost time for your next dose, you may either double the next dose or space the missed dose and the next dose one to two hours apart. Then go back to your regular dosing schedule.

Take all the penicillin V exactly as prescribed. If you still have symptoms of the infection after you have taken all the medication, contact your doctor.

After your doctor tells you to stop taking penicillin V, throw away any unused portion of it. Penicillin V may lose its effectiveness after a period of time and should not be saved to treat another infection. Because this medication was prescribed for your particular condition, do not allow anyone else to take your penicillin V.

Keep this medication in the container it came in. Keep liquid penicillin V in the refrigerator, but do not freeze it. You will find an expiration date on the container. Do not take the medication after that date. Throw it away and, if you need more, get a new supply. If you are not sure of the expiration date or have any questions about a refill, contact your pharmacist.

Keep this medication out of the reach of children.

TETRACYCLINES

Tetracyclines are systemic antibiotics commonly described as "broad spectrum" antibiotics. Broad spectrum implies that these drugs have a wide range of activity—that is, they fight infections caused by a variety of different organisms. These drugs are effective in treatment of infections caused by many kinds of bacteria and by some other less common organisms, such as spirochetes and rickettsia. Tetracyclines are not effective in the treatment of viral infections such as the common cold.

As with many other groups of drugs, there are many tetracyclines, all slight chemical modifications of the basic drug. The names of the individual drugs are demeclocycline, doxycycline, methacycline, minocycline, oxytetracycline and tetracycline. The more familiar names are the brand or trade names, which can be found in the discussions of the individual drugs.

The tetracyclines are the preferred drugs for treatment of only a few infections—and those infections are relatively uncommon. Because of their broad activity, however, tetracyclines often are used when the infecting organism is unknown. Also, a patient may be allergic to the antibiotic that is preferred for treatment of a particular infection; a tetracycline might be prescribed as the alternative or "second best" drug because it is active against so many different organisms.

Tetracyclines are most commonly prescribed for the treatment of infections of the respiratory tract such as pneumonia, tonsillitis, inflammation of the pharynx, bronchitis or whooping cough or for ear or sinus infections. Tetracyclines also are used to treat urinary tract infections, eye infections and infected abscesses, carbuncles, burns or wounds. They may be used following surgery if some infection is present. Tetracyclines also are prescribed for the treatment of some infections of the digestive tract, such as certain kinds of dysentery and salmonella infections. Rickettsial infections such as Rocky Mountain spotted fever, typhus and Q fever and some infections caused by spirochetal organisms such as yaws and syphilis also are susceptible to treatment by tetracyclines. In addition, tetracyclines have been used in the treatment of acne.

Many other infections may be treated successfully if a test of the infecting organism shows that a tetracycline will be effective.

Some organisms can become resistant to the tetracyclines, and the drugs then no longer effectively prevent their growth. Because the tetracyclines have been used so much over the past several years, many of the more common micro-organisms have become resistant to them. The usefulness of these drugs in treatment of "staph" infections, "strep throat" and pneumonia, for example, is rather limited for this reason.

Demeclocycline

(dem e kloe sye' kleen)

Brand name: Declomycin

Demeclocycline is one of the tetracycline antibiotics. It is used to treat a variety of infections, including pneumonia, bladder infections, Rocky Mountain spotted fever and acne. It can be used to treat infections caused by bacteria resistant to penicillin, but it is never the preferred drug for any "staph" infection.

Although penicillin is the preferred drug for treatment of "strep" infections and for the prevention of rheumatic fever, demeclocycline may be used to treat these infections in people who are sensitive or allergic to penicillin if dema-clocycline is known to be effective against the infecting strain of "strep."

(For more information, see **tetracyclines**, page 99.)

UNDESIRED EFFECTS

Allergic reactions, ranging from rash and hives to serious and sometimes fatal reactions, can occur in persons who have had allergic reactions to other tetracyclines, tetracycline combinations or tetracycline derivatives.

When you start to take demeclocycline, it may cause loss of appetite, diarrhea, nausea or vomiting. These effects tend to decrease or disappear as you continue to take it and as your body adjusts to the medication. Contact your doctor if they are severe or last more than two days.

If demeclocycline upsets your stomach or gives you abdominal or stomach cramps, take it with crackers or a light snack (no dairy products). Contact your doctor if these problems continue. In some people, this medication may cause a darkening or "furry" or black discoloration of the tongue. These changes are temporary and will go away when you stop taking demeclocycline.

Demeclocycline can allow an overgrowth of organisms that are not sensitive to tetracyclines. Some symptoms of overgrowth are itching of the rectal or genital areas, sore mouth or tongue or vaginal infection. If you have any of these effects, contact your doctor.

Demeclocycline frequently makes people more sensitive to sunlight than they are normally. Limit the amount of time you spend in sunlight. When you are in sunlight, cover your body with clothing, use a sunscreen preparation on exposed parts of your body and wear sunglasses. If you become severely sun-burned, contact your doctor or pharmacist. This sensitivity to sunlight may continue for two weeks to several months after you stop taking demeclocycline.

Demeclocycline can have bad effects on the kidneys when taken over a period of time. If you notice excessive thirst, unusual weakness or tiredness or a great increase in the frequency of urination or the amount of urine, stop taking the medication and contact your doctor.

Long-term therapy with demeclocycline may cause blood problems such as bone marrow depression or a decrease in one of the blood clotting factors. Contact your doctor if you notice any unusual bleeding or easy bruising, get painful sores in your mouth or throat or develop chills and fever.

PRECAUTIONS

Demeclocycline should not be taken by children under eight years of age, women past the first trimester of pregnancy or nursing mothers. It can discolor and pit the enamel of children's teeth. Demeclocycline is passed to the unborn child and to the nursing infant and can cause tooth discoloration and retard bone growth of fetuses and infants. Women who become pregnant while taking demeclocycline should contact their doctors.

Before you start taking demeclocycline, be sure to tell your doctor or pharmacist if you have ever had an allergic reaction to any other tetracyclines, tetracycline combinations or tetracycline derivatives. Your doctor should be told if you have kidney disease, liver disease or a history of allergies.

Certain medications and foods affect the way your body responds to demeclocycline and should not be taken at the same time you take it. Take demeclocycline one hour before or two hours after you consume antacids, laxatives, baking soda and dairy products such as milk, cheese and ice cream. Do not take iron preparations (many vitamin combinations contain iron) within two hours of the time at which you take demeclocycline.

Tell your doctor what other prescription or nonprescription drugs you are taking, especially antacids, laxatives, iron, anticoagulants (blood thinners), diuretics (water pills) or penicillins. If you do not know the names of the drugs or what they were prescribed for, bring them in their labeled containers to your doctor or pharmacist. While you are taking demeclocycline, do not start to take any other medications, including nonprescription medication unless you first contact your doctor or pharmacist.

Even if you feel better a few days after you start taking demeclocycline, take *all* the medicine your doctor has prescribed. This is particularly important if you have a "strep" infection. Serious heart problems can result later if the infection is not completely cured. Bacterial infections take several days to weeks to be cured completely. However, if your symptoms do not improve or if they become worse within a few days after you start taking demeclocycline, contact your doctor. He may want to change your medication.

Laboratory tests for liver or kidney function or blood tests may be ordered by your doctor. *Be sure to keep all appointments with your doctor and at the laboratory.*

If you have diabetes, demeclocycline can cause false results in some tests for sugar in your urine. Do not change your diet or the dosage of your diabetes medicine unless you first check with your doctor.

Demeclocycline also can affect the results of several blood tests that indicate kidney and liver function, as well as some urine tests. If you have such tests done, be sure the person responsible for reporting the results knows you have been taking demeclocycline.

Before having surgery with a general anesthetic, including dental surgery, tell the doctor or dentist in charge that you are taking demeclocycline.

DOSAGE AND STORAGE

Your doctor has determined how often you should take demeclocycline. Follow the instructions on your prescription label and ask your doctor or pharmacist to explain any part of the instructions you do not understand.

Doses of demeclocycline should be taken as far apart as possible during the day. If your doctor tells you to take it four times a day, take a dose every six hours *around the clock.*

Demeclocycline comes in capsules, tablets and liquid form. It should be taken on an "empty stomach," one hour before meals or two hours after eating. However, if this medication upsets your stomach, take it with crackers or a light snack (no dairy products).

The capsules and tablets should be taken with a full eight-ounce glass of water. The container of liquid should be shaken thoroughly before each use to mix the medication evenly. Use a specially marked measuring spoon to make sure the dose is accurate.

If you forget to take a dose, take it as soon as you remember. Then take any remaining doses for that day at evenly spaced intervals. Take all the demeclocycline exactly as prescribed. If you still have symptoms of the infection after you have taken all of it, contact your doctor.

When your doctor tells you to stop taking demeclocycline, throw away any unused portion of it. This drug may lose its effectiveness over a period of time and should not be saved to treat another infection. Old demeclocycline can cause dangerous effects. Do not allow anyone else to take your demeclocycline. It was prescribed for your particular condition.

Keep this medication in the container it came in, tightly closed and in a dry place. Keep it out of the reach of children.

Doxycycline
(dox i sye' kleen)

Brand name: Vibramycin, Vibra-tabs

Doxycycline is one of the tetracycline antibiotics. It is used to treat a variety of infections, including pneumonia, Rocky Mountain spotted fever, acne and venereal disease. Doxycycline can be used to treat infections caused by bacteria resistant to penicillin, but it is never the preferred drug for any "staph" infection.

Although penicillin is the preferred drug for "strep" infections and for the prevention of rheumatic fever, doxycycline may be used to treat these infections in people sensitive or allergic to penicillin if doxycycline is known to be effective against the infecting strain of "strep."

Doxycycline can be given to people with kidney disease with less risk of additional kidney problems than if other tetracyclines are taken. Food does not interfere with the absorption of doxycycline.

(For more information, see **tetracyclines**, page 99.)

UNDESIRED EFFECTS

Allergic reactions, ranging from rash and hives to serious and sometimes fatal reactions, can occur in persons who have had an allergic reaction to other tetracyclines, tetracycline combinations or tetracycline derivatives.

Doxycycline may cause loss of appetite, diarrhea, nausea or vomiting when you start to take it. These effects tend to decrease or disappear as you continue to take it and as your body adjusts to the medication. Contact your doctor if they are severe or last more than two days.

If doxycycline upsets your stomach or gives you abdominal or stomach cramps, take it with meals, milk or a carbonated beverage. Contact your doctor if these problems continue. In some people, this medication may cause a darkening or "furry" or black discoloration of the tongue. These changes are temporary and will go away when you stop taking doxycycline.

Doxycycline can allow an overgrowth of organisms that are not sensitive to tetracyclines. If you experience symptoms of overgrowth such as itching of the rectal or genital areas, sore mouth or tongue or vaginal infection, contact your doctor.

All tetracyclines can make some people more sensitive to sunlight than they normally are. This effect is rare with doxycycline, but you should limit the amount of time you spend in sunlight until you see how you react, especially if you sunburn easily. If you become severely sunburned, contact your doctor or pharmacist.

Long-term therapy with doxycycline may cause blood problems such as bone marrow depression or a decrease in one of the blood clotting factors. Contact your doctor if you notice any unusual bleeding or easy bruising, get painful sores in your mouth or throat, or develop chills and fever.

PRECAUTIONS

Doxycycline should not be taken by children under eight years of age, women past the first trimester of pregnancy or nursing mothers. It can discolor and pit the enamel of children's teeth. Doxycycline is passed to the unborn child and to the nursing infant and can cause tooth discoloration and retard bone growth of fetuses and infants. Women who become pregnant while taking doxycycline should contact their doctors.

Be sure to tell your doctor or pharmacist if you have ever had an allergic reaction to any other tetracyclines, tetracycline combinations or tetracycline derivatives. Your doctor should be told if you have liver disease or a history of allergies before you start taking doxycycline.

Certain medications can affect the way your body responds to doxycycline and should not be taken at the same time you take it. Take doxycycline one hour before or two hours after you consume antacids, laxatives or baking soda. Do not take iron preparations (many vitamin combinations contain iron) within two hours of the time you take doxycycline.

To help your doctor select the treatment best for you, tell him what other prescription or nonprescription drugs you are taking, particularly antacids, laxatives, iron, penicillins, sleeping pills, anticoagulants (blood thinners), diuretics (water pills) and medicine for seizures. If you do not know the names of the drugs or what they were prescribed for, bring them in their labeled containers to your doctor or pharmacist.

Take *all* the medicine your doctor has prescribed, even if you feel better a few days after you start taking doxycycline. This is particularly important if you have a "strep" infection. Serious heart problems can result later if the infection is not completely cured. Bacterial infections take several days to a week to be cured completely. However, if your symptoms do not improve within a few days after you start to take doxycycline or if they become worse, contact your doctor. He may want to change your medication.

If you have diabetes, doxycycline can cause false results in some tests for sugar in your urine. Do not change your diet or the dosage of your diabetes medicine unless you first check with your doctor.

Doxycycline also can affect the results of several blood tests that check liver function, as well as some urine tests. If you have such tests done, be sure the person responsible for reporting the results knows you have been taking doxycycline.

Your doctor may ask you to have laboratory tests to measure the effect of this drug on your blood, liver or kidney function. *Be certain to keep all appointments with your doctor and at the laboratory.*

If you intend to have surgery under a general anesthetic, including dental surgery, make certain your doctor or dentist knows you are taking doxycycline.

DOSAGE AND STORAGE

Doxycycline comes in capsules and in liquid form and usually is taken once or twice a day. Your doctor will determine how often you should take this medication. Follow the instructions on your prescription label and ask your doctor or pharmacist to explain any part of the instructions you do not understand.

The container of liquid doxycycline should be shaken before each use to mix the medication evenly. Use a specially marked measuring spoon to get an accurate dose of the liquid.

If you forget to take a dose, take it as soon as you remember. Then take any remaining doses for that day at evenly spaced intervals. Take *all* this medication exactly as prescribed. If you still have symptoms of the infection after you have taken all your doxycycline, contact your doctor.

When your doctor tells you to stop taking doxycycline, throw away any unused portion of your prescription. This drug may lose its effectiveness over a period of time and should not be saved to treat another infection. Old doxycycline can cause dangerous effects. Because this medication was prescribed for your particular condition, do not allow anyone else to take your doxycycline.

Keep this medication in the container it came in and store it at room temperature. You will find an expiration date on the container of liquid. Do not take the liquid after that date. Throw it away and, if you need more, get a new supply. If you are not sure of the expiration date or have any questions about a refill, contact your pharmacist.

Keep this medication out of the reach of children.

Methacycline
(meth a sye' kleen)

Brand name: Rondomycin

Methacycline is one of the tetracycline antibiotics. It is used to treat pneumonia, bladder infections, Rocky Mountain spotted fever and acne. Although it can be used against infections caused by bacteria resistant to penicillin, it is never the preferred drug for any kind of "staph" infection.

Penicillin is the preferred drug for "strep" infections and for the prevention of rheumatic fever, but methacycline may be used to treat these infections in people sensitive or allergic to penicillin if methacycline is known to be effective against the infecting strain of "strep."

(For more information, see **tetracyclines**, page 99.)

UNDESIRED EFFECTS

Allergic reactions, ranging from rash and hives to serious and sometimes fatal reactions, can occur in persons who have had allergic reactions to other tetracyclines, tetracycline combinations or tetracycline derivatives.

When you start to take methacycline, it may cause loss of appetite, diarrhea, nausea and vomiting. These effects tend to decrease or disappear as you continue to take it and as your body adjusts to the medication. Contact your doctor if they are severe or last more than two days.

If methacycline upsets your stomach or gives you abdominal or stomach cramps, take it with crackers or a light snack (no dairy products). Contact your doctor if these problems continue. Some people get a darkening or "furry" or black discoloration of the tongue when they take methacycline. These changes are temporary and will go away when you stop taking the medication.

An overgrowth of organisms that are not sensitive to tetracyclines can occur during methacycline therapy. Some symptoms of overgrowth are itching of the rectal or genital areas, sore mouth or tongue or vaginal infection. If you experience any of these effects, contact your doctor.

Some people who take methacycline may become more sensitive to sunlight than they are normally. When you start taking this medicine, limit the amount of time you spend in the sunlight until you know how you will react to it, particularly if you tend to sunburn easily. When you are in sunlight, keep your body covered with clothing, use a sunscreen preparation on the exposed parts of your body and wear sunglasses. If you become severely sunburned, contact your doctor or pharmacist.

Long-term therapy with methacycline may cause blood problems such as bone marrow depression or a decrease in one of the blood clotting factors. Contact your doctor if you notice any unusual bleeding or easy bruising, get painful sores in the mouth or throat or develop chills or fever.

PRECAUTIONS

Methacycline should not be taken by children under eight years of age, women past the first trimester of pregnancy and nursing mothers. It can discolor and pit the enamel of children's teeth. Methacycline is passed to the unborn child and to the nursing infant and can cause tooth discoloration and retard bone growth of fetuses and infants. Women who become pregnant while taking methacycline should contact their doctors.

Before you start taking methacycline, be sure to tell your doctor or pharmacist if you have ever had an allergic reaction to another tetracycline, tetracycline combinations or tetracycline derivatives. Your doctor should be told if you have kidney disease, liver disease or a history of allergies.

Certain medications and foods affect the way your body responds to methacycline and should not be taken at the same time you are taking methacycline. Take methacycline one hour before or two hours after you consume antacids, laxatives, baking soda and dairy products such as milk, cheese and ice cream. Do not take iron preparations (many vitamin combinations contain iron) within two hours of the time you take methacycline.

Tell your doctor or pharmacist what other prescription or nonprescription drugs you are taking, particularly antacids, laxatives, iron, penicillins, diuretics (water pills) and anticoagulants (blood thinners). If you do not know the names of the drugs or what they were prescribed for, bring them in their labeled containers to your doctor or pharmacist. Before you start to take any other medications while you are taking methacycline, contact your doctor or pharmacist.

Even if you feel better a few days after you start to take methacycline, take *all* the medicine your doctor has prescribed. This is particularly important if you have a "strep" infection. Serious heart problems can result later if a "strep" infection is not completely cured. Bacterial infections take several days to weeks to be cured completely. However, if your symptoms do not improve within a few days or become worse, contact your doctor. He may want to change your medication.

Your doctor may order laboratory tests of your kidney function, or blood tests. *Be sure to keep all appointments with your doctor and at the laboratory.*

If you have diabetes, methacycline can cause false results in some tests for sugar in your urine. Do not change your diet or the dosage of your diabetes medicine unless you first check with your doctor.

Methacycline can also affect the results of several tests for liver and kidney function. If you have such tests done, be sure the person responsible for reporting the results knows you have been taking methacycline.

If you need surgery with a general anesthetic, including dental surgery, be sure the doctor or dentist knows you are taking methacycline.

DOSAGE AND STORAGE

Your doctor has determined how often you should take methacycline. Follow the instructions on your prescription label and ask your doctor or pharmacist to explain any part of the instructions you do not understand.

Doses of methacycline should be taken as far apart as possible during the day. If your doctor instructs you to take it four times a day, take a dose every six hours *around the clock.*

Methacycline is best taken on an "empty stomach," one hour before meals or two hours after eating. However, if this medication upsets your stomach, take it with crackers or a light snack (no dairy products).

Methacycline comes in capsules, tablets and liquid form. The capsules and tablets should be taken with a full eight-ounce glass of water. The container of liquid should be shaken thoroughly before each use to mix the medication evenly. Use a specially marked measuring spoon to make sure you get an accurate dose.

If you forget to take a dose, take it as soon as you remember and then take any remaining doses for that day at evenly spaced intervals.

When your doctor tells you to stop taking methacycline, throw away any unused portion of it. This drug may lose its effectiveness over a period of time and should not be saved to treat another infection. Old methacycline can cause dangerous effects. Because this medication was prescribed for your particular condition, do not allow anyone else to take your methacycline.

Keep this medication in the container it came in and store it, tightly closed, at room temperature. Keep it out of the reach of children.

Minocycline
(mi noe sye' kleen)

Brand name: Minocin

Minocycline is one of the tetracycline antibiotics used to treat a variety of infections, including pneumonia, bladder infections, acne and venereal disease. Although minocycline is not used to treat meningitis, it is effective in eliminating the bacteria that cause meningitis from the nose and throat of "carriers" who spread the disease.

Penicillin is the preferred drug for "strep" infections and the prevention of rheumatic fever, but minocycline may be used to treat these infections in people sensitive or allergic to penicillin if minocycline is known to be effective against the infecting strain of "strep."

Food does not interfere with the absorption of minocycline.

(For more information, see **tetracyclines**, page 99.)

UNDESIRED EFFECTS

Allergic reactions, ranging from rash and hives to serious and sometimes fatal reactions, can occur in persons who have had an allergic reaction to other tetracyclines, tetracycline combinations or tetracycline derivatives.

When you start to take minocycline, it may cause loss of appetite, diarrhea, nausea or vomiting. These effects tend to decrease or disappear as you continue to take minocycline and as your body adjusts to it. Contact your doctor if they are severe or last more than two days.

If minocycline upsets your stomach or gives you abdominal or stomach cramps, take it with meals, milk or a carbonated beverage. Contact your doctor if these problems continue. In some people, this medication may cause a darkening or "furry" or black discoloration of the tongue. These changes are temporary and will go away when you stop taking the medication.

Minocycline therapy can allow an overgrowth of organisms that are not sensitive to tetracyclines. Contact your doctor if you experience symptoms of overgrowth such as itching of the rectal and genital areas, sore mouth or tongue or vaginal infection.

All tetracyclines can make some people more sensitive to sunlight than they are normally. This effect is rare with minocycline, but you should limit the amount of time you spend in sunlight until you see how you will react, especially if you sunburn easily. If you become severely sunburned, contact your doctor or pharmacist.

Minocycline can make some people dizzy, lightheaded or unsteady. Do not drive a car or operate dangerous machinery until you know how you react to this medicine.

Long-term therapy with minocycline may cause blood problems such as bone marrow depression or a decrease in one of the blood clotting factors. Contact your doctor if you notice any unusual bleeding or easy bruising, get painful sores in your mouth or throat or develop chills and fever.

PRECAUTIONS

Minocycline should not be taken by children under eight years of age, women past the first trimester of pregnancy and nursing mothers. It can discolor and pit the enamel of children's teeth. Minocycline is passed to the unborn child and to the nursing infant and can cause tooth discoloration and retard bone growth of fetuses and infants. Women who become pregnant while taking minocycline should contact their doctors.

Before you start to take minocycline, tell your doctor or pharmacist if you have ever had an allergic reaction to any other tetracycline, tetracycline combinations or tetracycline derivatives. Your doctor should be told if you have kidney disease, liver disease or a history of allergies.

Certain medications can affect the way your body responds to minocycline and should not be taken at the same time you take minocycline. Take minocycline one hour before or two hours after consuming antacids, laxatives or baking soda. Do not take iron preparations (many vitamin combinations contain iron) within two hours of the time you take minocycline.

To help your doctor select the best treatment for you, tell him what other prescription or nonprescription drugs you are taking, especially penicillins, antacids, laxatives, iron, anticoagulants (blood thinners) and diuretics (water pills). If you do not know the names of the drugs or what they were prescribed for, bring them in their labeled containers to your doctor or pharmacist. Do not start to take any other medications, including nonprescription medications while you are taking minocycline unless you first check with your doctor or pharmacist.

Even if you feel better in a few days, take *all* the medication your doctor has prescribed. This is particularly important if you have a "strep" infection.

Serious heart problems can result later if the infection is not completely cured. Bacterial infections take several days to weeks to be cured completely. However, if your symptoms do not improve within a few days after you start to take minocycline or if they become worse, contact your doctor. He may want to change your medication.

If you plan to have surgery with a general anesthetic, including dental surgery, be sure to tell the doctor or dentist that you are taking minocycline.

Your doctor may ask you to have laboratory tests performed to measure the effect of this drug on your blood or on your liver or kidney function. *Be sure to keep all appointments with your doctor or at the laboratory.*

If you have diabetes, minocycline can cause false results in some tests for sugar in your urine. Do not change your diet or the dosage of your diabetes medicine unless you first check with your doctor.

Minocycline will also affect the results of several blood tests for kidney and liver function. If you have such tests, be sure the person responsible for reporting the results knows you have been taking minocycline.

DOSAGE AND STORAGE

Minocycline comes in capsules and in liquid form and is usually taken twice a day. Your doctor will determine how often you should take this medication and how much you should take at each dose. Carefully follow the instructions on your prescription label and ask your doctor or pharmacist to explain any part of the instructions you do not understand.

The container of liquid minocycline should be shaken thoroughly before each use to mix the medication evenly. Use a specially marked measuring spoon to get an accurate dose of the liquid or syrup.

If you forget to take a dose, take it as soon as you remember. Then take any remaining doses for that day at evenly spaced intervals. Take all the minocycline exactly as prescribed. If you still have symptoms of the infection after you have taken all the minocycline, contact your doctor.

When your doctor tells you to stop taking minocycline, throw away any unused portion of it. This drug may lose its effectiveness over a period of time and should not be saved to treat another infection. Old minocycline can cause dangerous effects. Because this medication was prescribed for your particular condition, do not allow anyone else to take your minocycline.

Keep this medication in the container it came in and store it, tightly closed, at room temperature. Keep it out of the reach of children.

Oxytetracycline
(ox i te tra sye' kleen)

Brand names: Oxlopar, Oxy-Kesso-Tetra, Terramycin

Oxytetracycline is one of the tetracycline antibiotics used to treat pneumonia, bladder infections, Rocky Mountain spotted fever and acne. Oxytetracycline can be used in infections caused by bacteria resistant to penicillin, but it is never the preferred drug for any kind of "staph" infection.

Although penicillin is the preferred drug for "strep" infections and for the prevention of rheumatic fever, oxytetracycline may be used to treat these infections in people who are sensitive or allergic to penicillin if oxytetracycline is known to be effective against the infecting strain of "strep."

(For more information, see **tetracyclines**, page 99.)

UNDESIRED EFFECTS

Allergic reactions, ranging from rash and hives to serious and sometimes fatal reactions, can occur in persons who have had allergic reactions to other tetracyclines, tetracycline combinations or tetracycline derivatives.

Oxytetracycline may cause loss of appetite, diarrhea, nausea and vomiting when you start to take it. As you continue to take it and as your body adjusts to oxytetracycline, these problems tend to decrease or disappear. Contact your doctor if they are severe or last more than two days.

If this medication upsets your stomach or gives you abdominal or stomach cramps, take it with crackers or a light snack (no dairy products). Contact your doctor if these problems continue. Some people get a darkening or "furry" or black discoloration of the tongue when they take oxytetracycline. These changes are temporary and will go away when you stop taking the medication.

Oxytetracycline can allow an overgrowth of organisms that are not sensitive to tetracyclines. Itching of the rectal or genital areas, sore mouth or tongue or vaginal infection are some problems overgrowth can cause. Contact your doctor if you have any of these problems.

Some people who take oxytetracycline may become more sensitive to sunlight than they are normally. When you start taking this medicine, limit the amount of time you spend in sunlight until you know how you will react, particularly if you tend to burn easily. While in sunlight, keep your body covered with clothing, use a sunscreen preparation on the exposed parts of your body and wear sunglasses. Contact your doctor or pharmacist if you become severely sunburned.

Long-term therapy with oxytetracycline may cause blood problems such as bone marrow depression or a decrease in one of the blood clotting factors. If you notice any unusual bleeding or easy bruising, get painful sores in the mouth or throat or develop chills and fever, contact your doctor.

PRECAUTIONS

Oxytetracycline should not be taken by children under eight years of age, women past the first trimester of pregnancy or nursing mothers. It can discolor and pit the enamel of children's teeth. Oxytetracycline given to an expectant mother or nursing mother is passed to the baby and can discolor the teeth and retard bone growth of fetuses and infants. Women who become pregnant while taking oxytetracycline should contact their doctors.

Before you start taking oxytetracycline, be sure to tell your doctor if you have ever had an allergic reaction to another tetracycline, tetracycline combinations or tetracycline derivatives. To help your doctor select the best treatment for you, tell him if you have kidney disease, liver disease or a history of drug allergy.

Certain medications and food affect the way your body responds to oxytetracycline and should not be taken at the same time you take this medicine. Take oxytetracycline one hour before or two hours after your consume antacids, laxatives, baking soda and dairy products such as milk, cheese and ice cream. Do not take iron preparations (many vitamin combinations contain iron) within two hours of the time you take oxytetracycline.

Tell your doctor or pharmacist what other prescription or nonprescription drugs you are taking, especially antacids, laxatives, iron, penicillin, diuretics (water pills) and anticoagulants (blood thinners). If you do not know the names of the drugs or what they were prescribed for, bring them in their labeled containers to your doctor or pharmacist.

Take *all* the medicine your doctor has prescribed, even if you feel better after you have taken oxytetracycline for a few days. This is particularly important if you have a "strep" infection. Serious heart problems can result later if a "strep" infection is not completely cured. Bacterial infections take several days to weeks to be cured completely. However, if your symptoms do not improve within a few days after you start taking oxytetracycline or if they become worse, contact your doctor. He may want to change your medication.

Laboratory tests of your blood or for kidney or liver function may be ordered by your doctor. *Be certain to keep all appointments with your doctor or at the laboratory.*

If you have diabetes, oxytetracycline can cause false results in some tests for sugar in your urine. Do not change your diet or the dosage of your diabetes medicine unless you first check with your doctor.

Oxytetracycline can also affect the results of several tests for liver and kidney function. If you have such tests done, be sure the person responsible for reporting the results knows you have been taking oxytetracycline.

Before you have surgery with a general anesthetic, including dental surgery, tell the doctor or dentist that you are taking oxytetracycline.

DOSAGE AND STORAGE

Your doctor will determine how often you should take oxytetracycline and how much to take at each dose. Carefully follow the label instructions and ask your doctor or pharmacist to explain any part of the instructions you do not understand.

Doses of oxytetracycline should be taken as far apart as possible during the day. If your doctor instructs you to take it four times a day, take a dose every six hours *around the clock.*

Oxytetracycline should be taken on an "empty stomach." However, if this medication upsets your stomach, take it with crackers or a light snack (no dairy products).

Oxytetracycline comes in capsules, tablets and liquid form. The capsules and tablets should be taken with a full eight-ounce glass of water. The container of liquid should be shaken thoroughly before each use to mix the medication evenly. Use a specially marked measuring spoon to be sure you get an accurate dose.

If you forget to take a dose, take it as soon as you remember it. Take any remaining doses for that day at evenly spaced intervals.

When your doctor tells you to stop taking oxytetracycline, throw away any unused portion of it. This drug may lose its effectiveness over a period of time and should not be saved to treat another infection. Old oxytetracycline can cause serious problems. Because this medication was prescribed for your particular condition, do not allow anyone else to take your oxytetracycline.

Keep this medication in the container it came in and store it, tightly closed, at room temperature. Keep it out of the reach of children.

Tetracycline
(te tra sye′ kleen)

Brand names: Achromycin V, Cyclopar, Panmycin, Robitet, SK-Tetracycline, Sumycin, Tetracyn, Tetrex

Tetracycline is used to treat a variety of infections, including pneumonia, bladder infections, Rocky Mountain spotted fever and acne. Though tetracycline can be used against infections caused by bacteria resistant to penicillin, tetracycline is never the preferred drug for any kind of "staph" infection.

Penicillin is the preferred drug for treatment of "strep" infections and for the prevention of rheumatic fever, but tetracycline may be used to treat these infections in people sensitive or allergic to penicillin if tetracycline is known to be effective against the infecting strain of "strep."

(For more information, see **tetracyclines**, page 99.)

UNDESIRED EFFECTS

Allergic reactions, ranging from rash and hives to serious and sometimes fatal reactions, can occur in persons who have had allergic reactions to other tetracyclines, tetracycline combinations or tetracycline derivatives.

When you start to take tetracycline, it may cause loss of appetite, diarrhea, nausea and vomiting. These effects tend to decrease or disappear as you continue to take it and as your body adjusts to the medication. Contact your doctor if they are severe or last more than two days.

If tetracycline upsets your stomach or gives you abdominal or stomach cramps, take it with crackers or a light snack (no dairy products). Contact your doctor if these problems continue. Some people get a darkening or "furry" or black discoloration of the tongue when they take this medication. These changes are temporary and will go away when you stop taking tetracycline.

An overgrowth of organisms that are not sensitive to this drug can occur during tetracycline therapy. Some symptoms of overgrowth are itching of the rectal or genital areas, sore mouth or tongue or vaginal infection. Contact your doctor if you have any of these problems.

Some people who take tetracycline may become more sensitive to sunlight than they normally are. When you start taking this medicine, limit the amount of time you spend in sunlight until you know how you will react, particularly if you tend to burn easily. When you are in sunlight, keep your body covered with clothing, use a sunscreen preparation on the exposed parts of your body and wear sunglasses. If you get severely sunburned, contact your doctor or pharmacist.

Long-term therapy with tetracycline may cause blood problems such as bone marrow depression or a decrease in one of the blood clotting factors. Contact your doctor if you notice unusual bleeding or easy bruising, get painful sores in the mouth or throat or develop chills or fever. Problems of liver or kidney function can also occur.

PRECAUTIONS

Tetracycline should not be taken by children under eight years of age, women past the first trimester of pregnancy or nursing mothers. It can discolor and pit the enamel of children's teeth. Tetracycline taken by an expectant mother or a nursing mother is passed to the baby and can discolor teeth and retard bone growth of fetuses and infants. Women who become pregnant while taking tetracycline should contact their doctors.

Before you start taking tetracycline, be sure to tell your doctor or pharmacist if you have ever had an allergic reaction to another tetracycline, tetracycline combinations or tetracycline derivatives. Tell your doctor if you have kidney disease, liver disease or a history of drug allergy.

Certain medications and food affect the way your body responds to tetracycline and should not be taken at the same time you take this medication. Take tetracycline one hour before or two hours after you consume antacids, laxatives, baking soda and dairy products such as milk, cheese and ice cream. Do not take iron preparations (many vitamin combinations contain iron) within two hours of the time you take tetracycline.

Tell your doctor or pharmacist what other prescription or nonprescription drugs you are taking, especially antacids, laxatives, iron, penicillin, diuretics (water pills) and anticoagulants (blood thinners). If you do not know the names of the drugs or what they were prescribed for, bring them in their labeled containers to your doctor or pharmacist. Before you start taking any other medications while you are taking tetracycline, contact your doctor or pharmacist.

Even if you feel better a few days after you start taking tetracycline, take *all* the medicine your doctor has prescribed. This is particularly important if you have a "strep" infection. Serious heart problems can result later if a "strep" infection is not completely cured. Bacterial infections take several days to weeks to be cured completely. However, if your symptoms do not improve within a few days or become worse, contact your doctor. He may want to change your medication.

Your doctor may order laboratory tests for liver or kidney function or blood tests. *Keep all appointments with your doctor or at the laboratory.*

If you have diabetes, tetracycline can cause false results in some tests for sugar in your urine. Do not change your diet or the dosage of your diabetes medicine unless you first check with your doctor.

Tetracycline can also affect the results of several tests for liver and kidney function. If you have such tests done, be sure the person responsible for reporting the results knows that you have been taking tetracycline.

Before surgery with a general anesthetic, including dental surgery, tell the doctor or dentist that you are taking tetracycline.

DOSAGE AND STORAGE

Your doctor has determined how often you should take tetracycline and how much to take at each dose. Carefully follow the instructions on your prescription label and ask your doctor or pharmacist to explain any part of the instructions you do not understand.

Doses of tetracycline should be taken as far apart as possible during the day. If your doctor instructs you to take it four times a day, take a dose every six hours *around the clock.*

Tetracycline should be taken on an "empty stomach," one hour before meals or two hours after eating. However, if this medication upsets your stomach, take it with crackers or a light snack (no dairy products).

Tetracycline comes in capsules, tablets and liquid form. The capsules and tablets should be taken with a full eight-ounce glass of water. The container of liquid should be shaken thoroughly before each use to mix the medication evenly. Use a specially marked measuring spoon to make sure you get an accurate dose.

If you forget to take a dose, take it as soon as you remember it. Take any remaining doses for that day at evenly spaced intervals.

When your doctor tells you to stop taking tetracycline, throw away any unused portion of it. This drug may lose its effectiveness over a period of time and should not be saved to treat another infection. Taking old tetracycline can be dangerous. Because this medication was prescribed for your particular condition, do not allow anyone else to take your tetracycline.

Keep this medication in the container it came in and store it, tightly closed, at room temperature. Keep it out of the reach of children.

OTHER ANTIBIOTICS

Chloramphenicol

(klor am fen′ i kole)

Brand names: Amphicol, Chloromycetin

Chloramphenicol is an antibiotic. Because chloramphenicol can cause serious and sometimes fatal blood problems, its use is reserved for severe infections that do not respond to other safer antibiotics and for infections against which it is known to be particularly effective. It is the preferred drug for treating typhoid fever and is often used against severe cases of meningitis.

Chloramphenicol should not be used to treat mild or trivial infections; for colds, influenza, or sore throats; by people who have had problems with this drug in the past; or to prevent bacterial infection.

UNDESIRED EFFECS

The most serious side effects of chloramphenicol are blood problems, such as bone marrow depression and a decrease in one of the blood clotting components. Symptoms of these problems are unusual bleeding or bruising, unusual weakness or tiredness, fever, pale skin or sore throat. If you develop any of these symptoms, stop taking chloramphenicol and contact your doctor immediately. If you take chloramphenicol, you should be hospitalized during therapy so that you can be observed for these symptoms and so frequent blood tests can be done.

Blood problems may develop weeks or months after you stop taking chloramphenicol. Be alert for the symptoms of blood problems and contact your doctor immediately if they occur.

A less common but no less serious side effect is inflammation of the nerves of the eyes. It can result in blindness. If you experience eye pain, blurred vision or loss of vision, stop taking chloramphenicol and contact your doctor immediately.

Other indications that this medicine is having a bad effect on the nerves are numbness, tingling, burning pain or weakness in the hands or feet, headache and confusion. Stop taking the medicine and contact your doctor immediately if these symptoms occur.

Newborn and premature infants given chloramphenicol can develop a problem called "gray syndrome," which results from failure of the blood to circulate properly through the body. Though this problem is more common in infants, it can occur in children up to two years of age who are treated with the drug and in babies whose mothers are given chloramphenicol in the last stages of pregnancy or during labor.

If chloramphenicol is given to a baby and if the baby develops a gray skin color, low body temperature, bloated stomach, uneven breathing or drowsiness, stop the medicine and contact your doctor immediately.

Allergic reactions, ranging from rash and hives to a serious and sometimes fatal reaction, can occur with chloramphenicol. No one who has had an allergic reaction to this drug or who developed blood or nerve problems while taking it in the past should take chloramphenicol again.

Occasionally, chloramphenicol can cause nausea, vomiting or diarrhea. These effects usually occur when you start to take the drug and tend to disappear as you continue to take chloramphenicol and as your body adjusts to it. Contact your doctor if they continue or are bothersome.

As in therapy using other antibiotics, chloramphenicol therapy may result in an overgrowth of organisms against which chloramphenicol is not effective. If you have itching in the rectal or genital area, sore mouth or tongue or vaginal infection, contact your doctor.

PRECAUTIONS

Before you start taking chloramphenicol, tell your doctor if you have kidney or liver disease, have ever taken this drug before or have had problems with it in the past.

Certain other medications when taken with chloramphenicol can affect the way your body responds to this drug. These include anticoagulants (blood thinners), oral diabetes medicine, penicillin, lincomycin, clindamycin and medicine to prevent seizures. Chloramphenicol should not be taken with other drugs that can cause bone marrow depression, including anticancer medicines, colchicine, gold salts, phenylbutazone, oxyphenbutazone, and penicillamine.

Tell your doctor what other prescription or nonprescription drugs you are taking. If you do not know the names of the drugs or what they were prescribed for, bring them in their labeled containers to your doctor or pharmacist.

Take *all* the medicine your doctor has prescribed, even if you feel better a few days after you start taking chloramphenicol. Bacterial infections need to be completely cured before you stop taking the medicine, and this can take several days to weeks. However, if your symptoms do not improve in a few days or get worse, contact your doctor. He may want to change your medication.

Your doctor will want to check your progress regularly. *Be sure to keep all appointments with him.* Before you begin to take chloramphenicol and every few days during therapy, you should have blood tests performed. You may also be required to have liver and kidney function tests. Do not change your diet or the dosage of your diabetes medicine without first checking with your doctor.

Chloramphenicol should not be taken by mothers in the last few weeks of pregnancy or by mothers who are nursing a baby.

Dosage and Storage

Your doctor will determine how much chloramphenicol you should take and how often you should take it. Carefully follow the instructions on your prescription label and ask your doctor or pharmacist to explain any part of the instructions you do not understand.

Doses of chloramphenicol should be taken as far apart as possible during the day. If your doctor instructs you to take this medicine four times a day, take a dose every six hours. If you give chloramphenicol to a child, be sure he or she receives it around the clock, even if you have to wake the child for doses.

Chloramphenicol comes in capsules and in liquid form. It is best to take this medication on an "empty stomach," one hour before meals or two hours after eating.

The capsules should be taken with a full eight-ounce glass of water. The liquid should be measured in a specially marked measuring spoon to make sure of an adequate dose. Shake the container of liquid well before each use to mix the medication evenly.

If you forget to take a dose, take it as soon as you remember. Then take the remaining doses for that day at evenly spaced intervals.

Contact your doctor if you still have symptoms of the infection after you have taken all the medicine prescribed. When your doctor tells you to stop taking chloramphenicol, throw away any unused portion of it. Chloramphenicol may lose its effectiveness over a period of time and should not be saved to treat another infection. Do not allow anyone else to take your chloramphenicol, which was prescribed for your particular condition.

Keep this medication in the container it came in and store it at room temperature. Keep it out of the reach of children.

Clindamycin
(klin da mye' sin)

Brand name: Cleocin

Clindamycin is an antibiotic made from lincomycin and acts in a way similar to lincomycin to eliminate bacteria. Because clindamycin can cause serious and sometimes fatal bowel inflammation, its use is reserved for severe infections that would not respond to safer antibiotics and for infections against which it is particularly effective.

This drug is used to treat severe infections (such as abscesses) of the lungs, skin, abdomen, bone and female pelvis. *Clindamycin should not be used against mild infections or against colds, influenza or sore throats.*

UNDESIRED EFFECTS

The most serious side effect of clindamycin is inflammation of the bowel. Symptoms of this problem are fever; severe stomach cramps, pain and bloating; and severe, watery diarrhea, which may be accompanied by blood, mucus, pus or pieces of intestinal lining in the stool. *If you develop any of these symptoms, stop taking the medicine and contact your doctor immediately.*

If bowel inflammation occurs, symptoms usually develop two to nine days after you start taking clindamycin. However, they can also occur up to several weeks after you stop taking this medicine. Be alert for these symptoms even after you stop taking clindamycin, and contact your doctor *immediately* if they occur.

If clindamycin gives you diarrhea, do not take any diarrhea medicine without first checking with your doctor. These medicines, particularly those containing kaolin (for example, Kaopectate), can make the diarrhea worse or last longer. If diarrhea lasts longer than 24 hours, stop taking clindamycin and contact your doctor.

Clindamycin also can cause skin rash, abdominal pain, nausea or vomiting. These effects tend to lessen or disappear as you continue to take the drug and as your body adjusts to it. If these effects continue or are bothersome, contact your doctor.

Allergic reactions, ranging from rash and hives to a serious and sometimes fatal reaction, can occur with clindamycin. No one who has had an allergic reaction to clindamycin or lincomycin in the past should take clindamycin again.

As in therapy using other antibiotics, clindamycin therapy may result in an overgrowth of organisms against which clindamycin is not effective. Contact your doctor if you have itching in the rectal or genital areas, sore mouth or tongue or vaginal infection.

PRECAUTIONS

Before you start taking clindamycin, tell your doctor if you have ever had an allergic reaction to the drug or to lincomycin, if you have a history of stomach or bowel disease and if you have kidney or liver disease.

Certain other medications, such as chloramphenicol, erythromycins and medicines used to treat diarrhea, should not be taken when you are taking clindamycin. Tell your doctor what other prescription or nonprescription drugs you are taking. If you do not know the names of the drugs or what they were prescribed for, bring them in their labeled containers to your doctor or pharmacist.

Even if you feel better a few days after you start taking clindamycin, take *all* the medicine your doctor has prescribed. Your bacterial infections must be completely cured before you stop taking the medicine, and this can take several days to weeks. However, if your symptoms do not improve in a few days or get worse, contact your doctor. He may want to change your medication.

To help your doctor select the best treatment for you, tell him if you are pregnant or nursing a baby. The safe use of clindamycin for pregnant women has not been established, and the drug is passed to a nursing infant through the mother's milk.

Your doctor will want to check regularly the way you are responding to clindamycin and may order laboratory tests. *Be sure to keep all your appointments with him and at the laboratory.*

Before having surgery with a general anesthetic, including dental surgery, tell the doctor or dentist that you are taking clindamycin.

DOSAGE AND STORAGE

Your doctor will determine how much clindamycin you should take and how often you should take it. Carefully follow the instructions on your prescription label and ask your doctor or pharmacist to explain any part of the instructions you do not understand.

Doses of clindamycin should be taken as far apart as possible throughout the day. If your doctor instructs you to take this medicine four times a day, take a dose every six hours. If you give clindamycin to a child, make sure he or she receives it around the clock, even if you must wake the child for doses.

Clindamycin comes in capsules and in liquid form. Take this medication on an "empty stomach," one hour before meals or two hours after eating.

The capsules should be taken with a full eight-ounce glass of water to prevent irritation of the esophagus (the part of the digestive tract between the throat and stomach). The container of liquid should be shaken well before each use to mix the medication evenly. Measure doses of liquid with a specially marked measuring spoon to make sure of an accurate dose.

If you forget to take a dose, take it as soon as you remember. However, if it is almost time for the next dose, you may either double the next dose or space the missed dose and the next dose one to two hours apart. Then go back to your regular dosing schedule.

If you still have symptoms of the infection after you have taken all the clindamycin prescribed, contact your doctor. When he tells you to stop taking clindamycin, throw away any unused portion of it. This medication may lose its effectiveness over a period of time and should not be saved to treat another infection. Do not allow anyone else to take your clindamycin, which was prescribed for your particular condition.

Keep clindamycin in the container it came in and store it at room temperature. The liquid container will have an expiration date on it. Do not take the liquid after that date. Throw away the liquid and, if you need more, get a new supply. Contact your pharmacist if you are not sure of the expiration date or have questions about a refill.

Keep this medication out of the reach of children.

Colistimethate and Colistin
(koe list eh meth′ ate/koe list′ in)

Brand name: Coly-Mycin

Colistimethate and colistin are antibiotics that act in different ways on the body when they are given by injection or taken orally. Colistimethate, the injectable form, is used to treat bacterial infections of the urinary tract. Usually it is given in the hospital or at the physician's office. Colistin, which is given orally, is used to treat bacterial infections of the bowels, such as those that cause severe diarrhea.

UNDESIRABLE EFFECTS

The most frequent side effects of colistimethate are numbness, weakness and tingling of the hands and feet, the tongue and around the mouth. Less often, this medicine will cause itching all over the body, hives and changes in vision. If you experience any of these side effects after you have had an injection of this drug, contact your doctor.

Colistimethate makes some people dizzy, unsteady or less alert than usual. Do not drive a car or operate dangerous machinery until you know how this drug affects you.

The most serious side effect of colistimethate is kidney failure. Contact your doctor if you notice blood in your urine or a greatly decreased amount of urine.

Unlike the injectable form, colistin, the oral form, has few side effects.

Therapy with either colistimethate or colistin may result in an overgrowth of organisms against which they are not effective. Contact your doctor if you have itching in the rectal area or genital area or a sore mouth or tongue when you are taking either of these medicines.

PRECAUTIONS

Before you start to take colistimethate or colistin, tell your doctor if you have ever had an allergic reaction to these drugs or to similar antibiotics, including polymixin B, viomycin and bacitracin.

To help your doctor select the treatment best for you, tell him if you have kidney disease.

Certain medications, when given with colistimethate, increase the chance of side effects. Some of these are cephalothin, sodium citrate, muscle relaxants, kanamycin, streptomycin, polymixin B and neomycin. Tell your doctor what other prescription or nonprescription drugs you are taking. If you do not know the names of the drugs or what they were prescribed for, bring them in their labeled containers to your doctor or pharmacist.

If your symptoms do not improve in a few days or get worse, contact your doctor. He may want to change your medication or adjust the dosage.

Tell your doctor if you are pregnant or think you may be. The safe use of colistimethate for pregnant women has not been established.

Your doctor will want to check regularly on your response to colistimethate and may want to do kidney function tests. *Keep all appointments with him and at the laboratory.*

Before having surgery with a general anesthetic, including dental surgery, tell the doctor or dentist that you are taking colistimethate or colistin.

DOSAGE AND STORAGE

Colistimethate is given in an injection under a doctor's supervision.

Colistin is a liquid and usually is given three times a day. Your doctor will determine how often you should take colistin and how much you should take at each dose. Carefully follow the instructions on your prescription label and ask your doctor or pharmacist to explain any part of the instructions you do not understand.

The liquid should be measured in a specially marked measuring spoon to ensure an accurate dose. If you forget to take a dose, take it as soon as you remember and then take the remaining doses for that day at evenly spaced intervals. If you remember a missed dose when it is close to the time for another, omit the missed dose completely and take only the regularly scheduled dose. *Do not take a double dose.*

If you still have symptoms of the infection after you have taken all the medicine prescribed, contact your doctor. When your doctor tells you to stop taking colistin, throw away any unused portion of it. This medicine should not be saved to treat another infection, nor should anyone else be allowed to take it.

Keep colistin in the container it came in and store it out of the reach of children.

Gentamicin
(jen ta mye' sin)

Brand names: Apogen, Bristagen, Garamycin, U-Gencin

Gentamicin is an antibiotic used to treat serious infections of the bones and joints, the skin (including serious infections resulting from burns), the lungs and abdomen. It is given by injection only and is usually used in the hospital.

UNDESIRED EFFECTS

Gentamicin can cause serious kidney, ear and muscular problems. Symptoms of kidney problems are blood in the urine, excessive thirst, greatly decreased frequency of urination or amount of urine and loss of appetite.

Clumsiness or unsteadiness, dizziness, loss of hearing, a ringing or buzzing sound or a feeling of fullness in the ears or nausea or vomiting indicate that this drug may be damaging the nerves in your ears. Muscle problems will usually show up as difficulty in breathing, drowsiness or weakness. All of these problems should have medical attention and should be checked by your doctor.

PRECAUTIONS

If you have had a problem with gentamicin or any of the antibiotics similar to it (amikacin, kanamycin, neomycin, streptomycin and tobramycin), do not take gentamicin again. Tell your doctor if you have ever had a reaction to any of these drugs.

Before you start to take gentamicin, tell your doctor if you have ear problems, myasthenia gravis, Parkinson's disease or kidney disease. Gentamicin could make these conditions worse.

Several other drugs, when taken with gentamicin, may increase the chance of side effects. These are the antibiotics similar to gentamicin (see the list above), general anesthetics, medicine for neuromuscular diseases, capreomycin, cisplatin, diuretics (water pills), vancomycin, viomycin, cephaloridine and polymyxin.

Tell your doctor if you are pregnant or think you may be. Gentamicin can be passed from you to your baby and might result in the baby having hearing problems.

DOSAGE AND STORAGE

Gentamicin is given only by injection under a doctor's supervision.

Lincomycin
(lin koe mye' sin)

Brand name: Lincocin

Lincomycin is an antibiotic. Because lincomycin can cause serious and sometimes fatal bowel inflammation, its use is reserved for severe infections that would not respond to safer antibiotics and for infections against which it is particularly effective. Lincomycin is used to treat severe infections (such as abscesses) of the lungs, skin, abdomen, bone and female pelvis.

Lincomycin should not be used against mild infections or against colds, influenza or sore throats.

UNDESIRED EFFECTS

Inflammation of the bowel is the most serious side effect of lincomycin. Symptoms of this problem are fever; severe stomach cramps, pain and bloating; and severe, watery diarrhea, which may be accompanied by blood, mucus, pus or pieces of intestinal lining in the stool. *Stop taking the medicine and contact your doctor immediately if you develop any of these symptoms.*

Symptoms of bowel inflammation can also occur up to several weeks after you stop taking lincomycin. Be alert for them even after you stop taking lincomycin, and contact your doctor *immediately* if they occur.

If lincomycin gives you diarrhea, do not take any diarrhea medicine without first checking with your doctor. These medicines, particularly those containing kaolin (for example, Kaopectate), can make the diarrhea worse or last longer.

When you start to take lincomycin, you may get skin rash, mild diarrhea, nausea or vomiting. These effects tend to disappear as you continue to take lincomycin and as your body adjusts to it. Contact your doctor if these symptoms continue or are bothersome.

Allergic reactions, ranging from rash and hives to a serious and sometimes fatal reaction, can occur with lincomycin. No one who has had an allergic reaction to lincomycin or clindamycin in the past should take lincomycin again.

As in therapy using other antibiotics, lincomycin therapy may result in an overgrowth of organisms against which lincomycin is not effective. If you get itching in the rectal or genital area, sore tongue or mouth or vaginal infection, contact your doctor.

PRECAUTIONS

Lincomycin should not be given to newborn infants (those under one month of age).

Before you start taking lincomycin, tell your doctor if you have ever had an allergic reaction to this drug or to clindamycin, if you have a history of stomach or bowel disease and if you have kidney or liver disease.

Certain other medications, such as chloramphenicol, erythromycins and medicines used to treat diarrhea, should not be taken with lincomycin. Tell your doctor what other prescription or nonprescription drugs you are taking. If you do not know the names of the drugs or what they were prescribed for, take them in their labeled containers to your doctor or pharmacist.

Even if you feel better a few days after you start taking lincomycin, take *all* the medicine your doctor has prescribed. Your bacterial infections must be completely cured before you stop taking the medicine. It takes several days to weeks to cure bacterial infections completely. However, if your symptoms do not improve in a few days or get worse, contact your doctor. He may want to change your medication.

Tell your doctor if you are pregnant or are nursing a baby. This will help him select the best treatment for you and your baby. Safe use of lincomycin for pregnant women has not been established, and the drug is passed to a nursing infant through the mother's milk.

Your doctor will want to check regularly the way you are responding to lincomycin and may order laboratory tests. *Be sure to keep all your appointments with the doctor and at the laboratory.*

Before having surgery with a general anesthetic, including dental surgery, tell the doctor or dentist that you are taking lincomycin.

DOSAGE AND STORAGE

Your doctor has determined how much lincomycin you should take and how often you should take it. Carefully follow the instructions on your prescription label and ask your doctor or pharmacist to explain any part of the instructions you do not understand.

Doses of lincomycin should be taken as far apart as possible throughout the day. If your doctor instructs you to take this medication four times a day, take a dose every six hours. If you give lincomycin to a child, make sure he or she receives it around the clock, even if you must wake the child for doses.

Lincomycin comes in capsules and in liquid form. Take lincomycin on an empty stomach, one hour before meals or two hours after eating.

The capsules should be taken with a full eight-ounce glass of water to prevent irritation of the esophagus (the part of the digestive tract between the throat and the stomach). Doses of the liquid should be measured with a specially marked measuring spoon to ensure accuracy.

If you forget to take a dose, take it as soon as you remember. However, if it is almost time for the next dose, either double the next dose or space the missed dose and the next dose one to two hours apart. Then go back to your regular dosing schedule.

If you still have symptoms of the infection after you have taken all the lincomycin prescribed, contact your doctor. When he tells you to stop taking lincomycin, throw away any unused portion of it. This medication may lose its effectiveness over a period of time and should not be saved to treat another infection. Lincomycin was prescribed for your particular condition; do not allow anyone else to take your lincomycin.

Keep this medicine in the container it came in and store it at room temperature. Keep it out of the reach of children.

Neomycin
(nee oh mye' sin)

Brand names: Mycifradin, Neobiotic

Neomycin is an antibiotic used to treat infections of the bowels and to help lessen the symptoms of coma resulting from liver disease. It may be given before of after bowel surgery to help prevent infection.

UNDESIRED EFFECTS

The most common side effects of neomycin taken orally are nausea, vomiting and irritation or soreness of the mouth or rectal area. These effects tend to lessen or disappear as your body adjusts to the medication. If they continue or become bothersome, contact your doctor.

Neomycin may also cause diarrhea, excessive gas and light-colored, frothy, fatty-appearing stools. If these effects are severe or last more than a few days, contact your doctor.

Although serious side effects with oral neomycin are rare, long-term therapy with oral neomycin can result in damage to the inner ear or to the kidneys. Symptoms of ear problems when you are using oral neomycin are loss of hearing; a ringing, buzzing sound or feeling of fullness in the ears; clumsiness; dizziness or unsteadiness. Stop taking the medicine if you develop any of these symptoms, and contact your doctor as soon as possible.

If you notice excessive thirst or a greatly decreased frequency of urination or amount of urine, neomycin may be giving you kidney problems. Stop taking the medication and contact your doctor as soon as possible.

Allergic reactions, including rash, hives, itching and fever occur occasionally when you are taking neomycin. If you have had an allergic reaction to neomycin or to antibiotics similar to it (amikacin, gentamicin, kanamycin, streptomycin and tobramycin), do not take neomycin.

As in therapy using other antibiotics, neomycin therapy may result in an overgrowth of organisms against which neomycin is not effective. Contact your doctor if you have itching in the rectal or genital area, sore mouth or tongue or vaginal infection.

PRECAUTIONS

Before you start taking neomycin, tell your doctor if you have any of these medical problems: obstruction of the bowel, eighth-cranial-nerve disease (loss of hearing and/or balance), kidney disease, myasthenia gravis, Parkinson's disease or ulcers of the bowels.

Certain medications should not be taken with neomycin because they increase the possibility of serious ear and kidney problems. These are the antibiotics amikacin, capreomycin, cephaloridine, cephalothin, cisplatin, gentamicin, kanamycin, polymixin, streptomycin, tobramycin, vancomycin and viomycin, the diuretics (water pills), ethacrynic acid, furosemide and mercaptomerin.

Tell your doctor what other prescription or nonprescription drugs you are taking, including any of the above-mentioned drugs and anticoagulants (blood thinners) or digoxin. He may want to adjust the doses of the medications so they will work well together. If you do not know the names of the drugs you are taking or what they were prescribed for, bring them in their labeled containers to your doctor or pharmacist.

Even if you feel better a few days after you start taking neomycin, take *all* the medicine your doctor has prescribed. Your bacterial infections must be completely cured before you stop taking the medicine. This can take several days to weeks. However, if your symptoms do not improve in a few days or get worse, contact your doctor. He may want to change your medication or adjust the dosage.

Tell your doctor if you are pregnant or nursing a baby. This will help him select the best treatment for you and your baby. Safe use of neomycin for pregnant women has not been established.

Your doctor will want to check regularly the way you are responding to neomycin and may want tests for hearing and kidney function. *Be sure to keep all your appointments with him and at the laboratory.*

Before having surgery with a general anesthetic, including dental surgery, tell the doctor or dentist that you are taking neomycin.

DOSAGE AND STORAGE

Your doctor will determine how much neomycin you should take and how often you should take it. Carefully follow the instructions on your prescription

label and ask your doctor or pharmacist to explain any part of the instructions you do not understand.

Neomycin comes in tablets and in liquid form and can be taken without regard to meals. The tablets should be taken with a full eight-ounce glass of water. The liquid should be measured with a specially marked measuring spoon to make sure of an accurate dose.

If you forget to take a dose, take it as soon as you remember it and take the remaining doses for that day at evenly spaced intervals. If you remember a missed dose when it is close to the time for another, omit the missed dose completely and take only the regularly scheduled dose. *Do not take a double dose.*

If you still have symptoms of the infection after you have taken all the neomycin prescribed, contact your doctor. When your doctor tells you to stop taking neomycin, throw away any unused portion of it. Neomycin may lose its effectiveness over a period of time and should not be saved to treat another infection. Do not allow anyone else to take your neomycin.

Keep neomycin in the container it came in and store it at room temperature. Keep neomycin out of the reach of children.

Tuberculosis

Tuberculosis is an infection caused by bacteria. The type of bacterium is called a mycobacterium. In the past, patients with tuberculosis were isolated from the rest of society, usually in a sanatorium, to prevent the spread of TB. Now that health professionals have learned more about the causes and methods of transmitting infections in general and tuberculosis in particular, sanatoriums for tuberculosis patients have all but disappeared. Patients with tuberculosis rarely need to be hospitalized for treatment of TB.

The bacteria that cause TB can be present in the body for months or years without causing any health problem. This is called the "asymptomatic" stage. If not treated, the bacteria can become active, and "clinical" disease is present. Active disease usually is in the lungs (pulmonary tuberculosis) but also can be in other parts of the body.

The aims of treatment are to prevent the disease from advancing in the person who has TB and to prevent it from spreading to other people.

The TB bacteria in the body can be in a resting or harmless state, or they may be active and growing. To cure TB, treatment must be aimed at both resting and active bacteria. Tests of the bacteria must be done to determine their state and the drugs that might be effective in destroying them.

Usually more than one drug is used to treat TB and prevent relapse, especially if the disease is active and "clinical TB" is present. Tuberculosis can almost always be cured by drug therapy but, as with the use of any anti-infective drug, high enough doses of drugs must be taken for a long enough time for a cure. The time it takes to cure a patient is highly variable and depends on many factors, such as the type of disease, the age of the patient and the duration of the disease before therapy was begun. Usually 18 to 24 months of treatment are required.

Household members and personal contacts or other associates of a patient with active tuberculosis must also receive drug therapy. The assumption is that the associate probably has some inactive TB bacteria in his or her body and should be treated to prevent the inactive bacteria from becoming active. A positive sputum test, positive TB skin test or abnormal chest X ray would confirm the need for preventive drug therapy.

Any child younger than six who has a positive TB skin test should receive preventive drugs for a year, even if it is not known that he or she has been in contact with someone with an active TB infection.

Specimens (sputum, blood) must be taken before and during therapy to determine which drugs to use and to check on the patient's response to the drugs used.

The importance of taking the drugs exactly as prescribed for as long as ordered must be emphasized repeatedly.

ANTITUBERCULOSIS DRUGS
Ethambutol
(e tham' byoo tole)

Brand names: Myambutol

Ethambutol is an anti-infective drug used to treat tuberculosis. It is prescribed with one or two other antituberculosis drugs to quickly make the person treated unable to infect others. Ethambutol often must be taken for six months to a year in order to completely eradicate the infection.

UNDESIRED EFFECTS

Ethambutol may cause nausea, vomiting or loss of appetite when you start to take it. These effects tend to disappear as you continue to take it and as your body adjusts to it. If they continue over a long period of time or bother you a great deal, contact your doctor.

The most serious side effect of ethambutol is inflammation of an important nerve in the eye, the optic nerve. *This problem requires immediate medical attention.* Contact your doctor if you experience blurred vision, loss of vision, eye pain or inability to see the colors red and green.

Other undesired effects of ethambutol are allergic reactions, nerve problems and gout. Contact your doctor if you develop a rash or itching (allergic reaction); numbness, tingling, burning pain or weakness in the hands or feet (nerve problem); chills; swelling of the big toe, ankle or knee or hot skin over these joints (gout).

PRECAUTIONS

Because ethambutol can worsen certain medical problems, be sure to tell your doctor if you have gout, kidney disease, damage to nerves in the eyes or any other eye problems such as cataracts or recurring eye inflammations.

It is important that you take this medicine exactly as prescribed and continue to take it until your doctor tells you to stop. Even if you begin to feel better, your TB may not be completely cured. It may take a year or more to cure it.

If your symptoms do not improve within three weeks after you begin to take ethambutol, contact your doctor. He may wish to change your medication.

While you are taking ethambutol, your doctor may want to examine your eyes every three to six months to make sure the medicine is not having a bad effect on them. He may also do periodic blood counts and tests for kidney and liver function. *Keep all appointments with your doctor and at the laboratory.*

Before you start to take ethambutol, tell your doctor if you are pregnant or intend to become pregnant while you are taking this medicine. Although safe use of ethambutol in pregnant woman has not definitely been established, a combination of isoniazid and ethambutol usually is used to treat TB in pregnant women.

DOSAGE AND STORAGE

Ethambutol comes in tablets, usually taken once a day in the morning. Your doctor will determine when you should take this medicine and how much you should take at each dose. Carefully follow the instructions on your prescription label and ask your doctor or pharmacist to explain any part of the instructions you do not understand.

It is important that you do not miss any doses of this medicine. It may help you to remember to take your daily dose if you take ethambutol at the same time as you perform some other regular activity, such as brushing your teeth or eating your breakfast. Ethambutol can be taken with food if this drug upsets your stomach.

If you forget to take a dose, take it as soon as you remember. If you remember a missed dose when it is time to take the next one, omit the missed dose and take only the regularly scheduled dose. *Do not take a double dose.*

Keep ethambutol in the container it came in, and keep it out of the reach of children. Do not allow anyone else to take your ethambutol.

Isoniazid

(eye soe nye′ a zid)

Brand names: INH, Laniazid, Nydrazid, Panazid, Teebaconin

Isoniazid is an anti-infective drug used to treat or prevent tuberculosis. Isoniazid is considered one of the most effective antituberculosis drugs and is almost always included in the combination of medications used to treat active disease. In the prevention of tuberculosis in people who have been exposed to active disease or who have inactive TB bacteria in their bodies, isoniazid may be used alone.

Isoniazid eliminates only active (growing) bacteria that cause TB. Since many bacteria may exist that are resting (nongrowing), therapy with this and other drugs must be continued for a long time (usually six months to two years) to make sure the disease is cured.

UNDESIRED EFFECTS

When you start to take isoniazid, it may make you dizzy, upset your stomach or cause your breasts to enlarge. These effects tend to disappear as you continue to take isoniazid and as your body adjusts to it. However, if they continue to cause you great discomfort, contact your doctor.

Isoniazid can also decrease the level of vitamin B_6 in your body. If you experience clumsiness, unsteadiness or numbness, tingling or burning in your hands or feet, contact your doctor. He may want to prescribe pyridoxine (vitamin B_6) to counteract these effects.

Liver problems can result from isoniazid therapy. Stop taking the medicine and contact your doctor if you are unusually tired or weak or have a loss of appetite, nausea, vomiting or yellowing of the eyes or skin.

Contact your doctor if you get a skin rash, fever, swollen glands or other signs of allergy or if you experience blurred vision or loss of vision with or without eye pain.

PRECAUTIONS

To help your doctor select the treatment best for you, tell him if you have ever had an allergic reaction to isoniazid, have an alcohol problem or have seizures, diabetes, lupus erythematosus, liver disease or kidney disease.

Before you start taking isoniazid, tell your doctor what other prescription or nonprescription drugs you are taking, including antacids, anticoagulants (blood thinners), drugs to treat diabetes or high blood pressure, disulfiram (medicine to help curb drinking), phenytoin (medicine for seizures), sleeping medicines, stimulant drugs and rifampin (another antituberculosis drug). If you do not know the names of the drugs you are taking or what they were prescribed for, bring them in their labeled containers to your doctor or pharmacist.

It is very important that you take this medicine exactly as your doctor has prescribed and continue to take it until your doctor says you may stop. You may have to take it for as long as two years.

If your symptoms do not improve within three weeks after you start taking this medication or if they become worse, contact your doctor. He may wish to change your medication.

Do not drink alcoholic beverages while you are taking isoniazid. Regular use of alcohol can increase the possibility of liver problems and may make isoniazid less effective.

If you have diabetes, isoniazid can cause false results with some tests for urine sugar. Do not change your diet or the dosage of your diabetes medicine unless you first check with your doctor.

Tell your doctor if you are pregnant or plan to get pregnant while you are taking this medicine or if you are nursing a baby. He will need this information to select the treatment best for you.

Your doctor will want to check on your progress while you are taking isoniazid and may order laboratory tests or eye examinations. *Be sure to keep all your appointments with your doctor and at the laboratory.*

DOSAGE AND STORAGE

Isoniazid is usually taken once a day, in the morning. To avoid missing a dose, try to take this medicine at the same time you do something else every morning, such as brushing your teeth.

Isoniazid comes in liquid, powder and tablets to be taken orally. Your doctor will choose the form best for you and determine how often you should take isoniazid and how much to take each time. Follow the instructions on your prescription label carefully and ask your doctor or pharmacist to explain any part of the instructions you do not understand.

The container of liquid isoniazid should be shaken well before each use to distribute the medication evenly. Measure each dose with a specially marked measuring spoon to be sure of an accurate dose.

If you forget to take a dose, take it as soon as you remember. If you remember a missed dose at the time you are to take another one, take only the regularly scheduled dose. *Do not take a double dose.*

If your doctor prescribes pyridoxine (vitamin B$_6$) to prevent or lessen the side effects of isoniazid, take pyridoxine at the same time you take isoniazid. If you forget to take a dose of pyridoxine, take it as soon as possible and then go back to your regular dosing schedule.

Keep isoniazid in the container it came in and store it at room temperature. Keep it out of the reach of children and do not allow anyone else to take your isoniazid.

Rifampin
(rif′ am pin)

Brand names: Rifadin, Rimactane

Rifampin is an antibiotic used to treat tuberculosis. Rifampin usually is prescribed with one or two other antituberculosis drugs and often must be taken for three months to two years.

Rifampin also is used to eliminate meningitis bacteria from people who, though they are not sick, can spread meningitis to others.

UNDESIRED EFFECTS

The most frequent side effects of rifampin are stomach and bowel problems (loss of appetite, nausea, vomiting, stomach cramps or diarrhea), headache and muscle pain. These effects occur when you start to take the medicine, but they tend to lessen or disappear as your body adjusts to it. If they continue or bother you, contact your doctor.

While you are taking rifampin, your urine, stools, saliva, sputum, sweat or tears may have a red-orange color. This side effect is harmless, although soft contact lenses worn during rifampin therapy may be permanently stained. If rifampin causes a yellow discoloration of the skin, this effect should be reported to your doctor.

Rifampin can cause allergic reactions such as itching, hives, rash or sores on the skin or in the mouth. Contact your doctor if you have these effects. A more serious allergic reaction is a flulike illness with chills, fever, difficult breathing, dizziness, headache, shivering and muscle and bone pain. If you get these flulike symptoms, stop taking the medicine and contact your doctor.

Rifampin may cause disturbance of vision or impaired hearing. Rifampin rarely will cause kidney, liver or blood problems. Stop taking the medication and contact your doctor if you notice greatly decreased frequency of urination or amount of urine (kidney problem), unusual tiredness or weakness, vomiting or bleeding or sore throat (blood problem).

Some people get drowsy or dizzy when they take rifampin. Do not drive a car or operate dangerous machinery until you know how this drug affects you.

PRECAUTIONS

Before you start to take rifampin, tell your doctor if you have liver disease or an alcohol problem.

Several different medications can make rifampin less effective or can be made less effective by rifampin. Some of these are aminosalicylic acid (PAS) and isoniazid (other antituberculosis medicines), methadone, oral anticoagulants (blood thinners), birth control pills, probenecid (gout medicine) and oral diabetes medicines. Tell your doctor what other prescription or nonprescription drugs you are taking. If you do not know the names of the drugs or what they were prescribed for, bring them in their labeled containers to your doctor or pharmacist.

Birth control pills may not work as well if you take them while you are taking rifampin. Unplanned pregnancies, spotting and breakthrough bleeding can occur. You should use a different means of birth control while you are taking rifampin. Check with your doctor or pharmacist if you have any questions about this.

It is important that you take rifampin exactly as prescribed and continue to take it until your doctor tells you to stop. It may take from three months to two years to clear up your TB completely.

If your symptoms do not improve within three weeks after you begin to take rifampin, contact your doctor. It is important that your doctor check your progress while you are taking rifampin, and he may order laboratory tests for liver and kidney function, blood tests, or eye or hearing examinations. *Be sure to keep all your appointments with your doctor and at the laboratory.*

Do not drink alcoholic beverages while you are taking rifampin. Regular consumption of alcohol increases the possibility of liver problems and may make rifampin less effective.

To help your doctor select the treatment best for you, tell him if you are nursing a baby, are pregnant or intend to become pregnant while you are taking this medicine. If you become pregnant during treatment, contact your doctor.

DOSAGE AND STORAGE

Rifampin comes in capsules, usually taken once a day. Carefully follow the instructions on your prescription label and ask your doctor or pharmacist to explain any part of the instructions you do not understand.

Rifampin works best if it is taken on an "empty stomach," one hour before meals or two hours after eating. However, if you become nauseated when you take it on an "empty stomach," you may take it with a light snack.

If you are taking the drug PAS in addition to rifampin, you should take these two drugs at least eight hours apart.

You may find it easier to remember to take your daily dose of rifampin if you take it at the same time you do something else every day, such as when you brush your teeth in the morning or go to bed at night. If you forget a dose, take it as soon as you remember. If you remember a missed dose at the time you are to take the next one, omit the missed dose and take only the regularly scheduled dose. *Do not take a double dose.*

Keep this medicine in the container it came in. Keep it out of the reach of children.

URINARY TRACT INFECTIONS

The specific drug used to treat an infection of the urinary tract depends on the infecting organism and the location of the infection. Precise diagnosis is essential for good relief and permanent cure. Depending on the results of laboratory sensitivity testing, the drug used may be a sulfonamide (sulfa drug), an antibiotic or another urinary anti-infective (**Antibiotics** are discussed in the section beginning on page 63; sulfonamides and other urinary tract anti-infectives are described in this section.)

Resistance to drugs used to treat urinary tract infections develops frequently, and more than one drug or a series of drugs may be necessary to cure a urinary tract infection completely. A urinary tract infection is cured when a microscopic examination of laboratory culture tests show urine samples to be normal (infection-free) for three consecutive weeks after medication has been stopped.

URINARY TRACT ANTI-INFECTIVES
Co-trimoxazole
(koe trye mox′ a zole)

Brand names: Bactrim, Septa

Co-trimoxazole is trimethoprim combined with sulfamethoxazole, one of the sulfonamide or sulfa drugs. This combination is used to treat infections of the lungs, ears, urinary tract and bowels.

Together, trimethoprim and sulfamethoxazole seem to be more effective than either drug given separately. Co-trimoxazole presently is being studied for use against malaria and typhoid fever caused by bacteria resistant to other antibacterial drugs.

This combination of drugs should not be used for "strep throat," since the sulfa drugs may not eliminate the bacteria and it is possible that rheumatic fever might occur later.

UNDESIRED EFFECTS
Co-trimoxazole can cause nausea, vomiting, diarrhea and, once in a while, skin rash. These effects are more likely to occur with large doses or long-term therapy.

Some of the more serious side effects are caused by sulfamethoxazole in co-trimoxazole. These include allergic reactions, blood problems, kidney problems, liver problems, thyroid problems and an unusual sensitivity to sunlight. (See the section on **sulfamethoxazole**, page 142, for the symptoms of these problems and what to do about them.)

PRECAUTIONS
Before you start taking co-trimoxazole, tell your doctor if you have ever had an allergic reaction to any sulfa drug, a diuretic (water pill), oral diabetes medicine or oral medicine for glaucoma. Your doctor will need to know if you have G6PD deficiency (an inherited blood disease), porphyria, kidney disease or liver disease.

In order to help your doctor select the best treatment for you, tell him what other prescription or nonprescription drugs you are taking, including oral anticoagulants (blood thinners), oral diabetes medicine, penicillins, PABA (one of the B complex vitamins), isoniazid (antitubercular drug), methenamine (a urinary antiseptic), methotrexate (psoriasis or antitumor medicine), phenytoin (medicine for seizures), phenylbutazone or oxyphenbutazone (for arthritis), medicine for gout or any medicine to make your urine more alkaline. If you do not know the names of the drugs or what they were prescribed for, bring them in their labeled containers to your doctor or pharmacist.

Co-trimoxazole should not be taken by infants under two months of age, pregnant women or nursing mothers. Tell your doctor if you are nursing a baby, or pregnant or intend to become pregnant while taking this medicine.

Before having any surgery with a general anesthetic, including dental surgery, tell the doctor or dentist that you are taking co-trimoxazole.

Take *all* the medicine prescribed. Even if you feel better in a few days, the infection will not be completely cured and could return. Bacterial infections take several days to weeks to be cured completely. However, if your symptoms do not improve in a few days, contact your doctor. He may want to change your medication or adjust the dose.

It is important that you keep all your appointments with your doctor so he can check your response to this medicine with regular blood counts and urine tests.

DOSAGE AND STORAGE
Your doctor will determine how much of this medicine you should take and how often you should take it. Carefully follow the instructions on your prescription label and ask your doctor or pharmacist to explain any part of the instructions you do not understand.

Co-trimoxazole comes in tablets and in liquid form; it should be taken on an "empty stomach," one hour before meals or two hours after eating. While you are taking this medicine, drink at least eight full eight-ounce glasses of water or other liquids every day.

Both the tablets and the liquid should be taken with a full eight-ounce glass of water. The container of liquid should be shaken well before each use to distribute the medication evenly. Measure doses of liquid with a specially marked measuring spoon to be sure of an accurate dose.

If you forget to take a dose, take it as soon as you remember. However, if you remember a missed dose when it is close to the time for another, you may either double the next dose or space the missed dose and the next dose one or two hours apart. Then go back to your regular dosing schedule.

If you still have symptoms of the infection after you have taken all the medicine prescribed, contact your doctor. When your doctor tells you to stop taking the medicine, throw away any unused portion of it. This medicine should not be saved to treat another infection. Do not allow anyone else to take your co-trimoxazole, which was prescribed for your particular condition.

Keep this medicine in the container it came in and store it at room temperature. Keep it out of the reach of children.

Methenamine

(meth en′ a meen)

Brand names: Hiprex, Mandelamine, Urex and others

Methenamine is an anti-infective drug used to treat kidney and bladder infections. It will work properly only when the urine is very acid. The action of the acid on methenamine releases formaldehyde, which then eliminates bacteria from the urine.

Methenamine is never used alone against severe or "hot" infections. Its value against such infections is to keep the urinary tract free of bacteria after they have been eliminated by other antibacterial drugs. It is also used to prevent infection when parts of the urinary tract such as the bladder are examined by instruments.

UNDESIRED EFFECTS

Nausea and upset stomach are common side effects of methenamine. Taking the medicine with meals or a snack should relieve these problems; but if they continue or are severe, contact your doctor.

A skin rash, hives or itching may indicate that you are allergic to this medicine. Contact your doctor if you experience these effects.

Methenamine may cause kidney problems. Stop taking the medicine and contact your doctor if you notice blood in your urine, have pain in your lower back or experience pain or burning while urinating.

PRECAUTIONS

To help your doctor select the best treatment for you, tell him if you have kidney or liver disease,

Before you start taking methenamine, tell your doctor what other prescription or nonprescription drugs you are taking, particularly antacids, oral medicine for glaucoma, sulfa drugs, thiazide diuretics (water pills), vitamin C or any medicine to make your urine more alkaline. If you do not know the names of these drugs or what they are prescribed for, bring them in their labeled containers to your doctor or pharmacist. Do not take any other medications unless you first check with your doctor or pharmacist.

Your urine must be acid for this medicine to work well. Before you start taking methenamine, ask your doctor what you can do to maintain an acid urine and how to test your urine with special paper for that purpose.

Some changes in your diet may help keep your urine acid, but you should check first with your doctor if you are already on a special diet, such as one for diabetes. Do not drink milk or eat cheese or other dairy products. Do not take antacids. Try to eat more protein and foods such as cranberries (especially cranberry juice with added vitamin C), plums and prunes. If you have any questions about diet, or if these changes do not make your urine acid enough, check with your doctor.

To help cure your infection completely, take *all* the methenamine your doctor has prescribed. Symptoms of the infection may disappear before the infection is cured. Therefore, do not stop taking this medicine until your doctor tells you to do so.

Your doctor may conduct tests to determine if the infection is cured. Be sure to keep all your appointments so that your doctor can best decide when you may stop taking methenamine.

DOSAGE AND STORAGE

Your doctor will determine how much methenamine you should take and how often you should take it. Carefully follow the instructions on your prescription label and ask your doctor or pharmacist to explain any part of the instructions you do not understand.

Doses of methenamine should be taken as far apart as possible during the day. If your doctor instructs you to take this medicine twice a day, take one dose in the morning and another dose 12 hours later, in the evening. If you are to take it four times a day, take a dose every six hours.

While you are taking methenamine, drink at least eight full eight-ounce glasses of water or cranberry juice every day. This will help the medicine work better and will help prevent side effects.

Methenamine comes in tablets, liquid and powder and should be taken with a full glass of water or food. The tablets should be swallowed whole. *Do not break or crush them or take them if they are chipped.* The container of liquid should be shaken well before each use to distribute the medication evenly. Measure doses with a specially marked measuring spoon to make sure of an accurate dose.

The powder should be dissolved in two to four ounces of water. Then stir it well and take it immediately. Be sure to drink all the liquid in order to get the full dose of medicine.

If you forget a dose, take it as soon as you remember. However, if it is almost time for your next dose, you may either double the next dose or space the missed dose and the next dose one or two hours apart. Then go back to your regular dosing schedule.

If you still have symptoms of the infection after you have taken all the medicine prescribed, contact your doctor. When your doctor tells you to stop taking methenamine, throw away any unused portion of it. This medication may lose its effectiveness over a period of time and should not be saved to treat another infection.

Keep methenamine in the container it came in and store it out of the reach of children. Do not let anyone else take your methenamine.

Nalidixic Acid
(nal i dix′ ik ass′ id)

Brand name: NegGram

Nalidixic acid is an anti-infective drug that eliminates many kinds of bacteria from the urinary tract. Nalidixic acid is used to treat infections of the bladder and kidneys. However, its usefulness is limited by the tendency of infecting bacteria to become resistant to the drug.

UNDESIRED EFFECTS

Stomach problems such as nausea and vomiting as well as diarrhea may be avoided by taking this medicine with meals or milk. If these effects continue or get worse in spite of your precautions, contact your doctor. If you develop rash, hives or itching or have joint pain or swelling, you may be having an allergic reaction to nalidixic acid and should contact your doctor.

Nalidixic acid can cause eye, liver and blood problems that will need medical attention. If you experience blurred or decreased vision, double vision, changes in color vision, overbrightness of lights or halos around lights, contact your doctor. Symptoms of blood problems are unusual bleeding or bruising, unusual weakness or tiredness, fever, pale skin and sore throat. If you experience any of these effects or yellowing of the skin or eyes (liver problem), contact your doctor.

Other side effects are dark or amber urine, pale stools or severe stomach pain. Contact your doctor if you have these symptoms.

Nalidixic acid may cause some people to become drowsy or dizzy. Do not drive a car or operate dangerous machinery until you know how this medicine affects your alertness and vision.

Some people who take nalidixic acid may become more sensitive to sunlight than they normally are. Limit the time you spend in sunlight until you know how you react to this medicine, especially if you tend to burn easily. You may still be more sensitive to sunlight or sunlamps for up to a year after you stop taking this medicine. If you get severely sunburned, contact your doctor.

PRECAUTIONS

Before you start taking nalidixic acid, tell your doctor if you have kidney or liver disease, a history of seizures, Parkinson's disease, severe hardening of the arteries of the brain or any central nervous system (brain and spinal cord) damage.

To help your doctor select the treatment best for you, tell him what other prescription or nonprescription drugs you are taking, particularly oral antico-agulants (blood thinners), antacids, vitamin C and nitrofurantoin. If you do not know the names of the drugs or what they were prescribed for, take them in their labeled containers to your doctor or pharmacist.

Take *all* the medicine your doctor prescribes, even after you begin to feel better. If the infection is not completely cured, it can return. Bacterial infections take several days to weeks to be cured completely and even your doctor will need tests to determine whether the infection is cured.

If your symptoms do not improve in a few days, contact your doctor. He may want to do tests to find out whether the infecting bacteria are still sensitive to nalidixic acid, or he may want to adjust the dosage.

If you will be taking this medicine for more than two weeks, your doctor should check your progress with regular blood counts and tests for liver and kidney function. *Be sure to keep all appointments with your doctor and at the laboratory.*

Nalidixic acid should not be taken by infants under three months of age, pregnant women in the first three months of pregnancy or nursing mothers. Tell your doctor if you are nursing a baby, are in the first trimester of a pregnancy or intend to get pregnant while taking the drug.

Diabetics who use Clinitest, Benedict's solution or Fehling's solution to test their urine for sugar should be aware that nalidixic acid can affect the results of the test. If you use one of these tests, ask your doctor if you should use some other type of test.

DOSAGE AND STORAGE

Your doctor will determine how much nalidixic acid you should take and how often you should take it. Carefully follow the instructions on your prescription label and ask your doctor or pharmacist to explain any part of the instructions you do not understand.

Doses of nalidixic acid should be taken as far apart as possible during the day. If your doctor instructs you to take it four times a day, take a dose every six hours.

Nalidixic acid comes in tablets and in liquid form and is best taken on an "empty stomach," one hour before meals or two hours after eating. While you are taking this medicine, drink at least eight full eight-ounce glasses of water or other liquids every day. This will help prevent undesired effects.

Both the tablets and the liquid should be taken with a full eight-ounce glass of water. The container of liquid should be shaken before each use to distribute the medication evenly. Measure doses of liquid with a specially marked measuring spoon to be sure of an accurate dose.

If you forget to take a dose of nalidixic acid, take it as soon as you remember. Take any remaining doses for the day at evenly spaced intervals.

If you still have symptoms of the infection after you have taken all the medicine prescribed, contact your doctor. When he tells you to stop taking nalidixic acid, throw away any unused portion of it. Nalidixic acid may lose its effectiveness over a period of time and should not be saved to treat another infection. This medicine was prescribed for your particular condition; do not allow anyone else to take your nalidixic acid.

Keep this medicine in the container it came in and store it at room temperature. Keep it out of the reach of children.

Nitrofurantoin

(nye troe fyoor an' toyn)

Brand names: Furadantin, Furalan, Macrodantin, Trantoin

Nitrofurantoin is an anti-infective drug whose effect against bacteria is concentrated in the urinary tract. Nitrofurantoin is used to treat infections of the kidneys and the bladder.

UNDESIRED EFFECTS

The most common side effects of nitrofurantoin are diarrhea, loss of appetite, nausea and vomiting. These effects tend to disappear as you continue to take the drug and as your body adjusts to it. If they do not disappear of if they grow worse, contact your doctor. If diarrhea persists for longer than 24 hours, stop taking the drug and contact your doctor. To avoid stomach upsets, be sure to take nitrofurantoin with food or a glass of milk.

You may also notice that this medicine turns your urine rust-yellow or brown. This effect is harmless.

Nitrofurantoin can cause a severe allergic reaction with symptoms such as chest pain, chills, fever and cough or difficult breathing. If you have these symptoms, stop taking the medicine and contact your doctor. Less frequently, nitrofurantoin will cause headache, dizziness or drowsiness, weakness and tiredness. Stop taking the medicine and contact your doctor if you have these problems.

Nerve, liver and blood problems can result from nitrofurantoin therapy. If you experience numbness, tingling or burning of the face, mouth, fingers or toes (nerve problem), unusual weakness or tiredness, pale skin (blood problem) or yellowing of the eyes or skin (liver problem), stop taking the medicine and contact your doctor.

PRECAUTIONS

Before you start taking nitrofurantoin, tell your doctor if you have ever had an allergic reaction to this drug or to any of its related drugs, such as furazolidone and nitrofurazone.

To help your doctor select the best treatment for you, tell him if you have G6PD deficiency (an inherited blood disease), lung disease, nerve damage or kidney disease.

Tell your doctor what other prescription or nonprescription drugs you are taking, particularly nalidixic acid (another anti-infective drug) or gout medicines such as probenecid or sulfinpyrazone. If you do not know the names of the drugs or what they were prescribed for, bring them in their labeled containers to your doctor or pharmacist.

Avoid consuming alcoholic beverages while taking nitrofurantoin.

Nitrofurantoin should not be taken by infants under one month of age, pregnant women who are a few weeks away from delivery or nursing mothers. This medicine can cause anemia in newborn babies when given directly or passed to them through the mother. Tell your doctor if you are nursing a baby, are pregnant or intend to get pregnant while taking nitrofurantoin.

Be sure to take all of the nitrofurantoin your doctor prescribes. Symptoms of the infection may disappear before the infection is cured, but bacterial infections take several days to weeks to be cured completely.

Blood tests, laboratory tests for liver function or chest X rays may be ordered by your doctor while you are taking nitrofurantoin. *Be sure to keep all your appointments with him and the laboratory* so that he can do tests to determine when the infection is cured and when you may stop taking nitrofurantoin.

If your symptoms do not improve within a few days or get worse, contact your doctor. He may want to change your medication, adjust the dosage or treat an overgrowth of bacteria against which this drug is not effective.

If you have diabetes, nitrofurantoin can cause false results of urine sugar tests. Do not change your diet or the dosage of your diabetes medicine unless you first check with your doctor.

DOSAGE AND STORAGE

Your doctor will determine how much nitrofurantoin you should take and how often you should take it. Carefully follow the instructions on your prescription label and ask your doctor or pharmacist to explain any part of the instructions you do not understand.

Doses of nitrofurantoin should be taken as far apart as possible. If your doctor instructs you to take it four times a day, take a dose every six hours.

Nitrofurantoin comes in tablets and in liquid form, both of which should be taken with meals or with a full glass of water or milk. While you are taking this medicine, drink at least eight full eight-ounce glasses of water or other liquids (coffee, tea, soft drinks, milk, and fruit juice) every day. This practice will prevent side effects from taking nitrofurantoin.

Shake the container of the liquid form before each use to distribute the medication evenly. Measure the dose of the liquid with a specially marked measuring spoon to ensure an accurate dose. The liquid form may cause a temporary yellow discoloration of the teeth and may be mixed with water, milk, fruit juice or baby formula or lessen the chance of discoloring the teeth. All the liquid should be taken immediately after mixing.

If you forget to take a dose of nitrofurantoin, take it as soon as you remember. However, if you remember a missed dose when it is close to the time for another, you may either double the next dose or space the missed dose and the next dose one or two hours apart. Then go back to your regular dosing schedule.

If you still have symptoms of the infection after you have taken all the nitrofurantoin prescribed, contact your doctor. When your doctor tells you to stop taking nitrofurantoin, throw away any unused portion of it. Nitrofurantoin may lose its effectiveness over a period of time and should not be saved to treat another infection.

Keep this medicine in the container it came in and store it in a dark place. Do not let anyone else take your nitrofurantoin, and keep it out of the reach of children.

Oxolinic Acid

(ox o lin′ ik ass′ id)

Brand name: Utibid

Oxolinic acid is an anti-infective drug very similar to nalidixic acid. Oxolinic acid is used to treat bladder and kidney and other infections of the urinary tract. During therapy with oxolinic acid, bacteria against which it was originally effective may become resistant to the drug.

UNDESIRED EFFECTS

Oxolinic acid may cause some people to become drowsy or dizzy, or it may affect their vision. Do not drive or operate dangerous machinery until you know how this medicine affects your alertness and vision.

Other common side effects are stomach and bowel problems such as nausea, vomiting, diarrhea, loss of appetite and constipation. These effects tend to lessen or disappear as you continue to take oxolinic acid and as your body adjusts to it. If they are severe or last more than two days, contact your doctor.

Less frequently, oxolinic acid can cause sleeplessness, nervousness, headache, abdominal pain or cramps, restlessness, weakness or itching. If you have these effects and they bother you, contact your doctor.

Occasionally, oxolinic acid may cause swelling of the arms and legs, a prickling sensation in the fingers or toes, muscle pain, palpitation and shortness of breath, soreness of the mouth or gums, metallic taste, fever or an unusual sensitivity to sunlight. Contact your doctor if you experience these effects.

PRECAUTIONS

Before you start taking oxolinic acid, tell your doctor if you have kidney or liver disease, a history of seizures, severe hardening of the arteries of the brain or any central nervous system (brain or spinal cord) damage.

Tell your doctor what other prescription or nonprescription drugs you are taking, particularly anticoagulants (blood thinners), drugs to help you lose weight and nitrofurantoin. If you do not know the names of the drugs or what they were prescribed for, take them in their labeled containers to your doctor or pharmacist.

If your symptoms do not improve within two days after you start taking oxolinic acid or if they get worse, contact your doctor. This may indicate the bacteria have become resistant to oxolinic acid, and your doctor may want to change your medication.

Take *all* the medicine your doctor prescribes, even after you begin to feel better. If you are not completely cured of the infection, it can return. Bacterial infections take several days to weeks to cure completely, and even your doctor will need tests to determine whether the infection is cured.

While you are taking oxolinic acid, your doctor will want to check regularly on your progress and possibly may order laboratory tests. *Be sure to keep all your appointments for these checkups.*

Oxolinic acid should not be taken by infants and nursing mothers. Safe use for pregnant women has not been established, and oxolinic acid is not recommended for use in children under 12 years of age. Tell your doctor if you are pregnant or intend to become pregnant while taking this drug or if you are nursing a baby.

DOSAGE AND STORAGE

Your doctor will determine how much oxolinic acid you should take and how often you should take it. Carefully follow the instructions on your prescription label and ask your doctor or pharmacist to explain any part of the instructions you do not understand.

Oxolinic acid comes in tablets that are usually taken twice a day. It is best to take them on an "empty stomach," one hour before meals or two hours after eating. They should be taken with a full eight-ounce glass of water.

While you are taking this medicine, drink at least eight full eight-ounce glasses of water or other liquids (coffee, tea, milk, soft drinks and fruit juice) every day. This practice will help prevent undesired effects from taking oxolinic acid.

If you forget to take a dose of oxolinic acid, take it as soon as you remember. Take any remaining doses for the day at evenly spaced intervals. In order to prevent the development of resistant bacteria, it is particularly important that you skip no doses for the first few days of therapy.

If you still have symptoms of the infection after you have taken all the oxolinic acid prescribed, contact your doctor. When he tells you to stop taking oxolinic acid, throw away any unused portion of it. Oxolinic acid may lose its effectiveness over a period of time and should not be saved to treat another infection.

Keep this medication in the container it came in. Do not let anyone else take your oxolinic acid, and keep it out of the reach of children.

Phenazopyridine
(fen az oh peer' i deen)

Brand names: Aqua-Ton, Azo-100, Azodine, Azo Standard, DiAzo, Pryidium, Urodine and others

Phenazopyridine is a urinary analgesic used to relieve pain, burning, pressure and other discomfort caused by infection or irritation of the urinary tract. It is not an anti-infective drug and will not cure the infection itself. It is discussed here because it is used frequently with anti-infective medicines as part of the treatment for urinary tract infections.

UNDESIRED EFFECTS

Phenazopyridine can cause dizziness, headache, indigestion and stomach or abdominal pain or cramps. These effects may go away as you continue to take the drug and once the body adjusts to it. Check with your doctor if they continue or bother you.

Stop taking the medicine and contact your doctor if you notice yellowing of the eyes or skin.

Phenazopyridine will color your urine red or orange and may stain clothing. This effect is harmless.

PRECAUTIONS

Before taking phenazopyridine, tell your doctor if you have hepatitis (inflammation of the liver) or kidney disease or if you have ever had an allergic reaction to phenazopyridine in the past.

If you have diabetes, phenazopyridine may cause false test results of tests for sugar and ketones in your urine. Phenazopyridine also may interfere with tests for kidney and liver functions. If you have any questions about this, check with your doctor.

If you take phenazopyridine for a long period of time, your doctor may order laboratory tests for liver function or blood tests.

Tell your doctor if you are pregnant or are nursing a baby so he can decide on the best treatment for you with the least risk to your baby.

DOSAGE AND STORAGE

Your doctor will determine how much phenazopyridine you should take and how often you should take it. Carefully follow the instructions on your prescription label and ask your doctor or pharmacist to explain any part of the instructions you do not understand.

Phenazopyridine comes in tablets, which should be taken with a glass of water during or after meals to lessen stomach upset. *Do not chew or crush the tablets before swallowing them.*

If you forget to take a dose, take it as soon as you remember. If it is almost time for your next dose, do not take the missed dose at all and *do not double the next one.* Instead, go back to your regular dosing schedule.

When your doctor tells you to stop taking phenazopyridine, throw away any unused portion of it. It should not be saved to treat urinary tract problems in the future.

Keep this medication in the container it came in and store it out of the reach of children. Do not allow anyone else to take your phenazopyridine.

Sulfamethoxazole

(sul fa meth ox′ a zole)

Brand names: Gantanol, Methoxanal

Sulfamethoxazole is one of the sulfonamide anti-infectives or sulfa drugs that is used primarily to treat urinary tract infections and to prevent "strep" infections in people with a history of rheumatic fever. Sulfamethoxazole also can be used with penicillin or erythromycins for middle ear infections in children.

UNDESIRED EFFECTS

Sulfamethoxazole, like all sulfa drugs, can cause a number of undesired effects, including allergic reactions, and blood, kidney, liver or thyroid problems.

Early signs of allergic reaction are itching, rash and hives. Stop taking the medicine and contact your doctor if any of these effects occurs. Less frequently, sulfamethoxazole will cause fever; aching of the joints and muscles; difficulty in swallowing; or redness, blistering, peeling or loosening of the skin. If you experience any of these allergic reactions, stop taking the medicine and contact your doctor.

Symptoms of blood problems are unusual bleeding or bruising, unusual weakness or tiredness, fever, pale skin or sore throat. If you experience any of these symptoms, stop taking the medicine and contact your doctor. Also contact your doctor if you have yellowing of the eyes or skin (liver problems), and stop taking sulfamethoxazole.

Though kidney and thyroid problems are rarely caused by taking sulfamethoxazole, it can cause blood in the urine, lower back pain, pain or burning while urinating or swelling of the front part of the neck (goiter). If any of these problems occur, stop taking the medicine and contact your doctor.

Some people who take sulfamethoxazole may become more sensitive to sunlight than they are normally. Limit the amount of time you spend in the sunlight until you know how you react to sulfamethoxazole, especially if you tend to sunburn easily. You may still be more sensitive than you are normally to sunlight and sunlamps for many months after you stop taking sulfamethoxazole. If you become severely sunburned, contact your doctor.

When you start to take this medication, you may develop headache, loss of balance, ringing in the ears, dizziness, loss of appetite, nausea or vomiting or diarrhea. These effects tend to lessen or disappear as you continue to take sulfamethoxazole and as your body adjusts to the medication. If they continue or become bothersome, contact your doctor. If sulfamethoxazole upsets your stomach, take it after a meal or with a snack.

PRECAUTIONS

Before you start taking sulfamethoxazole, tell your doctor if you have ever had an allergic reaction to any sulfa drug, a diuretic (water pill), oral diabetes medicine or oral medicine for glaucoma. Tell your doctor if you have a history of allergy, hay fever or asthma.

If you have G6PD deficiency (an inherited blood disease), porphyria, kidney disease or liver disease, tell your doctor.

In order to help your doctor select the best treatment for you, tell him what other prescription or nonprescription drugs you are taking, including oral anticoagulants (blood thinners), oral diabetes medicine, penicillins, PABA (one of the B complex vitamins), isoniazid (an antitubercular drug), methenamine (a urinary antiseptic), methotrexate (a psoriasis or antitumor medicine), phenytoin (a medicine for seizures), probenecid or sulfinpyrazone (gout medicines), phenylbutazone or oxyphenbutazone (for arthritis) or any medicine to make your urine more alkaline, such as sodium bicarbonate or sodium citrate. If you do not know the names of the drugs you are taking or what they were prescribed for, bring them in their labeled containers to your doctor or pharmacist.

Sulfamethoxazole should not be taken by an infant under one month of age, pregnant women who are at term (ninth month) or nursing mothers. If you are nursing a baby, are pregnant or intend to become pregnant while taking this medicine, tell your doctor.

Alcoholic beverages should be consumed with caution while you are taking sulfamethoxazole, since the effects of alcohol may be increased by sulfa drugs.

Take *all* this medication exactly as prescribed. Even if you feel better in a few days, the infection will not be completely cured and could return. Bacterial infections take several days to weeks to cure completely. However, if your symptoms do not improve in a few days, contact your doctor. He may want to change your medication or adjust the dose.

It is important that you keep all appointments with your doctor so he can check your response to sulfamethoxazole with regular blood counts, urine tests and tests for thyroid, liver and kidney function.

Before having any surgery with a general anesthetic, including dental surgery, tell the doctor or dentist that you are taking sulfamethoxazole.

DOSAGE AND STORAGE

Your doctor will determine how much sulfamethoxazole you should take and how often you should take it. Follow the instructions on your prescription label carefully and ask your doctor or pharmacist to explain any part of the instructions you do not understand.

Sulfamethoxazole comes in tablets and in liquid form and should be taken with a full eight-ounce glass of water, on an "empty stomach," one hour before meals or two hours after eating. While you are taking this drug, drink at least eight full eight-ounce glasses of water or other liquids (coffee, tea, soft drinks, milk and fruit juice) every day.

The container of liquid should be shaken before each use to distribute the medication evenly. Measure doses of liquid with a specially marked measuring spoon to ensure an accurate dose.

If you forget to take a dose, take it as soon as you remember. However, if you remember a missed dose when it is close to the time for another, you may either double the dose or space the missed dose and the next dose one or two hours apart. Then go back to your regular dosing schedule.

If you still have symptoms of the infection after you have taken all the sulfamethoxazole prescribed, contact your doctor. When he tells you to stop taking sulfamethoxazole, throw away any unused portion of it. This medication may lose its effectiveness over a period of time and should not be saved to treat another infection. Do not allow anyone else to take your sulfamethoxazole, which was prescribed for your particular condition.

Keep this medicine in the container it came in and store it at room temperature. Keep it out of the reach of children.

Sulfisoxazole
(sul fi sox′ a zole)

Brand names: Gantrisin, Lipo Gantrisin, SK-Soxazole, Sosol, Sulfasox, Sulfizin and others

Sulfisoxazole is one of the sulfonamide anti-infectives or sulfa drugs. Because it is rapidly absorbed and quickly eliminated from the body, it often is the preferred sulfa for treating infections of the urinary tract and other infections. It can also be used to prevent "strep" infections in people with a history of rheumatic fever and, with penicillin or erythromycins, to treat middle ear infections in children.

UNDESIRED EFFECTS

Allergic reactions are the most common side effects of sulfisoxazole. Stop taking this medicine and contact your doctor if you develop a rash, hives and itching, which are early signs of allergic reaction. Less frequently, sulfisoxazole will cause more serious allergic reactions. If you get fever, aching of the joints or muscles, difficulty in swallowing or skin problems (redness, blistering, peeling or loosening of the skin), stop taking the medicine and contact your doctor.

Sulfisoxazole also can cause blood problems and liver problems. Stop taking the medicine and contact your doctor if you experience unusual bleeding or bruising, unusual weakness and tiredness, fever, pale skin or sore throat (symptoms of blood problems) or yellowing of the eyes or skin (symptoms of liver problems).

Sulfisoxazole may cause a brownish discoloration of the urine; this is harmless. Sulfisoxazole rarely will cause kidney or thyroid problems. If you notice blood in your urine, lower back pain, pain or burning while urinating or a swelling of the front part of the neck (goiter), stop taking the medicine and contact your doctor.

Some people who take sulfisoxazole may become more sensitive to sunlight than they are normally. Limit the amount of time you spend in sunlight until you know how you react to sulfisoxazole, especially if you tend to sunburn easily. You may still be more sensitive than you are normally to sunlight and sunlamps for many months after you stop taking sulfisoxazole. If you become severely sunburned, contact your doctor.

When you start to take sulfisoxazole you may get diarrhea, loss of appetite, abdominal pain, nausea or vomiting, dizziness and headache, loss of balance or ringing in the ears. These effects tend to lessen or disappear as you continue to take the drug and as your body adjusts to it. If they continue or are bothersome, contact your doctor. If this medication upsets your stomach, take it with a meal or a snack.

PRECAUTIONS

Before you start taking sulfisoxazole, tell your doctor if you have ever had an allergic reaction to any sulfa drug, a diuretic (water pill), oral diabetes medicine or oral medicine for glaucoma. Your doctor should also know if you have a history of allergy, hay fever or asthma.

To be able to select the best treatment for you, your doctor needs to know if you have G6PD deficiency (an inherited blood disease), porphyria, kidney disease or liver disease or if you have ever had anemia produced by a drug.

Certain other medicines, when taken with sulfisoxazole, will affect the way your body responds to this drug. Tell your doctor what other prescription or nonprescription drugs you are taking, including oral anticoagulants (blood thinners), oral diabetes medicines, penicillins, PABA (one of the B complex vitamins), isoniazid (an antituberculosis drug), methenamine (a urinary antiseptic), methotrexate (a psoriasis or antitumor medicine), phenylbutazone or oxphenbutazone (for arthritis), phenytoin (a medicine for seizures), probenecid or sulfinpyrazone (gout medicines) or any medicine to make your urine more alkaline, such as sodium bicarbonate or sodium citrate. If you do not know the names of the drugs you are taking or what they were prescribed for, bring them in their labeled containers to your doctor or pharmacist.

Alcoholic beverages should be taken with caution while you are taking sulfisoxazole, since the effects of alcohol may be increased by sulfa drugs.

Take *all* the sulfisoxazole your doctor prescribes, even after you begin to feel better. If the infection is not completely cured, it can return. Bacterial infections take several days to weeks to cure completely. However, if your symptoms do not improve in a few days, contact your doctor. He may want to change your medication or adjust your dose.

Sulfisoxazole should not be taken by infants under one month of age, pregnant women who are at term (ninth month) or nursing mothers. Tell your doctor if you are nursing a baby, are pregnant or intend to become pregnant while taking this medicine.

It is important that you keep all appointments with your doctor so he can check your response to this medicine with regular blood counts, urine tests and tests for thyroid, liver and kidney function.

Before having any surgery with a general anesthetic, including dental surgery, be sure to tell the doctor or dentist that you are taking sulfisoxazole.

DOSAGE AND STORAGE

Your doctor has determined how much sulfisoxazole you should take and how often you should take it. Carefully follow the instructions on your prescription label and ask your doctor or pharmacist to explain any part of the instructions you do not understand.

Sulfisoxazole comes in tablets and in liquid form and should be taken on an "empty stomach," one hour before meals or two hours after eating. While you are taking this medicine, drink at least eight full eight-ounce glasses of water or other liquids (coffee, tea, soft drinks, milk and fruit juice) every day. This will help protect your kidneys from problems sulfisoxazole can cause.

Both the tablets and the liquid should be taken with a full eight-ounce glass of water. The container of liquid should be shaken before each use to distribute the medication evenly. Measure doses of liquid with a specially marked measuring spoon to ensure an accurate dose.

If you forget to take a dose of sulfisoxazole, take it as soon as you remember. However, if you remember a missed dose when it is close to the time for another, you may either double the next dose or space the missed dose and the next dose one to two hours apart. Then go back to your regular dosing schedule.

If you still have symptoms of the infection after you have taken all the medicine prescribed, contact your doctor. When your doctor tells you to stop taking sulfisoxazole, throw away any unused portion of it. Sulfisoxazole may lose its effectiveness over a period of time and should not be saved to treat another infection. Because this medicine was prescribed for your particular condition, you should not allow anyone else to take your sulfisoxazole.

Keep this medicine in the container it came in and store it at room temperature. Keep it out of the reach of children.

Vaginal Infections

Drugs discussed in this section are used to treat vaginitis—an inflammation of the vagina characterized by an itching and/or burning sensation and excessive vaginal discharge. The more common types of vaginitis, named for the organisms causing infection, are trichomonal vaginitis and monilial vaginitis. Trichomonal vaginitis is caused by an organism called a protozoa, and monilial vaginitis is caused by a fungus. Bacteria such as a hemophilus, "staph" or "strep" organisms cause what is commonly referred to as nonspecific vaginitis.

VAGINAL ANTI-INFECTIVES
Iodochlorhydroxyquin

(eye oh dough klor hye drox ee quin)

Brand name: Vioform

Iodochlorhydroxyquin is an anti-infective drug applied directly to the site of infection and is used to treat infections in the vagina or on the skin. This drug is particularly effective in eliminating the protozoa (tiny single-celled organisms) that cause vaginal infection. The powder and suppository forms of this medication are used to treat infections; the lotion and cream forms are used on skin infections. Iodchlorhydroxyquin is 40 percent iodine.

Undesired Effects

Side effects with iodochlorhydroxyquin are rare. However, if you should develop irritation of the vagina not present before using this medicine contact your doctor.

Precautions

Use *all* of the iodochlorhydroxyquin your doctor has prescribed, even though you may think the infection has disappeared. Failure to use all the medicine can allow the infection to return.

Be sure to tell your doctor if you have ever had a reaction to iodochlorhydroxyquin previously or to any product containing iodine. You should not use this drug if you are allergic to it or to iodine.

Discuss with your doctor any questions you may have about douching or intercourse during treatment with iodochlorhydroxyquin. You may want to wear a sanitary napkin while using this medication to protect your clothes from staining.

You can help cure the infection and prevent reinfection if you wear only clean, freshly laundered cotton panties or panties and pantyhose with cotton crotches. Do not wear panties made of nylon, rayon or other synthetic fabrics. These garments do not allow air to flow freely around the vagina and help create the conditions favorable to growth of the infection-causing organism.

DOSAGE AND STORAGE

To treat vaginal infections, iodochlorhydroxyquin powder is sprayed or suppositories are inserted into the vagina each night at bedtime for a period of about six weeks. A vinegar douche (two to three tablespoonfuls of vinegar to a quart of warm water) should precede insertion of the suppositories. Continue to use the medication through your menstrual period but omit the douche during this time.

Your doctor will select the form best for you and will determine how much of this medication you should use and how often you should use it. Carefully follow the instructions on your prescription label and ask your doctor or pharmacist about any part of the instructions you do not understand.

Suppositories to be inserted in the vagina come with a special applicator to insert them. There are also instructions and diagrams for proper insertion. Wash the applicator with soap and water each time you finish using it.

Metronidazole
(me troe ni′ da zole)

Brand name: Flagyl

Metronidazole is an anti-infective drug that eliminates protozoa (tiny one-celled organisms) that cause infection. Metronidazole is used most often to treat infections of the genital-urinary tract, particularly vaginal infections.

To cure a vaginal infection completely and to prevent it from recurring, the woman and her male sexual partner are treated at the same time with the oral form of metronidazole. In addition, vaginal suppositories may be prescribed for women along with the oral medication.

UNDESIRED EFFECTS

The most common side effects of metronidazole are diarrhea, loss of appetite, nausea, vomiting and stomach pain. If stomach discomfort occurs, take this medicine with food. Usually these effects will lessen as you continue to take metronidazole and as your body adjusts to it. If they continue or are troublesome, contact your doctor.

Less frequently, metronidazole taken orally will give you constipation, headache, dizziness or lightheadedness, dryness of the mouth or unusual tiredness or weakness. If you experience these effects and if they are severe, contact your doctor.

Another side effect of this medicine taken orally is an unpleasant or sharp metallic taste in your mouth. Chew gum or suck mints to overcome this problem. This medicine can also cause a darkening of the urine. This effect is harmless and will go away when you stop taking the medicine.

If you experience any irritation, discharge or dryness of the vagina not present before you started taking this medicine orally, or if you notice a white, furry growth on your tongue, it may indicate that metronidazole is not working as it should, or you may have an overgrowth of fungus. Contact your doctor. He may want to change your medication and/or treat the fungal overgrowth.

More serious side effects of metronidazole, though they do not occur frequently, are allergic reactions, blood problems and nerve problems. Skin rash, hives and itching are signs of an allergic reaction. Contact your doctor if you experience these effects.

If you get a numbness, tingling, pain or weakness in the hands and feet or notice clumsiness or unsteadiness, mood or mental changes or seizures, contact your doctor. Metronidazole may be having a bad effect on your nerves.

Contact your doctor if you get a sore throat or fever, which can indicate blood problems. Your doctor may ask you to have some blood tests or other laboratory tests done while you are taking metronidazole.

Drinking alcoholic beverages while you are taking this medicine may cause stomach pain, nausea, vomiting, headache, flushing or redness of the face. *Do not drink alcoholic beverages while you are taking metronidazole.* If you have any questions about this, ask your doctor or pharmacist.

PRECAUTIONS

Metronidazole has been shown to cause cancer in animals. Before you start taking this medicine, discuss the use of this drug with your doctor.

Before you start taking metronidazole, tell your doctor if you have a blood disease or history of blood disease or if you have central nervous system disease.

Tell your doctor what other prescription or nonprescription drugs you are taking, including anticoagulants (blood thinners) and disulfiram (a drug to help curb drinking of alcohol). If you do not know the names of the drugs you are taking or what they were prescribed for, bring them in their labeled containers to your doctor or pharmacist.

When you are taking metronidazole, you should not douche unless your doctor specifically tells you to do so. Wear only clean, freshly laundered panties of cotton or panties and pantyhose with cotton crotches until the infection is cured. Do not wear panties made of silk, nylon, Dacron or other synthetic fabrics, since these garments do not allow air to flow freely around the vagina and help create conditions favorable to growth of infecting organisms in the vagina.

Be sure to take *all* the doses of metronidazole your doctor prescribes. Do not stop taking the medicine even though the symptoms of the infection disappear. You must take metronidazole for as long as your doctor tells you to or the infection may return. However, if your symptoms do not improve in a few days or become worse, contact your doctor.

If you are taking this medicine for a genital infection, your sexual partner should be treated at the same time, since the infection may spread to another person during sexual intercourse. If you have any questions about this, check with your doctor.

Metronidazole should not be taken by pregnant women in the first three months of pregnancy and should be used with caution by nursing mothers and children under the age of two. Tell your doctor if you are pregnant or intend to become pregnant while taking this medicine or if you are nursing a baby.

DOSAGE AND STORAGE

Metronidazole comes in tablets to be swallowed and suppositories to be inserted in the vagina. Your doctor will choose the form best for you and will instruct you in its use. If you have any questions about these instructions, check with your doctor or pharmacist.

Metronidazole tablets to be swallowed may be taken with meals or a light snack to avoid the possibility of stomach upset.

Suppositories to be inserted in the vagina come with a special applicator for inserting them along with instructions and a diagram showing how to insert them. Remove the paper wrapper from the suppository just before inserting, and wet the suppository with a little tap water. Wash the applicator with soap and warm water each time you finish using it.

If you miss a dose of the oral metronidazole, take it as soon as you remember it. Take any remaining doses for that day at evenly spaced intervals. *Do not take a double dose.*

Keep this medication in the container it came in and keep it out of the reach of children.

Miconazole
(mi kon' a zole)

Brand name: Micatin, Monistat

Miconazole is an antifungal agent applied as a cream directly to the site of infection and is used to treat fungal infections of the vagina. Another cream form of this medication is used to treat fungal infections of the skin such as athlete's foot and jock itch.

UNDESIRED EFFECTS

Side effects of miconazole are irritation and allergic reactions. If you experience vaginal itching, burning or irritation not present before using this medicine, contact your doctor.

Stop using miconazole and contact your doctor if you get pelvic cramps, skin rash, hives or headache (signs of an allergic reaction). Your doctor may want to change your medication.

PRECAUTIONS

Before you start using this medicine, tell your doctor if you are pregnant or think you may be. A small amount of miconazole is absorbed from the vagina and may affect the health of the fetus. If you become pregnant while using miconazole, contact your doctor immediately.

Use *all* the miconazole prescribed by your doctor, even though you may think the infection has disappeared. Failure to use all the medicine prescribed could allow the infection to return. Continue to use miconazole as prescribed even if you begin to menstruate during the time of treatment.

To help cure the infection and prevent reinfection, wear only clean, freshly laundered panties of cotton or panties and pantyhose with cotton crotches. Do not wear panties made of nylon, rayon or other synthetic fabrics. These garments do not allow air to flow freely around the vagina and help create the conditions favorable to growth of fungus in the vagina.

While you are using miconazole, do not douche unless your doctor tells you to. You may wish to wear a sanitary napkin while using this medicine to protect your clothing from stains.

DOSAGE AND STORAGE

Your doctor will determine how often you should use miconazole and how much to use at each dose. Carefully follow the instructions on your prescription label and ask your doctor or pharmacist to explain any part of the instructions you do not understand.

Miconazole vaginal cream usually is applied once a day at bedtime for at least two weeks. It comes with a special applicator and should be used in this way:

1. Fill the applicator to the level indicated.

2. Lie on your back with your knees drawn upward and spread apart (similar to the position for a vaginal examination).

3. Gently insert the applicator into the vagina and push the plunger to release the medication.

4. Discard the applicator if it is disposable. If not, clean it thoroughly with soap and warm water.

If you forget to insert a dose, apply it as soon as you remember. If you remember a missed dose at the time you are scheduled to apply the next one, omit the missed dose completely and use only the regularly scheduled dose.

Keep this medicine in the container it came in. Keep it out of the reach of children. Do not allow anyone else to use your miconazole.

Nystatin
(nye stat′ in)

Brand names: Candex, Mycostatin, Nilstat

Nystatin is an antifungal antibiotic that, in the form of tablets to be inserted in the vagina, is used to treat fungal infections of the vagina. Nystatin also is used to prevent fungal infections of the mouth in babies born of mothers with vaginal infections.

Other forms of nystatin that are available to treat other fungal infections are oral suspension for mouth infections and cream, powder and ointment for skin infections such as diaper rash and infections of the fingernails.

UNDESIRED EFFECTS:

Side effects with nystatin are rare. However, if you should develop irritation of the vagina not present before using this medicine, contact your doctor.

PRECAUTIONS

Use *all* the nystatin your doctor has prescribed, even though you may think the infection has disappeared. Failure to use all the medicine prescribed could allow the infection to return. Continue to use it as prescribed even if you begin to menstruate.

Be sure to tell your doctor if you have had any reaction to nystatin previously. You should not use this drug if you are allergic to it.

Discuss with your doctor any questions you may have about douching or sexual intercourse during treatment with nystatin. You may wish to wear a sanitary napkin while you are using this medicine to protect your clothing from stains.

You can help cure the infection and prevent reinfection if you wear only clean, freshly laundered cotton panties or panties and pantyhose with cotton crotches. Do not wear panties made of nylon, rayon or other synthetic fabrics. These garments do not allow air to flow freely around the vagina and help create the conditions favorable to growth of fungus in the vagina.

DOSAGE AND STORAGE

Your doctor will determine how often you should use nystatin and how much to use at each dose. Carefully follow the instructions on your prescription label and ask your doctor or pharmacist to explain any part you do not understand.

Nystatin tablets usually are inserted in the vagina once or twice a day, usually for two or three weeks. They come with a special applicator, instructions and a diagram showing how the tablets are inserted.

When using nystatin vaginal tablets, unwrap them just before inserting. Wash the applicator with soap and warm water each time you finish using it.

Keep nystatin vaginal tablets in the container they came in and store them in the refrigerator. Keep this medicine out of the reach of children.

Sulfanilamide
(sul fa nil' a mide)

Brand name: AVC

Sulfanilamide is a sulfa drug. It is combined with another antibacterial drug and a tissue-healing substance to treat infections of the vagina when it is not known if the infection is caused by protozoa, bacteria or fungi. However, where the infecting organism is known, a drug is preferred that is effective against it specifically.

UNDESIRED EFFECTS

Sulfanilamide vaginal cream and suppositories can cause vaginal irritations. If you experience vaginal burning, itching or discomfort not present before you used this medicine, contact your doctor.

Some sulfanilamide is absorbed through the vagina and can result in the side effects caused by all sulfa drugs, including allergic reactions, blood problems, kidney problems and thyroid problems.

If you develop itching, rash, fever, aching of the joints and muscles, difficulty in swallowing, or redness, blistering, peeling or loosening of the skin, you may be allergic to sulfanilamide. If you develop any of these symptoms, stop using sulfanilamide and contact your doctor.

Symptoms of blood problems are unusual bleeding or bruising, unusual weakness or tiredness, fever, pale skin or sore throat. If you develop any of these symptoms, stop using sulfanilamide and contact your doctor. Also contact your doctor if you experience yellowing of the eyes or skin (liver problems), and stop taking sulfanilamide.

Kidney and thyroid problems are rare side effects from taking sulfanilamide, but it can cause blood in the urine, lower back pain, pain or burning while urinating or a swelling of the front part of the neck (goiter). If you experience any of these side effects, stop using sulfanilamide and contact your doctor.

PRECAUTIONS

Before you start using sulfanilamide, tell your doctor if you ever have had an allergic reaction to any sulfa drug, a thiazide diuretic (water pill), oral diabetes medicine or oral medicine for glaucoma.

To help your doctor select the best treatment for you, tell him if you have G6PD deficiency (an inherited blood disease), porphyria, kidney disease or liver disease.

Because the sulfanilamide absorbed from the vagina might affect the health of your baby, tell your doctor if you are pregnant or think you may be. If you become pregnant while using sulfanilamide, contact your doctor at once.

If the infection does not improve within a few days, stop using this medicine and contact your doctor. Even though you may think the infection has disappeared after a few days of treatment, use all the sulfanilamide your doctor has prescribed. Failure to use all the medicine prescribed could allow the infection to return. Continue to use the sulfanilamide even if you begin to menstruate.

You may be asked to have laboratory tests of your blood or for kidney, liver or thyroid function while you are using this drug. *Keep all appointments with your doctor and at the laboratory.*

Check with your doctor about your douching or having sexual intercourse while you are using sulfanilamide. You may wish to wear a sanitary napkin while you are using this medicine to protect your clothing from stains.

To help cure the vaginal infection and prevent reinfection, wear only clean, freshly laundered cotton panties, or panties and pantyhose with cotton crotches. Do not wear panties made of nylon, rayon or other synthetic fabrics. These garments do not allow air to circulate freely around the vagina and help create the conditions favorable to the growth of infecting organisms.

DOSAGE AND STORAGE

Your doctor will determine how often you should use sulfanilamide cream or suppositories and how much to use at each dose. Carefully follow the instructions on your prescription label and ask your doctor or pharmacist to explain any part of the instructions you do not understand.

Sulfanilamide for vaginal infections comes in cream and suppositories which usually are used once or twice a day. Both forms come with a special applicator and instructions and a diagram showing how to use them. After inserting the cream or suppository, wash the applicator with soap and warm water.

Keep your sulfanilamide in the container it came in and keep it out of the reach of children.

Eye Infections

Drugs applied to the eye are called ophthalmic drugs.

Apply an ophthalmic *ointment* to your eye in the following way:
1. Use a mirror or have someone else apply the ointment.
2. Before applying the ointment, wash your hands thoroughly with soap and water.
3. Avoid touching the tip of the tube against the eye or against anything else.
4. Holding the tube between your thumb and index finger, place the tube as near as possible to your eyelid without touching it.
5. Brace the remaining fingers of this hand against your cheek or nose to steady your hand.
6. Tilt your head back.
7. With the index finger of your other hand, pull the lower lid of the eye down to form a pocket.
8. Place the proper amount of ointment into the pocket made by the lower lid and the eye.
9. Blink your eye gently.
10. Wipe off any excess ointment from the eyelid and lashes with a clean tissue.
11. Replace and tighten the cap right away.
12. Wash your hands again to remove any medicine.

Apply eye *drops* in the following way:
1. Use a mirror or have someone else put the drops in your eye.
2. Before using the drops, wash your hands thoroughly with soap and water.
3. Make sure there are no chips or cracks at the end of the dropper.
4. Avoid touching the dropper against the eye or against anything else.
5. Hold the dropper tip down at all times. This prevents the drops from flowing back into the bulb, where they may become contaminated.
6. Lie down or tilt your head back.
7. Holding the bulb of the dropper between your thumb and index finger, place the dropper as near as possible to your eyelid without touching it.
8. Brace the remaining fingers of this hand against your cheek or nose to steady your hand.
9. With the index finger of your other hand, pull the lower lid of the eye down to form a pocket.
10. Drop the prescribed number of drops into the pocket made by the lower lid and the eye. Placing drops on the surface of the eyeball can cause stinging.

11. Replace and tighten the cap or dropper right away. Do not wipe or rinse it off.
12. Press your finger against the inner corner of your eye for one minute. This prevents medication from entering the tear duct.
13. Close your eye gently and wipe off any excess liquid with a clean tissue.
14. Wash your hands again to remove any medicine.

Do not use eye makeup when you have an infection in one or both eyes. Eye makeup is a frequent source of cross contamination, spreading the infection from one eye to the other or from one person to another when eye makeup is shared.

Infections in the *outer* ear also can be treated with some of the drugs described in this section. In some cases, the ophthalmic ointment or solution is used in the ear; for other drugs, a special otic (ear) product is used.

To apply eardrops:

1. You can put a drop or drops in your ear yourself or have someone do it for you.
2. Before using the drops, wash your hands thoroughly with soap and water.
3. Make sure there are no chips or cracks at the end of the dropper.
4. Avoid touching the drops against the ear or against anything else.
5. Hold the dropper tip down at all times. This prevents the drops from flowing back into the bulb, where they may become contaminated.
6. Lie down on your side with the affected ear up, or tilt your head to the side.
7. To allow the drops to run in, hold the earlobe up and back.
8. Drop the prescribed number of drops in the ear.
9. Replace the dropper right away. Do not wipe or rinse it off.
10. Keep the ear tilted up for a few minutes, or insert a soft cotton plug, whichever has been recommended by your doctor or pharmacist.
11. Wash your hands again to remove any medicine.

OPHTHALMIC ANTI-INFECTIVES
Bacitracin
(bass i tray′ sin)

Brand name: Baciguent Ophthalmic

Bacitracin is an antibiotic that eliminates bacteria that cause certain types of eye infections. In addition to being used alone to treat eye problems, bacitracin also is combined with other antibiotics, such as neomycin and/or polymyxin (Mycitracin, Neopolycin, Neosporin, Polysporin) for eye infections.

UNDESIRED EFFECTS

Bacitracin, when used to treat the eyes, has few side effects. However, allergic reactions have occurred. If this medicine causes itching, burning or redness of the skin, stop using it and contact your doctor.

A more serious allergic reaction also can occur. Stop using this medicine and contact your doctor immediately if you experience itching all over your body, swelling of the lips and face or difficult breathing. You may need emergency treatment.

PRECAUTIONS
Before you start to use bacitracin, tell your doctor if you have any history of allergies such as asthma, hay fever or hives and if you have had an allergic reaction to bacitracin.

Do not apply bacitracin to areas of the body other than those indicated by your doctor. Do not apply more frequently than stated on your prescription label, and do not cover the medication with any dressing other than those your doctor has indicated.

If your eye infection appears to be worse after you start using bacitracin, contact your doctor. He may want to change your medication.

DOSAGE AND STORAGE
Your doctor will determine how often you should use bacitracin and how much to use at each application. Carefully follow the instructions on your prescription label and ask your doctor or pharmacist to explain any part of the instructions you do not understand.

(See page 156 for instructions on how to apply bacitracin ointment to your eye.)

If you forget to apply a dose, apply the ointment as soon as you remember it. Then go back to your regular dosing schedule. Do not apply a double dose to make up for the missed one.

When your doctor tells you that you may stop using bacitracin ointment, throw away any bacitracin ointment you have left. Do not save it for another infection and do not allow anyone else to use it.

Keep bacitracin in the container it came in and keep it out of the reach of children.

Chloramphenicol
(klor am fen′ i kole)

Brand names: AntiBiOpto, Chloromycetin, Chloroptic, Enconochlor

In addition to the oral and injectable forms of chloramphenicol used to treat serious infections within the body, this antibiotic also is available in solutions and ointments that are applied directly to the eye or outer ear to treat infections there. However, chloramphenicol should be used for infections caused by bacteria against which it is known to be effective, and then only when safer antibiotics have been tried and have not worked.

UNDESIRED EFFECTS
The most common side effects of chloramphenicol eye or ear medicines are allergic reactions. If you experience burning, itching, rash, redness, swelling or any other sign of irritation not present before you began to use this medicine, stop using it and contact your doctor.

When chloramphenicol is used over a long period of time or for repeated short periods of time, it can interfere with proper development of the bone marrow. There is also a chance that chloramphenicol will be absorbed into the body from the eye or ear and cause some of the serious blood problems associated with this medicine when it is taken by mouth or by injection. (See **chloramphenicol**, page 114, for more information.)

As with other antibiotics, use of chloramphenicol medicine for the eyes and ears may cause overgrowth of organisms against which it is not effective. If you develop another infection in addition to the one for which this medicine was prescribed, stop using it and contact your doctor.

PRECAUTIONS

Before you start to use this medicine, tell your doctor if you have ever had any problem with chloramphenicol in the past.

Use all the medicine your doctor has prescribed, even though your symptoms seem to improve in a few days. However, do not use chloramphenicol more often or for a longer period than your doctor has ordered. To do so may increase the chance of side effects.

Tell your doctor if you are pregnant or are breast-feeding a baby. Although problems are not likely, your doctor can select the treatment best for you and your baby if he has this information.

DOSAGE AND STORAGE

Your doctor will determine how often you should use chloramphenicol and how much you should use with each application. Carefully follow the instructions on your prescription label and ask your doctor or pharmacist to explain any part of the instructions you do not understand.

Chloramphenicol comes in drops and ointment for treating the eyes, and in drops for the ears. Before using any of these forms, wash your hands thoroughly with soap and water. Avoid touching the tip of the dropper of the ointment tube against anything.

To use the eyedrops. If the solution looks cloudy, shake the bottle for about 10 seconds. (See page 156 for instructions on how to apply eyedrops.)

To use the eye ointment. (See page 156 for instructions.)

To use the eardrops. Warm the drops to near body temperature by holding the bottle of drops in your hand for a few minutes. If the drops look cloudy, shake the bottle for about 10 seconds. (See page 157 for instructions on how to apply eardrops.)

If you miss a dose of this medicine, apply it as soon as possible. However, if it is almost time for another application, use only the regularly scheduled dose. Skip the missed dose entirely.

Keep chloramphenicol in the container it came in, and keep it out of the reach of children.

Erythromycin
(eh rith roe mye′ sin)

Brand name: Ilotycin Ophthalmic

Erythromycin, an antibiotic used to treat general systemic infections when given by mouth or injection, also is available as an ointment to treat bacterial infections of the eyes. (See **erythromycins**, page 71.)

UNDESIRED EFFECTS

No one who has ever had an allergic reaction to any of the erythromycins should use erythromycin ointment for the eyes. Although allergic reactions to the eye medication are rare, they can occur in people who are very sensitive to it.

The use of erythromycin to treat eye infections can result in an overgrowth of organisms against which it does not work. If you develop another infection or if your infection does not improve in a few days, contact your doctor.

PRECAUTIONS

Before you start to use this medicine, tell your doctor if you have ever had problems with erythromycin in the past.

Use all the medicine your doctor has prescribed, even though your symptoms seem to improve in a few days. It takes time for a bacterial infection to be cured completely. If it is not cured, it can return.

DOSAGE AND STORAGE

Your doctor will determine how often you should use erythromycin and how much you should use with each application. Carefully follow the instructions on your prescription label and ask your doctor or pharmacist to explain any part of the instructions you do not understand.

Erythromycin comes in ointment that is applied to the eye. (See page 156 for instructions on how to apply eye ointments.)

If you miss an application, apply the ointment as soon as you remember. If it is almost time for another application, use only the regularly scheduled dose. Skip the missed dose entirely. Then go back to your regular dosing schedule.

Keep erythromycin ointment in the container it came in. Keep it out of the reach of children, and do not allow anyone else to use it.

Gentamicin
(jen ta mye′ sin)

Brand names: Garamycin Ophthalmic, Genoptic

Gentamicin is an antibiotic available in injectable form to treat serious systemic infections, and as eyedrops and ointment to be applied directly to the eye to treat several kinds of bacterial infections.

UNDESIRED EFFECTS

When applied to the eye, gentamicin eyedrops or ointment may cause a temporary burning or stinging sensation.

Occasionally gentamicin will cause increased redness or tearing of the eye. If you experience these effects or any signs of irritation (redness, swelling or itching) you did not have before using this medicine, stop using it and contact your doctor.

If you use gentamicin according to your doctor's instructions and your symptoms do not improve or get worse, an overgrowth of organisms that this medicine does not work against may be occurring. Stop using gentamicin and contact your doctor.

PRECAUTIONS

Before you start using gentamicin, tell your doctor if you have had any problems with any form of gentamicin in the past.

Keep using this medicine for the full course of treatment your doctor has prescribed, even though your symptoms may disappear after a few days. Bacterial infections often take many days to cure completely. If they are not completely cured, they can return.

DOSAGE AND STORAGE

Your doctor will determine how often you should use gentamicin and how much you should use at each application. Carefully follow the instructions on your prescription label and ask your doctor or pharmacist to explain any part of the instructions you do not understand.

Gentamicin comes in eyedrops and in ointment to be placed in the eye. (See page 156 for instructions on how to apply these medicines.)

Keep gentamicin eyedrops in the container they came in. Keep both forms of this eye medicine out of the reach of children.

Idoxuridine
(eye dox yoor' i deen)

Brand names: Dendrid, Herplex, Stoxil

Idoxuridine is used to treat viral infections of the eye. It is considerably more effective against first infections than against recurrent or chronic infections.

UNDESIRED EFFECTS

Idoxuridine can cause pain, itching or swelling of the eye. If you experience these effects and they are mild, continue to use the medicine. Contact your doctor if these problems become severe.

While you are using idoxuridine your eyes may be more sensitive to light. Avoid exposing your eyes to bright lights, and when you are in sunlight wear sunglasses or a sunshade.

PRECAUTIONS

Before you start to use idoxuridine, tell your doctor if you have ever had problems with this medicine. No one who has had an allergic reaction to it should use it again.

Follow the treatment schedule prescribed by your doctor as closely as possible. If your eye infection has not improved within one week after you begin to use idoxuridine, contact your doctor. He may want to change your medication.

When the infected eye appears to be healed, continue to use the medicine for one more week unless your doctor specifically tells you to stop using it.

Do not use any other eye medications while you are using idoxuridine. If you have questions about this, discuss them with your doctor or pharmacist.

DOSAGE AND STORAGE

Your doctor will determine how often you should use idoxuridine and how much you should use at each dose. Carefully follow the instructions on your prescription label and ask your doctor or pharmacist to explain any part of the instructions you do not understand.

Idoxuridine comes as drops and as ointment to be used in the eyes. (See page 156 for instructions on how to apply the drops and the ointment.)

If you forget to apply a dose, apply it when you remember. Apply any remaining doses for that day at regularly spaced intervals. If you remember a missed dose at the time you are to apply another, omit the missed dose entirely and apply only the regularly scheduled dose. *Do not apply a double dose.* Then continue to follow your regular medication schedule.

When your doctor tells you to stop using idoxuridine, throw away any unused portion. Do not save it for use against another infection and do not allow anyone else to use it.

Keep idoxuridine eyedrops in the container they came in and store the container in the refrigerator. The ointment may be stored at room temperature. Keep these medicines out of the reach of children.

Neomycin
(nee oh mye′ sin)

Brand name: Myciguent Ophthalmic

Neomycin is an antibiotic that eliminates bacteria that cause certain infections of the eye and the outer ear. It is used alone or in combination with other antibiotics (Mycifradin, NeoPolycin, NeoSporin, Polyspectrin) or cortisone-type drugs (Cortisporin) to treat eye infections. In combination with other drugs, neomycin is used to treat outer ear infections. However, there is no substantial evidence that these combinations are effective against outer ear infections, and they carry a high risk of causing skin irritation.

UNDESIRED EFFECTS

The application of neomycin to the eyes and ears frequently causes allergic reactions. If you get swelling, burning, itching or redness from this medicine, stop using it and contact your doctor.

Neomycin ointment can also cause ear and kidney problems. Stop using the medicine and contact your doctor if you have any loss of hearing; a ringing, buzzing sound or a feeling of fullness in the ears; or clumsiness, dizziness or unsteadiness.

If you notice excessive thirst or a greatly decreased frequency of urination or amount of urine, neomycin may be giving you kidney problems. Stop using the medicine and contact your doctor.

PRECAUTIONS

Before you start using neomycin, tell your doctor if you have ever had an allergic reaction to neomycin or to other similar antibiotics (amikacin, gentamicin, kanamycin, streptomycin or tobramycin). No one who has had an allergic reaction to these drugs should use neomycin.

To help your doctor select the treatment best for you, tell him if you have inner ear disease, kidney disease, myasthenia gravis or Parkinson's disease.

Certain medications, if taken while you are using neomycin ointment, may increase the possibility of ear and kidney problems. They are the antibiotics amikacin, capreomycin, cephaloridine, cephalothin, gentamicin, kanamycin, polymyxin, streptomycin, tobramycin, vancomycin and viomycin, and the diuretics (water pills) ethacrynic acid, furosemide and mercaptomerin.

Tell your doctor what prescription or nonprescription drugs you are taking, including those named above and any anticoagulants (blood thinners) or digoxin (heart medicine). If you do not know the names of the drugs or what they were prescribed for, bring them in their labeled containers to your doctor or pharmacist.

If your symptoms do not improve within a few days or get worse, contact your doctor. This may mean that neomycin is not effective against the bacteria causing your infection or that overgrowth of bacteria against which it does not work has caused a second infection.

Tell your doctor if you are pregnant or think you may be while you are using neomycin. Safe use of this medicine in pregnant women has not been established.

DOSAGE AND STORAGE

Your doctor will determine how much neomycin ointment you should use and how much you should use for each application. Carefully follow the instructions on your prescription label and ask your doctor or pharmacist to explain any part of the instructions you do not understand.

Do not apply this medication to any other part of your body except that directed by your doctor. Do not apply more frequently than stated on the prescription label.

See page 156 for instructions on applying an ointment for the eye and page 157 for instructions on applying eardrops.

If you forget to apply a dose, apply it as soon as you remember. Then go back to your regular dosing schedule. *Do not apply a double dose to make up for a missed dose.*

When your doctor tells you to stop using neomycin ointment, throw away any unused portion. Do not save it for use against another infection and do not allow anyone else to use it.

Keep neomycin in the container it came in, and keep it out of the reach of children.

Polymyxin
(pol i mix' in)

Brand name: Aerosporin Otic

Polymyxin is an antibiotic that eliminates bacteria that cause certain types of eye and ear infections. It is used alone or in combination with other antibiotics or cortisonelike medication to treat infections of the eyes and ears. The names of some products containing polymyxin in combination with other antibiotics are Mycifradin, NeoPolycin, NeoSporin and Polyspectrin. Cortisporin is a combination of polymyxin and neomycin with a steroid.

UNDESIRED EFFECTS

When placed directly on eye infections, polymyxin has few side effects. It can irritate the eyes. If this effect is bothersome to you, contact your doctor.

Allergic reactions are rare with polymyxin. If you get itching, burning or redness, stop using the medication and contact your doctor.

PRECAUTIONS

Before you start using polymyxin, tell your doctor if you have ever had an allergic reaction to this medicine or to similar antibiotics such as colistin, viomycin or bacitracin.

If your eye infection appears to be worse after you start using polymyxin, contact your doctor. This may mean the medicine is not effective against the bacteria causing your eye infection, or the bacteria against which it does not work have overgrown and caused a second infection.

Do not apply polymyxin to areas of the body other than those indicated by your doctor. Do not apply more frequently than stated on your prescription label.

DOSAGE AND STORAGE

Your doctor will determine how often you should use polymyxin and how much to use at each application. Carefully follow the instructions on your prescription label and ask your doctor or pharmacist to explain any part of the instructions you do not understand.

(For instructions on how to use eyedrops or ointment, see page 156. See page 157 for instructions on how to use eardrops.)

If you forget to use polymyxin once, put it in your eye or ear as soon as you remember. Then go back to your regular dosing schedule. *Do not use a double dose to make up for a missed dose.*

When your doctor tells you to stop using polymyxin, throw away any unused portion. Do not save it for use against another infection and do not allow anyone else to use it.

Keep polymyxin in the container it came in, and keep it out of the reach of children.

Sulfacetamide

(sul fa see′ ta mide)

Brand names: Bleph-10 Liquifilm, Cetamide, IsoptoCetamide, Sulf-10, Sulamyd

Sulfacetamide is a sulfonamide (sulfa-type) antibacterial drug that stops the
growth of bacteria that cause certain kinds of eye infections. It is also used to
prevent infection after injury to the eyes. For more serious infections, it may
be necessary to give an oral antibacterial agent along with sulfacetamide eyedrops or ointment.

Sulfacetamide also is combined with cortisonelike drugs and with drugs that
narrow the blood vessels to treat certain eye problems.

UNDESIRED EFFECTS

Sulfacetamide may make your eyes red, sore or watery. Contact your doctor
if you have these effects.

Although very little sulfacetamide is absorbed into the body when it is applied
to the eye, there is always the possibility of an allergic reaction in a person
who is very sensitive to sulfa drugs. If you develop itching, rash, fever, aching
of the joints and muscles, difficulty in swallowing or redness, blistering, peeling
or loosening of the skin, you may be having an allergic reaction. Stop using
this medicine and contact your doctor.

PRECAUTIONS

Before you start using sulfacetamide, tell your doctor if you have ever had
an allergic reaction to any sulfa drug, a thiazide diuretic (water pill), oral
diabetes medicine or oral medicine for glaucoma.

Tell your doctor what prescription or nonprescription drugs you are taking.
If you do not know the names of the drugs or what they were prescribed for,
bring them in their labeled containers to your doctor or pharmacist.

If the infection for which sulfacetamide was prescribed has not improved
within two or three days after you start using it, contact your doctor. He may
want to change your medication or add another drug. The lack of improvement
in the infection also might indicate an overgrowth of bacteria against which
sulfacetamide does not work.

DOSAGE AND STORAGE

Your doctor will determine how often you should use sulfacetamide and how
much you should use at each application. Carefully follow the instructions on
your prescription label and ask your doctor or pharmacist to explain any part
of the instructions you do not understand.

Sulfacetamide comes in drops and ointment for the eyes. If the solution looks
cloudy, shake the bottle for about 10 seconds. (See page 156 for instructions
on using the eyedrops and the ointment.)

If you forget an application, apply the missed treatment when you remember

it. Apply any remaining treatment for that day at evenly spaced intervals. If
you remember a missed treatment at the time you are scheduled to apply the
next one, omit the missed dose completely and apply only the scheduled treatment. *Do not apply a double dose.* Then return to your regular dosing schedule.

When your doctor tells you to stop using sulfacetamide, throw away any of
the medicine that is left. Do not save it for use against another infection and
do not allow anyone else to use it.

Keep sulfacetamide in the container it came in, store it away from excess
heat and keep it out of the reach of children.

SKIN PROBLEMS

DRUGS USED TO TREAT SKIN PROBLEMS

Skin Infections

This section describes a few of the many medicines used to treat skin infections. Skin infections can be treated with "systemic" drugs (drugs that act throughout your body) or with drugs applied directly to the skin. Drugs applied directly to the skin are called "topical," and the drugs are said to be applied "topically."

Proper washing and care of the skin are extremely important in combating any skin disease. Always ask your doctor about proper hygienic practice for your particular situation and follow his advice about what kind of soaps (if any) to use and other precautions you should follow in caring for your skin.

Before beginning to use any medicine on your skin, discuss with your doctor or pharmacist the way to apply it (for example, rub it in, or lay it on), the methods of "dressing" the infected area (for example, leave it open, or cover it, and what to use to cover it) and finally the way to remove the medicine, if that is necessary.

Although many antibiotic creams, lotions and ointments are available to treat bacterial skin infections, most health professionals question the use of topical antibiotics except in treating infected burns. Minor skin infections usually heal without drug treatment if proper hygienic measures are followed. Serious or extensive bacterial skin infections require *systemic* anti-infective therapy. (Some examples of bacterial infections are erysipelas, impetigo, carbuncles and abscesses.) Casual use of antibiotics topically can lead to the development of strains of bacteria which are resistant to the antibiotic used and to similar antibiotics.

Culture and sensitivity tests should be done before any antibiotic is prescribed. Among the systemic antibiotics useful in treating bacterial infections of the skin are erythromycin, penicillins and tetracyclines.

Fungal infections of the skin or nails are treated with topical medicines and medicines taken orally that have a particular affinity for skin or nail tissue.

Specific parasiticides are available for topical application in the treatment of scabies, a scaly, itchy skin disease caused by the itch mite, and in the treatment of pediculosis, caused by lice.

ANTIBACTERIAL ANTI-INFECTIVES (TOPICAL)
Nitrofurazone
(nye troe fyoor' a zone)

Brand names: Furacin, Ni-Furin, Nisept, Nitrozone
Nitrofurazone is an antibacterial agent that is effective against a wide variety

[169]

of bacteria, including some that are resistant to antibiotic and sulfa drugs. Nitrofurazone is used to prevent and treat infections of second- and third-degree burns when there is a possibility that such an infection might be caused by resistant bacteria.

This medication is also used on skin grafts when bacteria on the grafts or at the donor site might cause graft rejection, particularly when the infection-causing bacteria are resistant to other anti-infectives.

UNDESIRED EFFECTS

Allergic skin reactions are the most common problems when you use nitrofurazone. Stop using this medication and contact your doctor if you experience redness, itching or burning of the skin, swelling, blisters or ulcers.

Nitrofurazone also can cause hives, peeling of the skin and a serious and sometimes fatal allergic reaction. If you have any of these symptoms contact your doctor immediately, because you may need emergency treatment.

During nitrofurazone therapy, bacteria and fungi against which this medicine is not effective may overgrow. If your condition does not improve within a few days, stop using nitrofurazone and contact your doctor.

PRECAUTIONS

Before using nitrofurazone, tell your doctor if you have ever had an allergic reaction to it.

Tell your doctor if you are pregnant or think you may be. Safe use of nitrofurazone in pregnant women has not been established.

DOSAGE AND STORAGE

Your doctor will determine how often you should apply nitrofurazone and how much to use at each application. Carefully follow the instructions on your prescription label and ask your doctor or pharmacist to explain any part of the instructions you do not understand.

Nitrofurazone comes in powder, liquid spray, ointment, cream and wet dressings. Your doctor will determine which form is best for you.

Nitrofurazone powder comes in a shaker-top vial and can be applied directly to the area to be treated. The liquid spray also can be applied directly to the burned area. If you are using the ointment or cream, you may put them directly on the area to be treated or apply them to the dressings to be used to cover the area.

The dressings that already contain nitrofurazone ointment or liquid are put directly on the area to be treated and then covered with dry gauze or a blanket to prevent drying or evaporation.

The frequency of application of nitrofurazone depends on your condition and the form used. If you are treating second- or third-degree burns, it usually is best to change the dressing every day. With second-degree burns that are oozing very little, the dressing may be left in place for four or five days. If you have any questions about the way to treat your burn or how long to leave dressings in place, contact your doctor.

Keep nitrofurazone in the container it came in and store it in a cool, dry place. Keep nitrofurazone out of the reach of children.

Silver Sulfadiazine
(sul fa dye' a zeen)

Brand name: Silvadene

Silver sulfadiazine is a combination of silver nitrate and sulfadiazine (one of the sulfa drugs) that is effective against a wide variety of bacteria. This cream is used to prevent and treat infections of second- and third-degree burns, usually in a hospital.

UNDESIRED EFFECTS

Occasionally, application of silver sulfadiazine will cause burning, rash or itching. Only if these effects are severe is it necessary to stop using the medicine.

Because significant amounts of silver sulfadiazine are absorbed into the body, it is possible that side effects caused by all the sulfa drugs can occur. These include allergic reactions, blood problems and kidney and liver problems. If you experience fever, aching of the joints or difficulty swallowing (symptoms of allergic reaction); unusual bleeding or bruising, unusual weakness or tiredness, fever, pale skin or sore throat (symptoms of blood problems); yellowing of the eyes or skin (symptoms of liver problems); or blood in the urine, low back pain or pain or burning while urinating (symptoms of kidney problems), contact your doctor.

PRECAUTIONS

To help your doctor select the treatment best for you, tell him if you have ever had an allergic reaction to silver sulfadiazine, methylparaben or any sulfa drug and if you have G6PD deficiency (an inherited blood disease) or kidney or liver disease.

Tell your doctor what other prescription or nonprescription drugs you are taking. If you do not know the names of the drugs or what they were prescribed for, bring them in their labeled containers to your doctor or pharmacist.

Tell your doctor if you are pregnant or think you may be. Silver sulfadiazine should not be used by pregnant women unless the burned area covers more than 20 percent of their bodies or the potential benefit to the mother would be greater than the possible risk to the baby. This medicine should not be used by pregnant women within two to three weeks of delivery, premature babies or infants under one month of age. It can cause harmful jaundice in newborn babies.

Do not stop using silver sulfadiazine until your doctor tells you to. Your burn must be sufficiently healed that the possibility of infection is no longer a problem.

DOSAGE AND STORAGE

Your doctor will determine how often you should use silver sulfadiazine and how much you should use for each application. Carefully follow the instructions on your prescription label and ask your doctor or pharmacist to explain any part of the instructions you do not understand.

Silver sulfadiazine cream usually is applied to the cleaned area of burn once or twice a day. First put on a sterile, disposable glove. Then apply the cream until it covers the burned area with a one-sixteenth-inch thickness of cream. *The burned area should be covered at all times.* If necessary, reapply the cream to any area from which your activity has removed it. Dressings usually are not required but may be used.

Keep silver sulfadiazine in the container it came in and store it at room temperature. Keep it out of the reach of children.

ANTIFUNGAL ANTIBIOTICS (TOPICAL)
Griseofulvin
(gri see oh ful′ vin)

Brand names: Fulvicin P/G, Fulvicin-U/F, Grifulvin V, Grisactin, Gris-PEG

Griseofulvin is an antifungal antibiotic that is taken orally to treat ringworm infections of the skin, hair, fingernails and toenails. Griseofulvin keeps the fungus infection from spreading to new skin or nails as they develop and takes from several weeks to several months to cure the infection completely.

UNDESIRED EFFECTS

Headache is the most common side effect of griseofulvin. If a headache occurs, it is usually when you start to take this medicine. Headaches tends to disappear as you continue to take griseofulvin and your body adjusts to the medicine. Contact your doctor if you continue to have headaches.

Upset stomach, diarrhea, nausea and vomiting, which can occur when you take griseofulvin, may be controlled if you take it after meals. If this medicine makes your mouth dry, you can suck lozenges or hard candies, chew gum or drink liquids.

Griseofulvin also can cause dizziness, insomnia and tiredness. Contact your doctor if you experience these effects and if they bother you.

More serious side effects of griseofulvin are allergic reactions, blood problems and infection of the mouth by fungi against which griseofulvin is not effective. Contact your doctor if you develop skin rash, hives or itching; mental confusion; soreness or irritation of the mouth; numbness, tingling, pain or weakness in the hands or feet; or sore throat or fever.

Some people who take griseofulvin become more sensitive to sunlight. Until you know how you will react to this medicine, limit the amount of time you spend in sunlight, particularly if you tend to sunburn easily. When you are in sunlight, keep your body well covered with clothing, use a sunscreen preparation and wear sunglasses. If you do become severely sunburned, contact your doctor.

PRECAUTIONS

Before you start taking griseofulvin, tell your doctor if you have ever had an allergic reaction to any of the penicillins. People who are sensitive to penicillin also may be sensitive to griseofulvin. Your doctor also will need to know if you have liver disease, porphyria or lupus erythematosus.

Tell your doctor what other prescription or nonprescription drugs you are taking, particularly sleeping pills and anticoagulants (blood thinners). If you do not know the names of the drugs or what they were prescribed for, bring them in their labeled containers to your doctor or pharmacist.

Do not drink alcoholic beverages while you are taking griseofulvin. The combination of alcohol and griseofulvin can make your heartbeat unusually fast and cause a flushing or redness of your face.

Be sure to take all doses of this medicine that your doctor tells you to and continue to take it until your doctor tells you to stop. It may be some time before your infection is completely cured—as much as two to six weeks for infections of the scalp or the skin on most parts of the body, from four to eight weeks for infections of the palms of the hands and the soles of the feet, from four to six months for fingernail infections and from six to 12 months for toenail infections. *Do not stop taking griseofulvin because you see signs of improvement. You must continue to take it until the infection is completely gone.*

Your doctor will want to check your progress while you are taking griseofulvin, particularly if treatment will continue for a long period. *Be sure to keep all appointments with your doctor so that he can do blood counts and tests for liver and kidney function on a regular basis.*

Griseofulvin should not be taken by pregnant women or by children under two years of age. Before taking this medicine, tell your doctor if you are pregnant or intend to become pregnant while taking griseofulvin. If you become pregnant while taking griseofulvin, contact your doctor.

DOSAGE AND STORAGE

Your doctor will determine how often you should take griseofulvin and how much you should take at each dose. Carefully follow the instructions on your prescription label and ask your doctor or pharmacist to explain any part of the instructions you do not understand.

Griseofulvin comes in tablets and in liquid form and should be taken with or right after meals to lessen stomach upset. This medicine works better if you eat high-fat meals. So be sure to include fats such as butter and vegetable oil in your diet every day. Your doctor can give you more information about your diet.

If you forget to take a dose of this medicine, take it as soon as you remember. Take the remaining doses for that day at evenly spaced intervals. *Do not take a double dose.*

If you take the liquid form of griseofulvin, be sure to shake the container well to distribute the medication evenly before removing each dose. Measure each dose with a specially marked measuring spoon to assure an accurate dose.

Keep griseofulvin in the container it came in. Keep your griseofulvin out of the reach of children and do not allow anyone else to take it.

Tolnaftate

(tole naf ' tate)

Brand names: Aftate, Tinactin

Tolnaftate is an antifungal agent that is applied to the skin to treat such fungal infections as athlete's foot, jock itch and body ringworm. This medicine is available without a prescription but it is best to use it according to a doctor's instructions for your particular problem.

UNDESIRED EFFECTS

Tolnaftate rarely causes undesired effects. However, if you get irritation of the skin that was not present before using this medicine, contact your doctor.

When you apply the spray liquid form of tolnaftate, you may notice a mild stinging sensation, which quickly goes away.

PRECAUTIONS

Tolnaftate preparations should not come in contact with the eyes.

Contact your doctor if your skin infection has not improved after you have used tolnaftate for four weeks. He may want to change your medication or supplement it with oral antifungal medicine.

Unless instructed otherwise by your doctor, continue to use tolnaftate for two weeks *after* the symptoms (burning, itching, etc.) disappear. It is important that your infection be cured completely.

Good health habits can help cure your skin infection and prevent reinfection. Wash all towels, sheets and clothing each day after they have come in contact with the infected area. After the period of treatment with tolnaftate, you may continue to use it to *prevent* reinfection. Apply the powder or aerosol powder form each day after you have bathed and dried carefully.

If you have used this drug in the past and know you are allergic to it, do not use it again.

DOSAGE AND STORAGE

Tolnaftate comes in cream, liquid, powder, gel, aerosol powder, aerosol liquid and spray liquid forms. Your doctor or pharmacist can help you choose the form best for your problem.

Tolnaftate must be used regularly to be effective. It should be applied twice a day until the infection is gone and then continued for another two weeks. Before applying tolnaftate, wash the area to be treated and dry it carefully. Then put on enough medicine to cover the area.

When you use the powder to treat your feet, sprinkle it between your toes, on the rest of your feet and in your socks and shoes.

Shake the aerosol powder well before each use. Then spray the affected area from a distance of six to 10 inches. On the feet, spray the powder between your toes, on the rest of your feet and in your shoes and socks. Do not inhale the powder and do not use it near heat, near an open flame or while smoking.

If tolnaftate liquid becomes solid, warming will melt it. To melt it, place the closed container in warm water.

If you are using the aerosol liquid, shake it well before each use. Then spray the infected area from a distance of six inches. To treat your feet, spray between your toes and over the rest of your feet. Do not inhale the vapors from the aerosol liquid. Do not use near heat, near an open flame or while smoking.

When you use the spray liquid, spray the infected area from a distance of four to six inches. As with other spray forms, do not use near heat, near an open flame or while smoking.

Aerosol cans should not be punctured, broken or burned.

Keep all forms of tolnaftate in a cool, dry place. Keep tolnaftate out of the reach of children.

PARASITICIDE
Lindane
(lin′ dane)

Brand names: GBH, Kwell

Lindane, formerly known as gamma benzene hexachloride, is applied to the skin or scalp to treat infections of lice and scabies. One application usually will kill these parasites and their eggs.

UNDESIRED EFFECTS

When you first apply lindane, it may make your skin itch. This itching should ease, but if it continues or grows worse, contact your doctor.

Lindane can cause allergic reactions. Contact your doctor if you develop irritation of the skin or a rash that was not present before using this medicine.

Lindane is absorbed through the skin and there is a chance that you may experience symptoms such as clumsiness or unsteadiness, convulsions or seizures, muscle cramps, unusual nervousness, restlessness or irritability, unusually fast heartbeat and vomiting. If you experience any of these side effects, contact your doctor.

If your skin has become sensitive to mites, itching may continue one to two weeks after treatment. This does not mean that treatment was a failure and is not necessarily a reason for further treatment. If you have any questions about this, contact your doctor.

PRECAUTIONS

Before taking this medicine, tell your doctor if you have ever had an allergic reaction to lindane (gamma benzene hexachloride). He also will need to know if you are presently using any other skin preparations such as lotions, ointments or oils. Use of other skin preparations along with lindane increases the chance of absorption of lindane through the skin and the chance of undesired effects.

Use lindane only as directed by your doctor. Do not use more, do not use it for a longer period of time and do not use it more often than your doctor has instructed. Using lindane exactly as prescribed will lessen the chance of serious side effects.

Do not put this medicine on your face and be sure to keep it away from your eyes. If you accidentally get lindane in your eyes, flush them thoroughly with water.

Because lindane is absorbed through the skin, it should be used with caution by pregnant women and for infants. To help your doctor select the treatment best for you, tell him if you are pregnant or think you may be. If you are treating a small child with lindane, be careful to prevent the child from getting any of the medicine in his mouth, as by thumb-sucking.

Take precautions to prevent reinfection or spreading the infection to other people. Boil or dry-clean any clothing, bedding, towels or other things in which the parasites that caused the problem may be living. Thoroughly clean all bathtubs, showers and toilets in your home with a solution of 70 percent alcohol. When the problem is head lice, combs and brushes can be cleaned with lindane shampoo, but they must be rinsed thoroughly with water to remove all the drug.

DOSAGE AND STORAGE

Lindane comes in lotion, cream and shampoo form. Your doctor will determine which form is best for you. Carefully follow the instructions on your prescription label and ask your doctor or pharmacist to explain any part of the instructions you do not understand.

If your doctor has prescribed cream or lotion for scabies, do the following:
1. Take a hot, soapy bath or shower.
2. Dry yourself well.
3. Apply the lotion or cream to all parts of your body from the neck down. Do not apply it to the face or head. Rub it in well.
4. Leave the cream or lotion on your body for 12 hours. Do not take a bath during this 12-hour period. Do not wash off any of the cream or lotion.
5. Dress in clean clothes. Wear the same clothes during the 12-hour period that the medicine is left on your skin. Do not change your clothes during the treatment.
6. When the 12-hour period is over, take another hot, soapy bath or shower.
7. Dry yourself well with a clean, dry towel.
8. Dress in freshly laundered or dry-cleaned clothing.

If your doctor prescribes cream or lotion for lice, do the following:
1. Apply enough medicine to cover only the affected areas, and rub well into the hair and skin.
2. Leave the cream or lotion on for 12 hours. Do not wash off any of the medicine.

3. After the 12-hour period is over, remove the cream or lotion in a hot, soapy bath or shower.
4. Put on freshly laundered or dry-cleaned clothing.

If your doctor has prescribed the shampoo, do the following:

1. Take a hot, soapy bath or shower. Shampoo your hair with your regular shampoo.
2. While your hair is still wet, apply one ounce (two tablespoonfuls) of the lindane shampoo. Lather the shampoo into your hair for a full five minutes.
3. Rinse your hair thoroughly with water. Dry it with a clean towel.
4. Comb through your hair with a fine-tooth comb.

Keep lindane at room temperature. Keep it out of the reach of children.

InflAMMATiON of ThE SkiN

The drugs described in this section are used to treat inflammation of the skin. Such inflammation may be a symptom of an allergic reaction or the result of other skin conditions such a eczema or psoriasis.

Steroids are used to treat a wide variety of inflammatory skin problems. In some cases, steroids are taken orally and used topically at the same time. Usually minor skin problems are treated with the topical ointments and creams, which help relieve the redness and itching.

The topical steroids come in cream, ointment and aerosol form. Your doctor will choose the form best suited to your condition and will give you specific instructions on how to use it.

TOPICAL STEROIDS
Betamethasone
(bay ta meth′ a sone)

Brand names: Celestone, Diprosone, Uticort, Valisone

Betamethasone is a steroid or cortisonelike medicine that is used to relieve the redness, itching and discomfort of many skin problems. Like all other drugs of this type, betamethasone helps control the skin disease but does not cure it.

UNDESIRED EFFECTS
When you apply this medicine, a mild temporary stinging can be expected.

Betamethasone can cause burning, itching, blistering or peeling of the skin not present before using this medicine. If you experience any skin reactions or signs of irritation or infection when you use betamethasone, contact your doctor.

PRECAUTIONS
Before you start to use betamethasone, tell your doctor if you have any kind of infection. This medicine can hide the symptoms of infection or make it worse.

If you are using this medicine on a baby's diaper area, do not use tightly fitting diapers or plastic pants on the baby. These can increase the chance that betamethasone will be absorbed through the skin. Such absorption can result in side effects and affect the child's growth. Whenever this medicine is used on a child, keep in touch with your doctor.

Use betamethasone exactly as prescribed by your doctor. Do not use it more often or longer than your doctor has ordered. If this medicine is applied too often, the chances of absorption through the skin and of side effects are increased. Using too much on thin skin areas such as the face, armpits or groin can result in thinning of the skin and stretch marks.

Unless directed by your doctor, do not bandage or otherwise wrap the area of skin being treated. Betamethasone is absorbed more quickly and in greater amounts when the treated area is covered. Check with your doctor or pharmacist if you have any questions about this.

Your doctor has prescribed this medicine for a specific skin problem. Do not apply it to other parts of your body or use it for other problems unless you have your doctor's permission. Using betamethasone other than as directed by your doctor can create problems. This medicine should not be used against many kinds of bacterial, viral or fungal skin infections. Do not apply cosmetics, lotions or any other kind of skin preparations to the area being treated unless you first check with your doctor.

To help your doctor select the best treatment for you and your baby, tell him if you are pregnant, plan to become pregnant or are breast-feeding.

DOSAGE AND STORAGE

Your doctor will determine how often you should use betamethasone and how much you should use for each application. Carefully follow the instructions on your prescription label and ask your doctor or pharmacist to explain any part of the instructions you do not understand.

Betamethasone comes in ointment, cream, gel, lotion and aerosol form. Before applying it, clean your skin. Then apply a small amount and rub it in gently. If you are using the aerosol form, avoid breathing in the vapors from the spray. Do not use the aerosol form near heat or an open flame or while smoking.

If you forget a dose, apply it as soon as you remember. Then use the other applications at evenly spaced intervals. *Do not use twice as much to make up for the missed application.*

When your doctor tells you to stop using betamethasone, throw away any unused portion of the medication. Do not puncture, break or burn the aerosol container.

Keep betamethasone in the container it came in. Store the aerosol form away from heat and direct sunlight. Keep this medicine out of the reach of children. Do not allow anyone else to use your betamethasone, since another person's skin problem may be very different from yours.

Fluocinolone and Fluocinonide
(floo oh sin' oh lone) (floo oh sin' oh nide)

Brand names for fluocinolone: Fluonid, Flurosyn, Synalar, Synemol; for fluocinonide: Lidex, Topsyn

Fluocinolone and fluocinonide are closely related steroids or cortisonelike drugs that are applied to the skin to help relieve the redness, itching and discomfort of many kinds of skin problems. The drugs control symptoms of the disease but do not cure it.

UNDESIRED EFFECTS

When you apply any forms of these medicines (ointment, cream, gel or solution), you can expect a mild temporary stinging.

The drug can cause burning, itching, blistering or peeling of the skin not present before using this medicine. Check with your doctor if you develop any skin reactions or signs of irritation or infection.

PRECAUTIONS

Before you start to use fluocinolone or fluocinonide, tell your doctor if you have any type of infection. These medicines can hide the symptoms of infection or make it worse.

If you are using either of these medicines on a baby's diaper area, do not use tightly fitting diapers or plastic pants on the baby. These can increase the chance that the medicine will be absorbed through the baby's skin. Such absorption can cause side effects and affect the baby's growth. Have your doctor check the baby frequently while you are using this medicine.

Do not use fluocinolone or fluocinonide more often or for a longer period of time than ordered by your doctor. If these medicines are applied too often, the chances of absorption through the skin are increased and side effects are more likely to occur. Thinning of the skin and stretch marks can occur if you use too much of these medicines on thin skin areas such as the face, armpits or groin.

Do not bandage or wrap the area of skin being treated, unless your doctor has told you to do so. These medicines are absorbed more quickly and in larger amounts when the treated area is covered. If you have any questions about this, check with your doctor or pharmacist.

Do not use these medicines for any problems except those for which they were prescribed; do not apply them to other parts of your body unless you have your doctor's permission. These medicines should not be used on many kinds of bacterial, viral or fungal skin infections, and only your doctor is qualified to determine the kind of skin problem you have. Do not apply cosmetics, lotions or any other kind of skin preparation to the area being treated unless you first check with your doctor.

Be sure to tell your doctor if you are pregnant or plan to become pregnant while you are using these medicines. He can then select the best treatment for both you and your baby.

DOSAGE AND STORAGE

Your doctor will determine how often you should use these medicines and how much you should apply at each dose. Carefully follow the instructions on your prescription label and ask your doctor or pharmacist to explain any part of the instructions you do not understand.

Fluocinolone and fluocinonide come in ointment, cream, gel or solution forms. Apply small amounts to clean skin and rub in gently. If your doctor has directed you to use a bandage or plastic film over the medicine, be sure you understand how to do this properly. Carefully follow your doctor's directions.

If you forget a dose, apply it as soon as you remember. Then apply the other doses at evenly spaced intervals. *Do not apply a double dose to make up for a missed one.*

If the skin problem for which either of these medicines was prescribed continues or gets worse, contact your doctor. When your doctor tells you to stop using these medicines, throw away any unused portions.

Keep fluocinolone and fluocinonide in the containers they came in. Keep them out of the reach of children. Do not allow anyone else to use your portions of these medicines, since another person's skin problem may be very different from yours.

Flurandrenolide
(flure an dren' oh lide)

Brand name: Cordran

Flurandrenolide is a steroid or cortisonelike medicine that is applied to the skin to help relieve the redness, itching and discomfort of many skin problems. It controls symptoms of skin disease but does not cure it.

UNDESIRED EFFECTS

When you apply the cream, lotion or ointment forms of this medicine, you probably will experience a mild temporary stinging.

Flurandrenolide can cause burning, itching, blistering or peeling of the skin not present before using this medicine. Contact your doctor if you have any skin reactions or signs of infection or irritation that were not present before you started to use flurandrenolide.

PRECAUTIONS

Before you start using flurandrenolide, tell your doctor if you have any kind of infection. This medicine hides the symptoms of infection and can make an infection worse.

If you are using this medicine on a baby's diaper area, do not use tightly fitting diapers or plastic pants on the baby. These can increase the chance that flurandrenolide will be absorbed through the baby's skin. Such absorption can cause side effects and affect your baby's growth. The baby should be checked regularly by the doctor to determine the effect the medicine is having.

Do not use flurandrenolide more often or longer than prescribed by your doctor. Applied too often, this medicine is more likely to be absorbed into the skin and cause side effects. If you use too much of this medicine on thin skin areas such as the face, armpits or groin, thinning of the skin and stretch marks may result.

Unless your doctor has told you to do so, do not bandage or wrap the area of skin being treated. When the treated area is covered, flurandrenolide is absorbed more quickly and in larger amounts. If you have any questions about this, check with your doctor or pharmacist.

Do not apply this medicine to areas of the body other than those your doctor has prescribed it for unless you have his permission. Flurandrenolide should not be used on many kinds of bacterial, viral and fungal infections. If you develop a problem on another part of your body, see your doctor. Check with him before you apply cosmetics, lotions or any other kind of skin preparation to the area being treated.

Before you start to use flurandrenolide, tell your doctor if you are pregnant or plan to become pregnant while you are using this medicine. The safe use of this medicine for pregnant women has not been established.

DOSAGE AND STORAGE

Your doctor will determine how often you should use this medicine and how much you should apply at each dose. Carefully follow the instructions on your prescription label and ask your doctor or pharmacist to explain any part of the instructions you do not understand.

Flurandrenolide comes in cream, lotion and ointment form and as a dressing tape. If you are using the cream, lotion or ointment, apply it to clean skin in small amounts and rub it in gently. The tape should be applied according to the directions. Do not use the tape under your arms, between your toes or in the groin area.

If you forget a dose, apply it as soon as you remember. Then apply the other doses at evenly spaced intervals. *Do not apply a double dose to make up for the missed one.*

When your doctor tells you to stop using flurandrenolide, throw away any unused portion. If your condition does not improve or if it gets worse, contact your doctor.

Keep flurandrenolide in the container it came in and keep it out of the reach of children. Do not allow anyone else to use your flurandrenolide, since another person's skin problem may be very different from yours and may require medical attention.

Hydrocortisone
(hye dro cor' ti sone)

Brand names: Aeroseb-HC, Acticort, Alphaderm, Anusol HC, Bactin, Carmol-HC, Cetacort, Cortaid, Cort-Dome, Cortef, Cortenema, Cortifoam, Cortiprel, Cortril, Cotacort, Cremesone, Delacort, Dermacort, Dermolate, Econsone, Eldecort, Epicort, Epifoam-HC, HC, Heb-Cort, Hexaderm, Hycort, Hytone, Kort, Lexocort, Microcort, My-Cort, Nutracort, Orabase HCA, Proctocort, Proctofoam-HC, Rectoid, Relecort, Texacort, Ulcort, Westcort and others

Hydrocortisone is a steroid or cortisonelike medicine that is applied to the skin to relieve the redness, itching and discomfort of many skin problems. The drug controls the skin disease but does not cure it.

The paste form of hydrocortisone is applied to inflamed areas of ulcers in the mouth to provide temporary relief. Hydrocortisone enema and hydrocortisone foam are used with other types of therapy to relieve the inflammation of mild to moderate ulcerative colitis. Hydrocortisone rectal suppositories help relieve the redness and swelling of hemorrhoids.

UNDESIRED EFFECTS

When applied to the skin, the cream, gel, lotion, solution or aerosol forms of hydrocortisone will cause a mild temporary stinging.

Hydrocortisone can cause burning, itching, blistering or peeling of the skin not present before using it. With all forms of this medicine, if you have any skin reaction or signs of irritation or infection, contact your doctor.

PRECAUTIONS

Before you start to use any form of hydrocortisone, tell your doctor if you have any kind of infection. This medicine may make the infection worse or hide an infection until it becomes a serious problem.

If you are using this medicine for a problem in your mouth, contact your doctor if your condition does not improve in one week or gets worse, or if you notice signs of a throat or mouth infection.

When you use this medicine on a baby's diaper area, do not use tightly fitting diapers or plastic pants, which can increase the chance of absorption through the baby's skin. Absorption of hydrocortisone can result in side effects and affect your baby's growth. The baby should be checked regularly by a doctor to determine the effect the medicine is having.

Use hydrocortisone exactly as directed by your doctor. Do not use it more often or longer than your doctor has ordered. If this medicine is used too often there is a greater chance that it will be absorbed through the skin and cause side effects. If too much of this medicine is used on areas with thin skin such as the face, armpits or groin, it can cause thinning of the skin and stretch marks.

Do not bandage or wrap the area of skin being treated unless your doctor has told you to do so. Covering the treated area can cause the medicine to be absorbed more quickly and in larger amounts. Contact your doctor or pharmacist if you have any questions about this.

Your doctor has prescribed hydrocortisone for a particular skin problem. Do not use it on other parts of your body. See your doctor if you develop a problem on another part of you body. This medicine should not be used against many kinds of bacterial, viral and fungal infections. Do not apply cosmetics, lotions or any other kind of skin preparation to the skin area being treated unless you have your doctor's permission.

Before you start to use hydrocortisone, tell your doctor if you are pregnant, plan to become pregnant or are breast-feeding.

DOSAGE AND STORAGE

Your doctor will determine how often you should use this medicine and how much you should apply at each dose. Carefully follow the instructions on your prescription label and ask your doctor or pharmacist to explain any part of the instructions you do not understand.

Hydrocortisone comes in cream, gel, lotion, solution and aerosol forms to be applied to the skin and in enema, foam and suppository forms to be placed in the rectum, as well as in oral paste form. Your doctor will select the best form for your particular problem.

Cream, gel, lotion or solution should be applied to clean skin in small amounts and rubbed in gently. If your doctor has directed you to use a bandage or plastic film over the medicine, be sure you understand how to do this properly. Carefully follow his instructions.

Aerosol spray should be used according to the directions that come with this form. It is important that you do not breathe in the vapors from the spray. Do not use the spray near heat, close to an open flame or while smoking.

The enema form comes with instructions that you should carefully read and follow. Lie on your left side while taking the enema and for 30 minutes afterward. Try to hold the enema for at least an hour or, better still, overnight. Keep in touch with your doctor while you are using the hydrocortisone enema so your progress can be checked and you can be told when to start using it less frequently.

Hydrocortisone rectal foam also comes with directions. Carefully read them before you use this form. A special applicator is provided and always should be used to apply the foam. *Do not insert any part of the aerosol container into the rectum.* After using the applicator, pull it apart and clean it thoroughly with warm water.

To use the rectal suppositories, remove the foil wrapper and dip the tip of the suppository into water. Lie on your side, draw your top knee up to your chest and insert the suppository. Push it well up into the rectum with your finger and hold it there for a few moments. If the suppository is too soft to insert because it has been stored in a warm place, chill it in the refrigerator for 30 minutes or run cold water over it before removing the foil wrapper.

If you are using the oral paste form, press but do not rub a small amount of paste onto the area to be treated until the paste sticks and forms a smooth, slippery film. Apply hydrocortisone film at bedtime (so the medicine can work overnight) and after meals.

If you forget to apply a dose of hydrocortisone, do so as soon as you remember and then apply the other doses at evenly spaced intervals. *Do not apply a double dose to make up for a missed dose.*

When your doctor tells you to stop using hydrocortisone, throw away any unused portions. Do not puncture or burn the aerosol can.

Keep hydrocortisone in the container it came in. Store the aerosol container away from heat and direct sunlight. Keep this medicine out of the reach of children.

Do not allow anyone else to use your hydrocortisone, since another person's skin problem may be very different from yours and may require medical attention.

Other Skin Problems

TOPICAL ANESTHETIC
Benzocaine
(ben′ zoe kane)

Brand names: Americaine, Dermacoat, Dermoplast

Benzocaine is an anesthetic that is a common ingredient in preparations to relieve sore throat, hemorrhoids, arthritis pain, pain in the mouth, toothache and cold sores. When applied to the skin, benzocaine relieves the pain or itching of insect bites, prickly heat, chafed skin, sunburn and minor cuts and scrapes. It also relieves rectal and genital itching.

Undesired Effects
In people who are sensitive to benzocaine, it can cause an allergic reaction. If you have signs of irritation not present before you began to use this medicine, stop using it and contact your doctor.

Precautions
If you have ever had an unusual reaction to benzocaine, do not use any preparation containing this medicine. Check the labels of nonprescription drugs carefully. If you have any questions about this, ask your doctor or pharmacist. Do not use benzocaine near your eyes, or for a long period of time.

Dosage and Storage
Because most benzocaine preparations are nonprescription anesthetics, carefully follow the instructions on the package. If you have any questions about how to use these preparations, ask your pharmacist. Aerosol spray and foam preparations have special instructions. Be sure you know how to use them properly.

Keep benzocaine preparations in the containers they came in and keep them out of the reach of children.

ASTHMA AND OTHER BREATHING PROBLEMS

DRUGS USED TO TREAT ASTHMA AND OTHER BREATHING PROBLEMS

See also Steroids under
Drugs Used to Treat Arthritis

ASTHMA

Asthma is a condition characterized by repeated attacks of wheezing, shortness of breath, difficulty in breathing and occasionally pain in the chest. During an attack of asthma, the air passages—primarily the bronchi in the lungs—narrow and go into spasm. The spasms occur in response to stimulation or irritation by, for example, pollen from trees or flowers or from emotional stress, excitement or any number of other causes. When the air passages are in spasm, air flow is partially obstructed, causing wheezing, shortness of breath and difficult breathing.

Narrowing of the air passages also occurs in bronchial infection and pulmonary emphysema and in some kinds of congestive heart failure. It is often difficult even for a doctor to diagnose asthma and to distinguish it from other conditions that cause breathing problems.

Drugs used to treat asthma are called bronchodilators. They relax the muscle spasm in the air passages and relieve shortness of breath. Relief usually is quick—within an hour for tablets taken orally and within 20 minutes for products used by inhalation. If a bronchodilator does not provide excellent and rapid relief from an asthma attack, the patient should seek medical attention immediately.

Some drugs are useful only in *preventing* attacks of asthma and will not help to stop an attack once it has started. Other drugs can be used to stop an attack once it is under way.

Drugs described here, with the exception of cromolyn (page 203), are used in the treatment and prevention of asthma, chronic bronchitis, emphysema and other lung diseases. Cromolyn is not a bronchodilator and is used only to prevent asthma.

Steroids may be used to treat bronchial asthma in the form of an inhalation or tablets taken orally. By injection, steroids also can be used to treat acute episodes of asthma. Prolonged treatment of asthma with steroids should be reserved for patients with disabling asthma that is not responsive to other drugs.

BRONCHODILATORS
Aminophylline
(am in off' i lin)

Brand names: Aminodur, Lixaminol, Panamin, Somphyllin and others
Note: Similar drugs in the same chemical family and having similar uses, undesired effects and precautions are: dyphylline, brand names Airet, Dilor, Lufyllin, Neothylline; oxtriphylline, brand name Choledyl; theophylline, brand names Bronkodyl, Elixophyllin, Slo-Phyllin, Somophyllin, Theo-Dur, Theolair;

and theophylline sodium glycinate, brand name Synophylate. There are many products containing aminophylline or one of these similar drugs in combination with other drugs. A few of the brand names are: Brondecon, Mudrane, Quibron, Theokin.

Aminophylline is a bronchodilator, which means it opens air passages in the lungs to make it easier to breath. It is particularly effective when wheezing, shortness of breath and other breathing problems are caused by spasm of the air passages. It is used primarily to treat bronchial asthma, chronic bronchitis, emphysema and other lung problems.

UNDESIRED EFFECTS

One of the most common side effects of aminophylline is irritation of the stomach and bowels. When you start to take this medicine, you may experience nausea, vomiting, stomach pain, abdominal cramps, loss of appetite and, rarely, diarrhea. These effects can be relieved by taking the medicine with meals or a light snack. If you continue to have these problems, contact your doctor.

Aminophylline also stimulates the central nervous system and can cause headache, irritability, nervousness, restlessness, trouble sleeping and dizziness or lightheadedness. These effects usually are more severe in children than in adults. If you experience these effects and they do not lessen or disappear as you continue to take aminophylline and as your body adjusts to it, contact your doctor. He may want to adjust the dose or change your medication.

Other effects, which are usually temporary, are flushing or redness of the face and fast breathing.

If you get a skin rash or hives from aminophylline, it means you are allergic to it. Stop taking it and contact your doctor.

Overdose can be a problem with aminophylline, particularly with the rectal suppository form. Some signs of overdose are cloudy urine, increased urination, mental confusion, muscle twitching, unusual thirst, unusual tiredness or weakness, unusually fast or irregular heartbeat, bloody or black stools and vomiting up blood or material that looks like coffee grounds. Contact you doctor at once if you have any of these effects.

PRECAUTIONS

If you have ever had an unusual reaction to aminophylline, caffeine, dyphylline, oxtriphylline or theophylline, tell your doctor before you start to take this medicine.

Aminophylline can make certain medical problems worse. Be sure to tell your doctor if you have an enlarged prostate, heart or blood vessel disease, high blood pressure, kidney or liver disease, overactive thyroid, porphyria or stomach ulcer.

Certain medications should not be taken while you are taking aminophylline. Tell your doctor what other prescription or nonprescription drugs you are taking, including erythromycins, lithium, other medicine for your heart or for asthma or other breathing problems, propranolol (medicine for high blood pressure), clindamycin and lincomycin. If you do not know the names of the drugs or what they were prescribed for, bring them in their labeled containers to your doctor or pharmacist.

Many nonprescription medicines for relief of asthma or breathing problems contain theophylline—a drug closely related to aminophylline. Taking theophylline and aminophylline together can cause upset stomach, nausea and vomiting or overdose (see **undesired effects**.) To avoid taking these drugs together without realizing it, *carefully check the labels of nonprescription medicines you are taking to make sure they do not contain theophylline*. If you have any questions about this, ask your doctor or pharmacist.

Beverages that also stimulate the central nervous system, such as tea, coffee, cocoa and colas, should not be consumed in large amounts while you are taking aminophylline.

Take aminophylline exactly as your doctor has directed. It can be harmful if you take more of it, take it more often or take it for a longer time than ordered by your doctor.

Your doctor will want to check your response to this drug, especially for the first few weeks after you begin to take it. *Be sure to keep all your appointments with your doctor*.

Aminophylline has been used by pregnant women without harm to the unborn child. However, it should not be used by women who are breast-feeding babies. Be sure to tell your doctor if you are nursing a baby.

DOSAGE AND STORAGE

Aminophylline comes in tablets, extended-release tablets, liquid to be taken orally, rectal suppositories and solution for enema.

Your doctor will determine which form is best for you and will instruct you how often to take this medicine and how much to take at each dose. Carefully follow the instructions on your prescription label and ask your doctor or pharmacist to explain any part of the instructions you do not understand.

The tablets should be swallowed whole. Do not break, crush or chew them before swallowing them. They are best taken with a full glass of water 30 minutes to one hour before meals. However, if the tablets upset your stomach, take them with meals or a snack.

Measure the oral liquid with a specially marked measuring spoon to ensure an accurate dose.

Rectal suppositories should be stored in the refrigerator. Take special care to keep them in a part of the refrigerator where they cannot be reached by small children and be sure the suppositories will not be mistaken for food either by adults or children. Aminophylline suppositories can be harmful if they are chewed or swallowed, especially by small children.

The suppositories come with directions for their use. Carefully follow these directions. Take the suppositories out of the refrigerator a few minutes before using them and let them warm at room temperature. If you are to use only part of a suppository, cut it lengthwise to the right size before inserting it. Remove the wrapper and dip the tip of the suppository in water. Lie on your side, draw your top knee up to your chest and insert the suppository well into the rectum with your finger. Hold it there for a few moments, then get up and resume your usual activities. Try not to have a bowel movement for at least an hour after inserting the suppository. If burning or other irritation of the rectal area occurs after you use the suppository and if it continues or becomes worse, contact your doctor.

The solution for enema comes with directions. Follow these directions carefully; if you have any questions about the use of this form, ask your pharmacist. If crystals form in the solution, dissolve them by placing the closed container of solution in warm water.

If you forget to take a dose of aminophylline, take it as soon as you remember and take any remaining doses for that day at evenly spaced intervals. *Do not take a double dose to make up for a missed dose.*

Keep all forms of aminophylline in the containers they came in. Store aminophylline suppositories in the refrigerator out of the reach of children. Keep all forms of this medicine out of the reach of children in a place away from excessive heat and moisture. Do not allow anyone else to take this medicine.

Ephedrine
(e fed′ rin)

Brand names: Ectasule Minus, Ephedsol and others

Brand names of some of the many products containing ephedrine in combination with other bronchodilators and other drugs are: Amesec, Bronkolixir, Bronkotabs, Marax, Mudrane, Quadrinal, Quibron, Tedral and others.

Ephedrine is used as a bronchodilator to relax the nerves of the lungs and enlarge the air passages to relieve wheezing, shortness of breath and difficult breathing. It is used in the prevention and treatment of asthma, chronic bronchitis, emphysema and other lung diseases. It also will relieve nasal congestion caused by hay fever and other allergies and is found in some colds products.

The injectable form of ephedrine is used to treat severe asthma attacks and, along with other measures, to treat shock. The oral forms often are used with other drugs to relieve the symptoms of myasthenia gravis.

UNDESIRED EFFECTS

The most common side effects of ephedrine are nervousness, restlessness and trouble sleeping. If you take the last dose for the day a few hours before bedtime, you should be able to sleep. Nervousness and restlessness may go away as you continue to take this medication and as your body adjusts to it. If these problems are persistent or severe, contact your doctor. He may want to adjust the dosage or change your medication.

Less often, ephedrine may cause difficult or painful urination, dizziness or lightheadedness, a feeling of warmth, headache, loss of appetite, nausea or vomiting, trembling, troubled breathing, increase in sweating, paleness, fast or pounding heartbeat or weakness. If you experience these effects, contact your doctor.

More serious effects of ephedrine are chest pain and irregular heartbeat. Stop taking the medicine and contact your doctor if you experience these effects.

High doses of ephedrine may give you hallucinations (seeing, hearing or feeling things that are not there) and mood or mental changes. If you have any of these problems, stop taking the medicine and contact your doctor.

PRECAUTIONS
Before you start to take a product containing ephedrine, tell your doctor or pharmacist if you have diabetes, an enlarged prostate, glaucoma, heart or blood vessel disease or an overactive thyroid. Ephedrine can make these conditions worse and should be taken only under a doctor's supervision.

Tell your doctor or pharmacist what prescription or nonprescription drugs you are taking. Ephedrine can increase or decrease the effects of amphetamines, digitalis drugs (heart medicine), medicine for high blood pressure such as propranolol, guanethidine or reserpine, other medicine for asthma, other medicine for hay fever or allergies, medicine to decrease bleeding after delivery of a baby (ergonovine or methylergonovine) and medicine for depression. If you do not know the names of the drugs you are taking or what they were prescribed for, bring them in their labeled containers to your doctor or pharmacist.

Because many of the products containing ephedrine are available without a prescription, be sure to use them only as directed on the package label or as instructed by your doctor. Do not take ephedrine more often than recommended on the label. If you have any questions about this, check with your doctor or pharmacist.

No one who has ever had an unusual reaction to medicines chemically similar to ephedrine (amphetamines, epinephrine, isoproterenol, metaproterenol, norepinephrine, phenylephrine, phenylpropanolamine, pseudoephedrine or terbutaline) should take ephedrine or products containing ephedrine.

Do not use ephedrine or products containing ephedrine if you are breastfeeding a baby. It will be passed to the baby through your milk. If you are pregnant, do not use any products containing ephedrine unless your doctor tells you to.

DOSAGE AND STORAGE
If your doctor has prescribed ephedrine, he has determined how often you should take this medicine and how much you should take at each dose. Carefully follow the instructions on your prescription label and ask your doctor or pharmacist to explain any part of the instructions you do not understand. If you have obtained ephedrine or a product containing it without a prescription, follow the instructions on the label or in the package.

Ephedrine comes in capsules, extended-release capsules, tablets and liquid form (all to be taken orally) and as a nasal solution and spray. If you are taking the extended-release capsules, be sure to swallow them whole. Do not crush, break or chew them before swallowing. If the capsule is too large to swallow, empty the contents into applesauce, jelly, honey or syrup. Stir to mix and then swallow without chewing.

Measure doses of the liquid with a specially marked measuring spoon to make sure you have an accurate dose.

If you forget to take a dose of ephedrine, take it as soon as you remember and then take the remaining doses for that day at evenly spaced intervals. If it is almost time for another dose, omit the missed dose and take only the regularly scheduled dose. *Do not take a double dose to make up for the missed dose.*

Keep ephedrine in the container it came in and keep it out of the reach of children. Do not allow anyone else to take your ephedrine.

Epinephrine
(ep i nef′ rin)

Brand names: Adrenalin, Bronkaid, Medihaler-Epi, microNEFRIN, Primatene, Sus-Phrine, S-2, Vaponefrin and others

Epinephrine is used as a bronchodilator to treat asthma, chronic bronchitis, emphysema and other lung diseases. It acts on the muscles and blood vessels of the lungs to open air passages by relieving muscle spasm, swelling and congestion. As a result, wheezing, shortness of breath and difficult breathing are relieved.

Epinephrine injection is used frequently in the *emergency* treatment of allergic reactions to insect stings, medicines, food and other substances. Some inhalation preparations of epinephrine are available without a prescription.

Undesired Effects

Use of inhaled epinephrine can cause dryness of the mouth and throat. If you rinse your mouth with water after using this medicine, you may be able to prevent this dryness. Coughing and other signs of bronchial irritation can occur after inhaling epinephrine. If these effects are severe, contact your doctor. He may want to change the strength of the solution you are using.

With the injectable form of epinephrine and sometimes with the inhalation form (because this medicine can be absorbed into the body through the tissues of the air passages), other effects may occur. The following effects usually decrease as you continue to use epinephrine and as your body adjusts to it: dizziness or lightheadedness; flushing or redness of the face or skin; headache; nausea or vomiting; nervousness, restlessness or trouble sleeping; trembling; troubled breathing; increase in sweating; paleness or weakness; and fast or pounding heartbeat. Contact your doctor if any of these effects are persistent or severe.

More serious side effects of epinephrine that may require medical attention are chest pain and irregular heartbeat. If you experience either of these, stop using the medicine and contact your doctor.

Precautions

Do not take epinephrine if you have ever had an unusual reaction to epinephrine or any of the medicines similar to it, such as amphetamines, ephedrine, isoproterenol, metaproterenol, norepinephrine, phenylephrine, phenylpropanolamine, pseudoephedrine or terbutaline.

Before you start to use epinephrine, tell your doctor or pharmacist if you have diabetes, glaucoma, brain damage, heart or blood vessel disease, high blood pressure or an overactive thyroid. This medicine can make these conditions worse.

Tell your doctor or pharmacist what prescription or nonprescription drugs you are taking, including any of the epinephrinelike drugs (see above), oral medicine for diabetes, insulin, medicine for high blood pressure (such as guanethidine, propranolol or reserpine), medicine for pheochromocytoma or blood vessel disease (such as phenoxybenzamine, phentolamine or tolazoline), medicine for angina attacks (such as nitroglycerin), other medicine for asthma or breathing problems, sedatives or tranquilizers, medicine for depression, medicine to decrease bleeding after delivery of a baby (ergonovine or methylergonovine) and antihistamines. If you do not know the names of the drugs you are taking or what they were prescribed for, bring them in their labeled containers to your doctor or pharmacist.

Do not use the solution for inhalation or for injection if it has turned pinkish to brownish in color or if it is cloudy. This means the epinephrine has deteriorated and may no longer be effective.

Do not use the inhalation form of epinephrine without a doctor's prescription unless a doctor has diagnosed your problem as asthma. If you still have trouble breathing 20 minutes after using the inhalation form or if your condition gets worse, stop using the medicine and check with your doctor.

Use epinephrine exactly as directed. Do not use any more of it and do not use it any more often than recommended on the label. *Keep all appointments for checkups.*

If you have diabetes, epinephrine may cause your blood sugar levels to rise. Contact your doctor if you notice a change in the results of your urine sugar test.

Tell your doctor if you are pregnant or are nursing a baby. Epinephrine should not be used by women who are pregnant or think they may be or by women who are breast-feeding babies.

DOSAGE AND STORAGE

Your doctor will determine how often you should use epinephrine and how much you should use at each dose. Carefully follow the instructions on your prescription label and ask your doctor or pharmacist to explain any part of the instructions you do not understand.

Epinephrine comes in three forms—inhalation, aerosol inhalation and injection. If you use the inhalation form in a nebulizer or a combination nebulizer and respirator, be sure you understand exactly how to use it. If you have any questions, check with your doctor or pharmacist.

If you use the aerosol form, keep the spray away from your eyes. Do not take more than two inhalations at one time, unless directed otherwise by your doctor. Wait one or two minutes after the first inhalation to determine if you need a second one. Save your applicator because refill units of this medicine may be available.

If you use the injection form and plan to give yourself injections, be sure you know how to do this properly. If you have any questions about this, check with your doctor or pharmacist.

Keep all forms of epinephrine in the containers they came in and store them away from heat and direct sunlight. Do not puncture, break or burn the aerosol container.

Keep epinephrine out of the reach of children. Do not allow anyone else to use it.

Isoproterenol

(eye soe proe ter' e nole)

Brand names: Aerolone, Iprenol, Isuprel, Medihaler-Iso, Norisodrine, Proterenol, Vapo-N-Iso

Isoproterenol is used as a bronchodilator to relieve wheezing, shortness of breath and troubled breathing caused by asthma, chronic bronchitis, emphysema or other lung diseases. It does this by relaxing the muscles in the air passages in the lungs and by counteracting histamine, one of the body's natural substances that can cause spasm of the airways.

Isoproterenol is also used to treat certain heart disorders.

UNDESIRED EFFECTS

The most common effects of isoproterenol are dryness of the mouth and throat, nervousness, restlessness and trouble sleeping. You can experience dryness of the mouth and throat after using one of the inhalation forms of this medicine; the dryness can be relieved by rinsing your mouth with water after each inhalation. The other effects, which can result after you take any form of isoproterenol, tend to decrease as you continue to take it and as your body adjusts to it. If they continue or bother you, contact your doctor.

Less often, isoproterenol will cause dizziness or lightheadedness, flushing or redness of the face or skin, headache, nausea or vomiting, trembling, increase in sweating, fast or pounding heartbeat, or weakness. Contact your doctor if these effects are severe. He may want to adjust your dosage or change your medication.

More serious side effects, which require medical attention if they occur, are chest pain and irregular heartbeat. Stop using isoproterenol and contact your doctor if you experience either of these effects.

Isoproterenol may cause your saliva to turn pink or red. This effect is harmless and happens only because isoproterenol turns red when it is exposed to air.

Contact your doctor if your sputum (the matter you spit up during an asthma attack) becomes thickened or changes color from clear white to yellow, green or gray. These changes may be signs of an infection that requires immediate treatment.

PRECAUTIONS

Before you start to take isoproterenol, tell your doctor if you have ever had an unusual reaction to this drug or to similar drugs, including amphetamines, ephedrine, epinephrine, metaproterenol, norepinephrine, phenylephrine, phenylpropanolamine, pseudoephedrine or terbutaline.

Isoproterenol can make certain medical conditions worse. Be sure to tell your doctor if you have diabetes, heart or blood vessel disease, high blood pressure or an overactive thyroid.

Tell your doctor what prescription or nonprescription drugs you are taking, including amphetamines, any of the isoproterenollike drugs, other medicines for your heart or for asthma or other breathing problems, or propranolol (medicine for high blood pressure). If you do not know the names of the drugs or what they were prescribed for, bring them in their labeled containers to your doctor or pharmacist.

Do not use more than two inhalations of isoproterenol at one time. If, after you have used the inhalation form as instructed, you still have trouble breathing or your condition gets worse, contact your doctor at once.

Use this medicine only as you have been directed by your doctor. Do not use more of it and do not use it more often than instructed. *Keep all appointments for checkups.*

If you are using the inhalation form of isoproterenol, do not use the solution if it has turned pinkish or brownish in color or if it has become cloudy.

If you are pregnant or are nursing a baby, tell your doctor. He can then select the isoproterenol treatment that is best for both you and your baby.

DOSAGE AND STORAGE

Your doctor will determine how often you should take isoproterenol and how much you should take at each dose. Carefully follow the instructions on your prescription label and ask your doctor or pharmacist to explain any part of the instructions you do not understand.

Isoproterenol comes in a solution for inhalation, aerosol inhalation, tablets to be swallowed and tablets to be dissolved under the tongue. If you use the inhalation solution in a nebulizer, be sure you know exactly how to use it. With the dropper provided, place in the nebulizer only that amount of solution needed for a single day's treatment. If you have any questions about this, ask your doctor or pharmacist.

If you use the aerosol form, turn the inhaler upside down to use it. Place the mouthpiece in your mouth and close your lips and teeth around it. Breathe out as much air through your nose as you possibly can. Then take a deep breath through the mouthpiece and at the same time press down on the container. Be sure the mist goes into your throat and is not blocked by your teeth or tongue.

Hold your breath for five seconds, remove the inhaler and exhale through your nose. Wait one to five minutes to see whether you need another inhalation. Do not take more than two inhalations at one time.

If you give a treatment to a young child, it may be best to hold the child's nose closed to be sure the medication goes into his or her throat.

If you take the under-the-tongue tablets, do not chew or swallow the tablets. This medicine is absorbed through the lining of the mouth as it dissolves slowly under your tongue. Do not swallow until the tablets have dissolved completely.

If you take isoproterenol extended-release tablets, be sure to swallow the tablets whole. Do not break, crush or chew these tablets before swallowing them.

Keep isoproterenol in the container it came in and store it away from heat and direct sunlight. Save the aerosol container; refill units of this medicine may be available. Do not puncture, break or burn the aerosol container.

Keep this medicine out of the reach of children. Do not allow anyone else to take it.

Metaproterenol
(met a proe ter' e nole)

Brand names: Alupent, Metaprel

Metaproterenol is used as a bronchodilator to relax and increase the size of the air passages in the lungs and make it easier to breathe. It is used to relieve the wheezing, shortness of breath and difficult breathing associated with asthma, bronchitis, emphysema and other lung diseases.

Although metaproterenol is similar to isoproterenol, metaproterenol works for a longer period of time and is more effective when taken as a tablet.

UNDESIRED EFFECTS
The most common side effects of metaproterenol are nervousness and restlessness. Generally these effects tend to decrease as you continue to take metaproterenol and as your body adjusts to it. If they continue or are severe, contact your doctor. Using the inhalation form of metaproterenol may make your mouth and throat dry. To relieve this problem, rinse your mouth with water after each treatment.

You also may notice a bad taste in your mouth. This effect is harmless and will go away when you stop taking metaproterenol.

Less often, metaproterenol will cause dizziness or lightheadedness; headache; muscle cramps in the arms, hands or legs; nausea or vomiting; trembling; increase in sweating; fast or pounding heartbeat; or weakness. If you experience these effects and they are severe, contact your doctor.

More serious side effects are chest pain and irregular heartbeat. If these occur, they require medical attention. Stop taking the medicine and contact your doctor.

If your sputum (the matter you spit up during an asthma attack) becomes thick or changes color from clear white to yellow, gray or green, contact your doctor. These changes may be signs of an infection that requires immediate treatment.

PRECAUTIONS
People who have had an unusual reaction to metaproterenol in the past or to any of the drugs like metaproterenol should not take this medicine. Tell your doctor if you have had a reaction to amphetamines, ephedrine, epinephrine, isoproterenol, norepinephrine, phenylephrine, phenylpropanolamine, pseudoephedrine or terbutaline.

Before you start to take metaproterenol, tell your doctor if you have diabetes, heart or blood vessel disease, high blood pressure or an overactive thyroid. Metaproterenol may make these conditions worse.

Tell your doctor what prescription or nonprescription drugs you are taking, including amphetamines, other medicine for your heart or for asthma or other breathing problems, or propranolol (medicine for high blood pressure). If you do not know the names of the drugs or what they were prescribed for, take them in their labeled containers to your doctor or pharmacist.

Take this medicine exactly as directed. Do not take more of it and do not take it more often than your doctor has ordered. If you still have trouble breathing after you have used metaproterenol as directed, or if your condition gets worse, contact your doctor. *Keep all appointments for checkups.*

Metaproterenol should not be taken by children under the age of six or by pregnant women or nursing mothers. Be sure to tell your doctor if you are pregnant or think you may be or if you are breast-feeding a baby. This will help him select the best treatment for you and your baby.

DOSAGE AND STORAGE

Your doctor will determine how often you should take metaproterenol and how much you should take at each dose. Carefully follow the directions on your prescription label and ask your doctor or pharmacist to explain any part you do not understand.

Metaproterenol comes in a metered dose inhaler, and in tablets and liquid to be taken by mouth. If you are using the inhaler, turn it upside down and place the mouthpiece in your mouth. Close your lips and teeth around the mouthpiece and breathe out as much as possible through your nose. Then take a deep breath through the mouthpiece and at the same time press down on the container to spray the medication into your mouth. Hold your breath for five seconds. Remove the inhaler from your mouth and exhale through your nose or mouth. Wait one full minute to decide whether you need another treatment. Do not take more than two inhalations at one time.

If you take tablets or liquid on a regular basis and forget to take a dose, take it as soon as you remember. Take any remaining doses for that day at evenly spaced intervals. If you remember a missed dose at the time you are to take another, take only the regularly scheduled dose. Omit the missed dose entirely. *Do not take a double dose to make up for the missed one.*

Keep metaproterenol in the container it came in. Store it away from heat and direct sunlight. Keep it out of the reach of children. Do not allow anyone else to take your metaproterenol.

Terbutaline
(ter byoo′ ta leen)

Brand names: Brethine, Bricanyl
Terbutaline is used as a bronchodilator to relax the muscles of the air passages in the lungs, making it easier to breathe. It is used to relieve the wheezing, shortness of breath and other breathing problems caused by asthma, bronchitis

and emphysema. Terbutaline begins to work in 30 minutes and continues to work for four to eight hours.

UNDESIRED EFFECTS

Nervousness, restlessness and trembling are the most common effects of terbutaline. These effects tend to decrease or disappear as you continue to take terbutaline and as your body adjusts to it. If they persist or are severe, contact your doctor. He may want to adjust the dose or change your medication.

Other effects that do not require medical treatment unless they are severe are dizziness or lightheadedness, drowsiness, headache, muscle cramps or twitching, nausea or vomiting, increase in sweating, fast or pounding heartbeat and weakness.

PRECAUTIONS

If you have had an unusual reaction to terbutaline or to drugs like it, you should not take terbutaline. Before you start to take terbutaline, tell your doctor if you have ever had a reaction to amphetamines, ephedrine, epinephrine, isoproterenol, metaproterenol, norepinephrine, phenylephrine, phenylpropanolamine or pseudoephedrine.

If you have diabetes, heart disease, high blood pressure, an overactive thyroid or a history of seizures, tell your doctor before you start to take terbutaline.

Tell your doctor what prescription or nonprescription drugs you are taking, including amphetamines, other medicine for your heart or for asthma or other breathing problems, and propranolol (medicine for high blood pressure). If you do not know the names of the drugs you are taking or what they were prescribed for, bring them in their labeled containers to your doctor or pharmacist.

Take terbutaline exactly as your doctor has directed. Do not take more of it and do not take it more often than your doctor has told you. If you still have trouble breathing after using terbutaline, or if your condition becomes worse, contact your doctor at once. *Keep all appointments for checkups.*

If you are breast-feeding a baby or are pregnant or think you may become pregnant while taking terbutaline, tell your doctor. While problems have not been reported, your doctor will want to consider the benefit of this treatment to you against the possible risk to your baby.

DOSAGE AND STORAGE

Your doctor will determine how often you should take terbutaline tablets and how much you should take at each dose. Carefully follow the instructions on your prescription label and ask your doctor or pharmacist to explain any part of the instructions you do not understand.

If you forget to take a dose of terbutaline, take it as soon as you remember and take any remaining doses for that day at evenly spaced intervals. If you remember a missed dose when it is close to the time for you to take another, omit the missed dose and take only the regularly scheduled dose. *Do not take a double dose to make up for the missed dose.*

Keep terbutaline in the container it came in and keep it out of the reach of children. Do not allow anyone else to take your terbutaline.

OTHER DRUGS FOR ASTHMA
Corticosteroids
(kore ti kos' ter oids)

The body produces a number of hormones that are essential to good health. When too little of these hormones (cortisones) is produced, corticosteroids may be prescribed to help make up the difference.

In addition, corticosteroids are used to reduce inflammation, redness and swelling in various parts of the body and to relieve allergic reactions.

The oral forms (capsules, tablets and liquid) are used to relieve the symptoms of arthritis, asthma, severe allergies and skin problems. There is also a form that is injected directly into the joint for the treatment of arthritis.

Included in this group of medicines are both the natural hormone (hydrocortisone) and substances made in the laboratory (dexamethasone, prednisone, triamcinolone) that act in the body like the natural hormone.

UNDESIRED EFFECTS

The most common side effect of corticosteroids is stomach upset (heartburn, indigestion and stomach pain). Take the medicine with meals or a snack and contact your doctor if stomach upsets continue in spite of this precaution.

Other side effects, which may go away as your body adjusts to the medicine, are a false sense of well-being, increase in appetite, nervousness, restlessness, trouble in sleeping and weight gain. Contact your doctor if these effects are severe.

Short-term therapy: Serious side effects requiring medical attention are rare. However, you should contact your doctor if you have decreased or blurred vision, frequent urination, increased thirst or skin rash.

Long-term therapy: In addition to the above side effects, a corticosteroid can cause a number of other serious problems when it is taken over a long period of time. Contact your doctor if you develop acne or other skin problems, back or rib pain, bloody or black stools, continuing stomach pain or burning, depression, fever or sore throat, irregular heartbeats, menstrual problems, mood or mental changes, puffiness of the face, muscle cramps or pains, muscle weakness, nausea or vomiting, seeing halos around lights, swelling of the feet or lower legs, unusual tiredness or weakness.

If you take a corticosteroid over a period of time, your body may need time to adjust after you stop taking this medicine. During this period of adjustment, be alert for side effects. Contact your doctor if you have fever, dizziness or fainting, muscle or joint pain, nausea or vomiting, loss of appetite for several days, shortness of breath, unusual tiredness or weakness or unusual weight loss.

PRECAUTIONS

Because a corticosteroid can make certain medical conditions worse, tell your doctor if you have bone disease, colitis, diabetes, diverticulitis, glaucoma, heart disease, herpes simplex of the eyes, high blood pressure, high cholesterol levels, fungal infection, kidney disease or kidney stones, liver disease, myasthenia gravis, stomach ulcer or other stomach problems, tuberculosis (positive skin test, partially healed TB or a history of TB) or underactive thyroid.

Before you start to take a corticosteroid, tell your doctor what prescription or nonprescription drugs you are taking, including amphotericin B, anticoagulants (blood thinners), aspirin or other salicylates, oral diabetes medicine, digitalis, diuretics (water pills), medicine for high blood pressure, other arthritis medicines, insulin, phenobarbital, phenytoin, rifampin and somatropin.

If you do not know the names of the drugs you are taking or what they were prescribed for, bring them in their labeled containers to your doctor or pharmacist.

A corticosteroid must be taken regularly to be effective. Take it exactly as prescribed by your doctor. Do not take more of it, do not take it more often and do not take it for a longer period of time than your doctor has ordered.

Keep in touch with your doctor while you are taking this medicine. He may want to adjust the dose as he checks your response to the corticosteroid. *Keep all your appointments with your doctor.*

Do not stop taking this medicine without first checking with your doctor. He may want you to reduce gradually the amount you are taking before you stop completely. When your doctor tells you to stop taking this medicine, throw away any unused portion.

Your doctor may instruct you to weigh yourself every day. Be sure to report any unusual weight gain and follow his instructions about cutting down on your intake of calories. He also may want you to follow a low-salt or potassium-rich diet.

Tell every doctor or dentist who treats you that you are taking a corticosteroid. You should wear a Medic-Alert bracelet or some other kind of identification in case of accident or other kind of medical emergency. Ask your pharmacist how to get this kind of identification.

Do not have a vaccination, other immunization or any type of skin test while you are taking a corticosteroid unless your doctor specifically tells you that you may.

If you have diabetes, this medicine may cause blood sugar levels to rise. If you notice a change in the results of your urine sugar test or if you have any questions, check with your doctor.

While you are taking a corticosteroid, do not take aspirin, Anacin, Excedrin or Bufferin unless you ask your doctor how many of these tablets you may take.

Because a corticosteroid can harm the growth of an unborn child and a nursing baby, be sure to tell your doctor if you are pregnant or are breast-feeding a baby before you take a corticosteroid. If you become pregnant while taking this medicine, notify your doctor immediately.

Cromolyn
(kroe' moe lin)

Brand names: Aarane, Intal

Cromolyn is used to prevent asthma attacks that occur when small cells in the body known as mast cells release materials that irritate the airways and make it difficult for persons with asthma to breathe. Cromolyn coats the mast cells so they cannot release these materials.

This medicine is used only to *prevent* asthma attacks. It will not help against an asthma attack that has already started.

UNDESIRED EFFECTS

The most common side effects of cromolyn are cough, hoarseness, dryness of the mouth and throat irritation. Gargling or rinsing your mouth after inhaling this medicine may help to prevent these effects. If these effects continue or are bothersome, contact your doctor.

More serious effects, which may require medical attention, are tightness in the chest, wheezing, troubled breathing or swallowing, difficult or painful urination, frequent urge to urinate, dizziness, joint pain or swelling, muscle pain or weakness, nausea or vomiting, headache, skin rash or itching and swelling of the lips and eyes. If you experience any of these effects, stop using cromolyn and contact your doctor.

PRECAUTIONS

Because cromolyn is available only mixed with lactose powder, tell your doctor if you have ever had an unusual reaction to lactose, milk or milk products. You should not take cromolyn if you are allergic to it or to milk.

Before you start taking cromolyn, tell your doctor if you have kidney disease or liver disease. Cromolyn may make these conditions worse.

Do not use cromolyn during an asthma attack because it may make the attack worse. If you have any questions about this, check with your doctor.

If you are also using a bronchodilator inhaler to help your breathing, use the bronchodilator first, wait several minutes, and then use the cromolyn inhaler. If you also are taking a steroid such as cortisone or prednisone for your asthma along with cromolyn, do not stop taking the steroid even if your asthma seems better.

It may take up to four weeks for you to feel the benefits of cromolyn. However, if your symptoms do not improve or if your condition gets worse, contact your doctor. *Keep all appointments for checkups.*

Children under five years of age and pregnant women should not use cromolyn. Safe use of this drug during pregnancy has not yet been established, although problems have not been reported.

DOSAGE AND STORAGE

Cromolyn usually is used four times a day. Your doctor will determine how often you should use it. Carefully follow the instructions on your prescription

label and ask your doctor or pharmacist to explain any part of the instructions you do not understand.

Cromolyn comes in a capsule and is used with a special inhaler. Directions are included with the inhaler. Carefully read the directions before using this medicine. Proper use will lessen the possibility of throat and mouth irritation from the powder.

Do not swallow the capsules. This medicine must be inhaled every day in regularly spaced doses as prescribed by your doctor for it to be effective.

Clean your inhaler at least once a week. Take the inhaler apart and rinse it in clean, warm water. *Do not use soap.* Allow the inhaler to dry in the air before you use it again. If properly cared for, the inhaler should last about six months.

If you forget to take a dose of cromolyn, take the missed dose as soon as you remember it. Take any remaining doses for that day at regularly spaced intervals. *Do not take a double dose.*

Keep cromolyn capsules in the container they came in and store them away from moisture and temperatures of more than 100 degrees Fahrenheit. Keep cromolyn out of the reach of children and do not allow anyone else to take it.

ALLERGIES, COLDS AND COUGHS

MEDICATIONS FOR ALLERGIES, COLDS AND COUGHS

Allergies, Colds and Coughs

The common cold is caused by a number of different viruses that are spread only by contact with persons who are already infected. Although chill and dampness do not cause colds, they may make a person more susceptible to catching one.

Symptoms of a cold usually begin one to four days after contact with the virus. They include nasal congestion and discharge, sneezing, sore throat, headache, chills and cough. In some cases, a mild fever may occur.

In healthy persons, the symptoms last five to seven days and complications are rare. Children and the elderly are more likely to develop complications such as sinus infection, ear infections and pneumonia. It is for this reason that antibiotics sometimes are prescribed for individuals with the common cold. Antibiotics are ineffective against the cold itself but they do prevent bacterial infections.

Cough results from irritation of the throat by postnasal drip. Cough is one of the body's natural reflexes that serves to keep the airways clear. Two types of medications are used to treat coughs—cough suppressants and expectorants. The cough suppressants are best used for dry coughs. Expectorants are used to thin phlegm and make it easier to cough up. In either case, it is very helpful to drink a lot of fluids. In severe cases, a humidifier may be used to keep the throat moist.

The symptoms of allergies are similar to those of the common cold. Nasal congestion, running nose, sneezing and itching, watery eyes usually are present. Pollens are the most common causes of allergic reactions and the seasonal appearance of symptoms is directly related to the amount of pollen in the air. Although pollens are the most common causes of allergic reactions, dust, animal dander, feathers and many other things can cause allergic reactions.

Several types of medications are used to treat allergies, including antihistamines and decongestants. Both types help relieve nasal congestion. Antihistamines act to prevent part of the allergic reaction itself, while the decongestants relieve symptoms after they occur. Many combination products are available that contain both types of medication.

MEDICATIONS FOR ALLERGIES

ANTIHISTAMINES

Histamine is a natural substance that is present throughout the body. It remains stored in cells until something that produces an allergic reaction (for example, pollen) comes in contact with the body. When this happens, histamine is released to produce allergy symptoms such as itching, watery eyes, rashes and runny nose.

Antihistamines are drugs that relieve allergy symptoms by counteracting the effects of histamine. These ingredients are present in many nonprescription cough medicines and cold products. Because drowsiness is a common side effect of some antihistamines, they are used in some nonprescription sleep aids.

When used correctly at recommended dosages, antihistamines rarely cause serious side effects. They may cause drowsiness, dryness of the mouth and stomach upset. These effects usually are minor, but if they are severe or persistent, you should contact your doctor or pharmacist.

Use of alcohol, tranquilizers, sleeping pills, narcotics and medications for seizures may increase the drowsiness caused by antihistamines. Check with your doctor or pharmacist before taking antihistamines with these other medications.

Because antihistamines can cause drowsiness, you should not drive or operate dangerous machinery until you know how antihistamines will affect you.

If you have an enlarged prostate, heart disease, high blood pressure, glaucoma, thyroid problems or ulcers, check with your doctor or pharmacist before taking antihistamines.

Women who are pregnant or breast-feeding should check with their doctor before using antihistamines.

Brompheniramine
(brome fen eer' a meen)

Brand names: B.P.E., Dimetane, Puretane, Rolabromophen, Spentane, Steraphenate, Veltane and others

Brand names of some products containing brompheniramine: Brocon, Dimetapp, Dynohist, Histapp, Phenatapp, Poly-Histine, Puretapp and others

Brompheniramine is one of a group of drugs called antihistamines. These drugs are used to counteract the effects of histamine, one of the body's natural substances. Antihistamines relieve the symptoms of allergy such as itching, watery eyes and runny nose by counteracting histamine. Antihistamines also are used for allergic reactions to bee stings, poison ivy and poison oak. Brompheniramine is available alone or in combination with decongestants, cough medicine, expectorants and pain medicine.

UNDESIRED EFFECTS
One common effect of brompheniramine is dryness of the mouth. This can be relieved by chewing gum, sucking hard candies or drinking fluids.

Brompheniramine also can upset your stomach. If it does, take it with meals or a snack. Contact your doctor if this does not help or if the upsets are severe.

Brompheniramine causes some people to become dizzy or drowsy. Do not drive a car or operate dangerous machinery until you know how this medicine will affect you. With children, the effect can be just the opposite and they may become nervous or restless or have trouble sleeping.

Other side effects include blurred vision, difficult or painful urination, headache, loss of appetite, skin rash, unusual increase in sweating and unusually fast heartbeat. If you experience any of these effects, contact your doctor or pharmacist.

PRECAUTIONS

Before you start taking brompheniramine, tell your doctor if you have an enlarged prostate, heart disease, high blood pressure, glaucoma, overactive thyroid, stomach ulcer or urinary tract blockage. People with these conditions should not take antihistamines such as brompheniramine. If you are considering using one of the products that can be obtained without a prescription, discuss this with your pharmacist.

Tell your doctor or pharmacist what prescription or nonprescription drugs you are taking, including barbiturates, medicine for seizures, narcotics, other medicine for hay fever or allergies, prescription medicine for pain, sedatives, tranquilizers, medicine to help you sleep and medicine for depression. If you do not know the names of the drugs you are taking or what they were prescribed for, bring them in their labeled containers to your doctor or pharmacist.

Do not start to take any of the drugs listed above while you are taking brompheniramine unless you first check with your doctor or pharmacist.

Do not drink alcoholic beverages while you are taking brompheniramine. Alcohol can increase the chance or severity of drowsiness and dizziness.

Antihistamines are used to relieve or prevent the symptoms of allergy and should be used only as directed. Do not take more of this medicine than your doctor or label instructions prescribe.

If you are pregnant or are breast-feeding a baby, do not take brompheniramine unless your doctor prescribes it for you and is aware of your pregnancy or the fact that you are breast-feeding.

DOSAGE AND STORAGE

If your doctor prescribes brompheniramine or a product containing this drug, he will tell you how often to take it and how much to take at each dose. Carefully follow the instructions on your prescription label and ask your doctor or pharmacist to explain any part of the instructions you do not understand. If you obtain brompheniramine without a prescription, follow the instructions on the label or in the carton carefully. If you have any questions about this, check with your pharmacist. Do not give brompheniramine to infants without your doctor's approval.

Brompheniramine is available in liquid, tablets and extended-release tablets. If you are taking the extended-release tablets, be sure to swallow them whole. Do not break, crush or chew them before swallowing.

Keep brompheniramine in the container it came in, and keep it out of the reach of children.

Carbinoxamine
(kar bi nox' a meen)

Brand names: Clistin, Clistin R-A

Brand names of products containing carbinoxamine: Clistin Expectorant, Clistin C, Rondec, Rondec DM

Carbinoxamine is an antihistamine used alone or with cough suppressants, decongestants, expectorants or pain medicine to relieve the symptoms of colds and allergies.

UNDESIRED EFFECTS

Drowsiness is the most common side effect. Do not drive a car or operate dangerous machinery until you know how carbinoxamine will affect you. Often drowsiness will disappear after a few days when your body has adjusted to carbinoxamine. If drowsiness continues or is severe, contact your doctor. He may want to adjust your dose or change your medicine.

Carbinoxamine also can cause dizziness, poor coordination and muscle weakness, particularly in older people. In children, the effect often is just the opposite, making them restless, nervous and unable to sleep. Contact your doctor if these effects are severe or continue for a period of time.

If carbinoxamine upsets your stomach or gives you stomach pain, take it with meals or a snack. If your mouth is dry, chew gum or suck candy.

Other effects of carbinoxamine are blurred vision, difficult or painful urination, headache, loss of appetite, skin rash, unusual increase in sweating and unusually fast heartbeat. Contact your doctor if you experience these effects.

PRECAUTIONS

Some products containing carbinoxamine are available without a prescription, but it is wise to get medical advice before you start to take these medicines. Tell your doctor or pharmacist if you have medical problems such as an enlarged prostate, heart disease, high blood pressure, glaucoma, an overactive thyroid, stomach ulcer or urinary tract blockage. Use of carbinoxamine may make these problems worse.

Certain medications can increase the possibility or the severity of carbinoxamine's side effects. Tell your doctor or pharmacist if you are taking barbiturates, medicine for seizures, narcotics, medicine for allergy, prescription medicine for pain, sedatives, tranquilizers, medicine to help you sleep or medicine for depression. If you do not know the names of the drugs you are taking or what they were prescribed for, bring them in their labeled containers to your doctor or pharmacist.

While you are taking carbinoxamine, do not drink alcoholic beverages or start to take any of the drugs listed above unless you first check with your doctor or pharmacist.

Carbinoxamine is used to relieve the symptoms of your medical problem and should be used with care. Do not take any more of it and do not take it more often than you have been directed.

Before having surgery with a general anesthetic, including dental surgery, tell the doctor or dentist that you are taking carbinoxamine.

To help your doctor select the best treatment for you and your baby, tell him if you are pregnant or are breast-feeding a baby.

DOSAGE AND STORAGE

If carbinoxamine was prescribed for you, your doctor has determined how often you should take it and how much you should take at each dose. Carefully follow the directions on your prescription label and ask your doctor or pharmacist to explain any part of the directions you do not understand. If you have obtained carbinoxamine without a prescription, check with your pharmacist on the proper way to use it.

Carbinoxamine comes in liquid, tablets and extended-release tablets. If you are taking the extended-release tablets, be sure to swallow them whole. Do not crack, crush or chew them. Take the tablets with a full eight-ounce glass of water. Use a specially marked measuring spoon to measure the liquid to ensure a proper dose.

Keep carbinoxamine in the container it came in, and keep it out of the reach of children. Do not allow anyone else to take your carbinoxamine.

Chlorpheniramine
(klor fen eer′ a meen)

Brand names: Allerbid, AL-R, Chloramate, Chlor-Span, Chlortab, Chlor-Trimeton, Ciramine, Histaspan, Histex, Panahist, Phenetron, T.D. Alermine, Teldrin and others.

Brand names of some of the many products containing chlorpheniramine: Anamine, Anatuss, Chlorfed, Codimal, Colrex, Comhist, Comtrex, Coricidin, Corilin, Coryban-D, CoTylenol, Decon-Aid, Deconamine, Decon-Tuss, Demazin, Extendryl, 4-Way Cold Tablets, Fedahist, Guistrey, Histabid, Hista-Clopine, Histadyl, Histalet, Historal, Isoclor, Korigesic, Kronohist, Naldecon, Napril, Nasalspan, Neotep, Nilcol, Nolamine, Norel Plus, Novafed, Novahistine, Ornade, P-V-Tussin, Pediacof, Probacon, Pseudo-Hist, Quelidrine, Rhinex, Romex, Ru-Tuss, Ryna, Rynatan, Rynatuss, Singlet, Sinovan, Sinulin, Sudafed-Plus, Triaminic, Tusquelin, Tussar, Tussi-Organidin, Tuss-Ornade and others.

Chlorpheniramine is an antihistamine that causes less drowsiness and more central nervous system stimulation than some antihistamines. It is particularly suited for daytime relief of the symptoms of colds and allergies. In addition to being used alone, chlorpheniramine is combined with pain medicine, other antihistamines, cough suppressants, decongestants, expectorants and bronchodilators.

UNDESIRED EFFECTS

One of the most common effects of chlorpheniramine is dryness of the mouth. This can be relieved by sucking hard candies, chewing gum or drinking fluids.

Chlorpheniramine may upset your stomach or give you stomach pains. If you take the medicine with a glass of milk, a snack or at mealtime, these problems may be helped. If they continue or are severe, contact you doctor.

Chlorpheniramine may make some people drowsy or dizzy. Do not drive a car or operate dangerous machinery until you know how this medicine will affect you. This effect is more common with older people. Children, on the other hand, may become restless and nervous and have trouble sleeping after they have been taking chlorpheniramine. If these effects continue for a period of time or are bothersome, contact your doctor.

Other side effects of chlorpheniramine include blurred vision, difficult or painful urination, headache, loss of appetite, skin rash, unusual increase in sweating and unusually fast heartbeat. If you experience these effects, contact your doctor.

PRECAUTIONS

If you have certain medical conditions you probably should not take chlorpheniramine or other antihistamines because these medicines can make the conditions worse. Since several of the products containing chlorpheniramine are available without a prescription, you should have medical advice concerning their use if you have an enlarged prostate, heart disease, high blood pressure, glaucoma, overactive thyroid, stomach ulcer or urinary tract blockage. Check with your doctor or pharmacist if you have any of these conditions.

Tell your doctor or pharmacist what prescription or nonprescription drugs you are taking, particularly barbiturates, medicine for seizures, narcotics, other medicines for allergy, medicine for pain, sedatives, tranquilizers, medicine to help you sleep, medicine for depression and MAO (monoamine oxidase) inhibitors. If you do not know the names of the drugs or what they were prescribed for, bring them in their labeled containers to your doctor or pharmacist.

While you are taking chlorpheniramine, do not drink alcoholic beverages or start to take any of the drugs listed above unless you first check with your doctor or pharmacist. All of these drugs can increase the chance or severity of drowsiness or dizziness.

Because chlorpheniramine is intended only to relieve the symptoms of your medical problem, it should be used with care. Do not take more than recommended and do not take it more often than prescribed by your doctor or directed on the package label.

Before having surgery (including dental surgery) with a general anesthetic, tell the doctor or dentist in charge that you are taking chlorpheniramine.

To help your doctor select the best treatment for you and your baby, tell him if you are pregnant or are breast-feeding. This drug can be passed to your unborn baby or breast-fed baby and also may decrease the quantity of your milk.

DOSAGE AND STORAGE

Carefully follow the instructions of your doctor or pharmacist or those on the package of chlorpheniramine products that you purchase without a prescription.

If you have any questions about the instructions, check with your pharmacist.

Do not give chlorpheniramine to infants without your doctor's approval. Chlorpheniramine is available in liquid, tablets, extended-release tablets and extended-release capsules. If you are taking the extended-release tablets or capsules, be sure to swallow them whole. Do not crack, crush or chew them. Take all tablets and capsules with a full glass of water, or with food if they upset your stomach. To ensure an accurate dose of liquid, use a specially marked measuring spoon.

Keep chlorpheniramine in the container it came in, and keep it out of the reach of children.

Cyproheptadine
(si proe hep' ta deen)

Brand name: Periactin

Cyproheptadine, an antihistamine, is used to relieve the symptoms of hay fever, bee stings, poison ivy, poison oak and colds. It also is used to treat some types of migraine headaches and, in some cases, to help gain weight.

UNDESIRED EFFECTS
One of the most common side effects of cyproheptadine, dryness of the mouth and throat, can be relieved by sucking on hard candy, chewing gum or drinking fluids.

Cyproheptadine may upset your stomach when you first begin to take it. To lessen this problem, take the medicine with milk or solid food.

Cyproheptadine makes some people drowsy or dizzy. Do not drive a car or operate dangerous machinery until you know how this medicine will affect you.

These effects may go away as your body adjusts to the medicine. If they continue or are severe, contact your doctor.

Other side effects of cyproheptadine include blurred vision, difficult or painful urination, headache, increased appetite or weight gain, nervousness, restlessness or trouble sleeping (especially in children), skin rash, unusual increase in sweating and unusually fast heartbeat. If you experience these effects and they are troublesome, contact your doctor.

PRECAUTIONS
Before you start to take cyproheptadine, tell your doctor if you have an enlarged prostate, heart disease, high blood pressure, glaucoma, an overactive thyroid, a stomach ulcer or urinary tract blockage. Cyproheptadine can make these conditions worse.

Tell your doctor what prescription or nonprescription drugs you are taking. Certain other drugs should not be taken with cyproheptadine, including medicine for seizures, narcotics, other medicines for allergy, prescription medicine for pain, sedatives, tranquilizers, medicine to help you sleep and medicine for depression. If you do not know the names of the drugs you are taking or what they were prescribed for, bring them in their labeled containers to your doctor or pharmacist.

Do not start to take any of the drugs listed above while you are taking cyproheptadine unless you first check with your doctor. Before you have surgery with a general anesthetic, including dental surgery, tell the doctor or dentist in charge that you are taking cyproheptadine.

Take this medicine exactly as directed. Do not take more of it and do not take it more often than your doctor has indicated.

Do not drink alcoholic beverages while you are taking cyproheptadine, because alcohol can increase the chance and severity of drowsiness.

To help your doctor select the best treatment for you and your baby, tell him if you are pregnant or are breast-feeding. Cyproheptadine can be passed to your unborn child or your breast-fed baby. It also can decrease the amount of your milk.

DOSAGE AND STORAGE

Your doctor will determine how often you should take cyproheptadine and how much you should take at each dose. Carefully follow the instructions on your prescription label and ask your doctor or pharmacist to explain any part of the instructions you do not understand.

Cyproheptadine comes in liquid and tablets. Take the tablets with a full eight-ounce glass of water or, if this medicine upsets your stomach, with a glass of milk or solid food. Use a specially marked measuring spoon to ensure a liquid dose that is accurate.

If you forget to take a dose, take it as soon as you remember it and take the remaining doses for the day at evenly spaced intervals. *Do not take a double dose to make up for the missed dose.*

Keep cyproheptadine in the container it came in, and keep it out of the reach of children. Do not allow anyone else to take your cyproheptadine.

Dexbrompheniramine
(dex brome fen eer' a meen)

Brand names: Disophrol, Drixoral

Dexbrompheniramine is an antihistamine very closely related to brompheniramine in chemical structure and in action. However, dexbrompheniramine is almost twice as effective as brompheniramine. Dexbrompheniramine is available only in combination with the decongestant pseudoephedrine. This combination is used to relieve the symptoms of respiratory allergies.

UNDESIRED EFFECTS

Two common effects of dexbrompheniramine are dryness of the mouth and throat and upset stomach. Dryness can be relieved by chewing gum, sucking on hard candy or drinking fluids. Stomach upset is less likely if you take this medicine with a glass of milk or with food. If these effects are severe or continue in spite of what you do, check with your doctor.

Although dexbrompheniramine causes less drowsiness than some other antihistamines, it can make some people drowsy or dizzy, particularly older people.

Do not drive a car or operate dangerous machinery until you know how this medicine will affect you. Drowsiness or dizziness may decrease or disappear as your body adjusts to dexbrompheniramine. If it does not or is severe, contact your doctor.

Dexbrompheniramine can have just the opposite effect on children, making them nervous or restless and making it difficult for them to sleep. If these effects occur, contact your doctor. He may want to adjust the dose or change the medication.

Other effects of dexbrompheniramine include blurred vision, difficult or painful urination, headache, loss of appetite, skin rash, unusual sweating or unusually fast heartbeat. Contact your doctor if these effects are severe.

PRECAUTIONS

Before you start to take one of the products containing dexbrompheniramine, tell your doctor if you have an enlarged prostate, heart disease, high blood pressure, glaucoma, an overactive thyroid, a stomach ulcer or urinary tract blockage. Dexbrompheniramine can make these conditions worse.

Tell your doctor what prescription or nonprescription drugs you are taking, especially barbiturates, medicine for seizures, narcotics, other medicines for allergy, prescription medicine for pain, sedatives, tranquilizers, medicine to help you sleep and medicine for depression. If you do not know the names of the drugs you are taking or what they were prescribed for, bring them in their labeled containers to your doctor or pharmacist.

Do not drink alcoholic beverages while you are taking dexbrompheniramine. They can increase the chance of or the severity of drowsiness. Do not start to take any of the drugs listed above until you first check with your doctor.

Before you have surgery with a general anesthetic, including dental surgery, tell the doctor or dentist that you are taking dexbrompheniramine.

Take dexbrompheniramine exactly as prescribed by your doctor. Do not take more of it and do not take it more often than instructed.

If you are pregnant or breast-feeding, check with your doctor before using dexbrompheniramine.

Products containing dexbrompheniramine should not be given to children under the age of 12.

DOSAGE AND STORAGE

Your doctor will determine how often you should take a product containing dexbrompheniramine and how much you should take at each dose. Carefully follow the instructions on your prescription label and ask your doctor or pharmacist to explain any part of the instructions you do not understand.

Dexbrompheniramine and pseudoephedrine are combined in tablets and extended-release tablets. If you are taking the extended-release tablets, be sure to swallow them whole. They should not be broken, crushed or chewed before being swallowed.

If you forget to take a dose of the medicine, take it as soon as you remember and then take the remaining doses for that day at evenly spaced intervals. *Do not take a double dose to make up for a missed dose.*

Keep dexbrompheniramine in the container it came in, and keep it out of the reach of children. Do not allow anyone else to take your dexbrompheniramine.

Dexchlorpheniramine
(dex klor fen eer′ a meen)

Brand name: Polaramine

Dexchlorpheniramine is an antihistamine that is similar in chemical structure and effect to chlorpheniramine. However, dexchlorpheniramine is much stronger than chlorpheniramine, and only about half as much dexchlorpheniramine is needed to achieve the same relief of symptoms of hay fever, bee stings, poison oak and poison ivy as chlorpheniramine.

UNDESIRED EFFECTS

Dexchlorpheniramine may make your mouth and throat dry. If this occurs, chew gum, suck hard candy or drink fluids. Dexchlorpheniramine also can cause stomach upsets, which usually decrease if you take this medicine with a glass of milk or food. If stomach upsets continue in spite of these precautions, contact your doctor.

Dexchlorpheniramine makes some people drowsy or dizzy. Do not drive a car or operate dangerous machinery until you know how this medicine will affect you. These problems are more likely to occur in older people. On the other hand, children may become nervous or restless or have trouble sleeping. When these effects are severe, contact your doctor.

Other side effects that dexchlorpheniramine can cause include blurred vision, difficult or painful urination, headache, loss of appetite, skin rash, unusual increase in sweating or unusually fast heartbeat. These effects usually decrease as your body adjusts to the medicine. However, if they are persistent or severe, contact your doctor.

PRECAUTIONS

Before you start to take dexchlorpheniramine, tell your doctor if you have an enlarged prostate, heart disease, high blood pressure, glaucoma, an overactive thyroid, a stomach ulcer or urinary tract blockage. This medicine could make such conditions worse.

Certain medications, when you take them with dexchlorpheniramine, can increase the chance of or the severity of side effects. Some of these are barbiturates, medicine for seizures, narcotics, other medicines for allergy, prescription medicine for pain, sedatives, tranquilizers, medicine to help you sleep and medicine for depression. Tell your doctor what prescription or nonprescription drugs you are taking. If you do not know the names of the drugs or what they were prescribed for, bring them in their labeled containers to your doctor or pharmacist.

Do not drink alcoholic beverages while you are taking dexchlorpheniramine because alcohol can make drowsiness more severe. Do not start to take any of the drugs listed above unless you first check with your doctor.

Take dexchlorpheniramine exactly as directed by your doctor. Do not take more of it and do not take it more often than instructed.

To help your doctor select the best treatment for you and your baby, tell him if you are pregnant or are nursing a baby.

DOSAGE AND STORAGE

Your doctor will determine how often you should take dexchlorpheniramine and how much you should take at each dose. Carefully follow the instructions on your prescription label and ask your doctor or pharmacist to explain any part of the instructions you do not understand.

Dexchlorpheniramine comes in liquid, tablets and extended-release tablets. If you are taking the extended-release tablets, be sure to swallow them whole. They should not be broken, crushed or chewed before they are swallowed.
• Tablets may be taken with a glass of milk or food if this medicine upsets your stomach. Use a specially marked measuring spoon to ensure an accurate dose of liquid.

If you forget to take a dose of dexchlorpheniramine, take it as soon as you remember. Then take the other doses for that day at evenly spaced intervals. *Do not take a double dose to make up for a missed dose.*

Keep dexchlorpheniramine in the container it came in, and keep it out of the reach of children. Do not allow anyone else to take your dexchlorpheniramine.

Diphenhydramine
(dye fen hye′ dra meen)

Brand names: Allerben, Benadryl, Bendylate, Benylin, Fenylhist, SK-Diphenhydramine, Tussat, Valdrene

Diphenhydramine is an antihistamine with many more uses than other drugs of this type. In addition to being used to treat the symptoms of allergy (itchy, watery eyes and runny nose), it is also used to prevent motion sickness, to induce sleep and to decrease the stiffness and tremors of Parkinson's disease.

UNDESIRED EFFECTS

Drowsiness, dizziness and lack of coordination are the most common side effects of diphenhydramine. While they are desired effects when this medicine is used to induce sleep, they can be problems when your activities require mental alertness. Do not drive a car or operate dangerous machinery until you know how this medicine will affect you.

Older people are more likely to experience drowsiness after they take diphenhydramine and may require a smaller dose. Young children, however, may have the opposite effect with restlessness, nervousness and difficulty sleeping. Contact your doctor if these effects are severe. He may want to adjust the dose or change the medication.

Diphenhydramine causes less upset stomach than other antihistamines and may even be used to stop vomiting. However, if you should experience stomach upset or pain, take this medicine with a glass of milk or food. If stomach upsets continue or are severe, contact your doctor.

Other effects of diphenhydramine include blurred vision, difficult or painful urination, dryness of the mouth and throat, headache, loss of appetite, skin rash, unusual increase in sweating and unusually fast heartbeat. Contact your doctor if these effects continue beyond the first few days you take this medicine.

PRECAUTIONS
Because diphenhydramine can make some medical problems worse, tell your doctor if you have an enlarged prostate, heart disease, high blood pressure, glaucoma, an overactive thyroid, a stomach ulcer or urinary tract blockage.

Certain medications, when you take them with diphenhydramine, can increase the chance of or severity of side effects. These include medicine for seizures, narcotics, other medicines for allergy, prescription medicines for pain, sedatives, tranquilizers, medicine to help you sleep and medicine for depression. Tell your doctor what prescription or nonprescription drugs you are taking. If you do not know the names of the drugs or what they were prescribed for, bring them in their labeled containers to your doctor or pharmacist.

Do not drink alcoholic beverages while you are taking diphenhydramine. They will increase the drowsiness and dizziness. Do not start to take any of the drugs listed above unless you have permission from your doctor.

Take diphenhydramine exactly as directed by your doctor. Do not take more of it and do not take it more often than instructed.

Before having surgery with a general anesthetic, including dental surgery, tell the doctor or dentist in charge that you are taking diphenhydramine.

Diphenhydramine should not be taken by pregnant women or by nursing mothers. Be sure to tell your doctor if you are pregnant or if you are breast-feeding.

DOSAGE AND STORAGE
Your doctor will determine how often you should take diphenhydramine and how much you should take at each dose. Carefully follow the instructions on your prescription label and ask your doctor or pharmacist to explain any part of the instructions you do not understand.

Diphenhydramine comes in capsules, tablets and liquid. Use a specially marked measuring spoon to measure a dose of liquid so that your dose will be accurate.

If you forget to take a dose of this medicine, take it as soon as you remember. Then take the remaining doses for that day at evenly spaced intervals. *Do not take a double dose to make up for a missed dose.*

Keep diphenhydramine in the container it came in, and keep it out of the reach of children. Do not allow anyone else to take your diphenhydramine.

Phenyltoloxamine
(fen ill toe lox' a meen)

Brand names of products containing phenyltoloxamine: Naldecon, Sinubid, Norel Plus, Poly-Histine-D

Phenyltoloxamine is an antihistamine that is combined with other antihistamines, decongestants or pain medicines to relieve sinus congestion resulting from allergy, colds or infection.

UNDESIRED EFFECTS

Phenyltoloxamine can cause upset stomach, diarrhea or stomach pain. If you have any of these effects, take phenyltoloxamine with solid food or with a glass of milk.

Phenyltoloxamine causes some people to become drowsy, dizzy or less alert than usual. This is especially true for older people. Do not drive a car or operate dangerous machinery until you know how this medicine will affect you.

Children often have effects that are just the opposite—trouble sleeping, nervousness, unusually fast heartbeat, weakness and even convulsions.

Dryness of the mouth, nose or throat occurs frequently after taking phenyltoloxamine. Chewing gum or sucking on hard candies can relieve this.

Other side effects of phenyltoloxamine are blurred vision, difficult or painful urination and hives. If you experience these effects they often will disappear as your body adjusts to the medication. If they are persistent or severe, contact your doctor.

PRECAUTIONS

Before you start to take any product containing phenyltoloxamine, tell your doctor if you have heart disease, high blood pressure, an enlarged prostate, glaucoma, an overactive thyroid, a stomach ulcer or urinary tract blockage.

There are several drugs that you should not take with phenyltoloxamine because they increase the possibility of side effects. These include barbiturates; medicine for seizures; narcotics; other antihistamines or medicine for hay fever, other allergies or colds; prescription pain medicine; sedatives; tranquilizers; medicine to help you sleep and medicine for depression.

Tell your doctor what other prescription or nonprescription drugs you are taking. If you do not know the names of the drugs or what they were prescribed for, bring them in their labeled containers to your doctor or pharmacist. Be sure not to start to take any of the drugs mentioned above while you are taking a product with phenyltoloxamine in it unless you first check with your doctor.

Alcohol will increase the drowsiness caused by phenyltoloxamine and should be used sparingly or not at all while you are taking this medicine. If you have any questions about this, check with your doctor or pharmacist.

Tell your doctor if you are pregnant or think you might be or if you are breast-feeding. This will help your doctor select the best treatment for you and your baby.

DOSAGE AND STORAGE

Your doctor will determine how often you should take a product containing phenyltoloxamine and how much to take at each dose. Carefully follow the instructions on your prescription label. Do not take more than prescribed nor more often than recommended. If you have questions about your prescription instructions, ask your doctor or pharmacist.

Keep a product containing phenyltoloxamine in the container it came in. Keep it out of the reach of children.

Promethazine
(proe meth' a zeen)

Brand names: Phenergan, Quadnite, Remsed, ZiPAN

Promethazine is a very versatile antihistamine. In addition to relieving symptoms of allergy, it is used as a sedative or tranquilizer before surgery and may be combined with medicine for pain for greater relief of pain. In addition, promethazine can be used to prevent and treat nausea from anesthesia and motion sickness.

UNDESIRED EFFECTS

The most common effects of promethazine are drowsiness and mental confusion. Do not drive a car, operate dangerous machinery or perform other tasks that require mental alertness until you know how this medicine will affect you.

If promethazine makes your mouth and throat dry, suck hard candies, chew gum or drink fluids.

Promethazine also can cause blurred vision, difficult or painful urination, headache, loss of appetite, nervousness, restlessness or difficulty sleeping (especially in children), skin rash, unusual sweating or unusually fast heartbeat. If you experience these effects, they should decrease as you continue to take promethazine and as your body adjusts to it. However, if they are persistent or severe, contact your doctor.

Rarely, a person who takes promethazine will be unusually sensitive to sunlight. Restrict the amount of time you spend in sunlight until you know whether this will happen to you. If you experience a severe sunburn, contact your doctor.

Occasionally promethazine may affect the facial muscles or make swallowing difficult. If either of these effects occurs, contact your doctor.

PRECAUTIONS

Promethazine can make certain medical problems worse. To help your doctor select the treatment best for you, tell him if you have seizures, blood disorders, an enlarged prostate, heart disease, high blood pressure, glaucoma, an overactive thyroid, a stomach ulcer or urinary tract blockage.

When taken with promethazine, certain medications can increase the chance of or the severity of side effects. Tell your doctor what prescription or non-prescription drugs you are taking, including barbiturates, medicine for seizures, narcotics, other medicine for allergy, prescription medicine for pain, sedatives, tranquilizers, medicine to help you sleep and medicine for depression. If you do not know the names of the drugs or what they were prescribed for, bring them in their labeled containers to your doctor or pharmacist.

Do not drink alcoholic beverages while you are taking promethazine; this will increase your drowsiness. Do not start to take any of the drugs listed above until you first check with your doctor.

Take promethazine exactly as your doctor prescribes. Do not take more of it and do not take it more often than instructed.

It is not known whether promethazine can be passed from a mother to her unborn baby or whether it is passed through the milk to a nursing baby. However, it would be wise to tell your doctor if you are pregnant or are breast-feeding a baby before you start to take this medicine.

DOSAGE AND STORAGE

Your doctor will determine how often you should take promethazine and how much you should take at each dose. Carefully follow the instructions on your prescription label and ask your doctor or pharmacist to explain any part of the instructions you do not understand.

Promethazine comes in capsules, tablets, liquid and suppositories. It is best to take capsules and tablets with a full eight-ounce glass of water. Liquid doses, to be accurate, should be measured with a specially marked spoon.

Suppositories should be used in the following way. Remove the wrapper or covering from the suppository and dip the tip of the suppository in water. Lie on your left side and raise your right knee to your chest. Insert the suppository into the rectum and hold it there for a few moments. You may then get up and resume your normal activities. Try to avoid having a bowel movement for about one hour after inserting the suppository. If you have any questions about this, check with your doctor or pharmacist.

If you forget to take a dose, take it as soon as you remember. Take any remaining doses for that day at evenly spaced intervals. If you remember a missed dose when it is time for you to take another, omit the missed dose entirely and take only the regularly scheduled dose. *Do not take a double dose to make up for the missed dose.*

Keep promethazine in the container it came in, and keep it out of the reach of children. Do not allow anyone else to take your promethazine.

Tripelennamine
(tri pel enn′ a meen)

Brand name: PBZ

Tripelennamine is an antihistamine used to prevent or relieve the symptoms of hay fever, bee stings, poison oak and poison ivy. Tripelennamine counteracts the effects of histamine, one of the body's natural substances, which causes some of the symptoms of allergy such as itchy, watery eyes and runny nose.

Undesired Effects

Upset stomach and stomach pain are two common side effects of tripelennamine. If this medicine upsets your stomach, take it with a glass of milk or with solid food. Contact your doctor if upsets continue or are severe. Tripelennamine also can make your mouth and throat dry. To relieve this, suck on hard candies, chew gum or drink fluids.

Tripelennamine makes some people drowsy or dizzy. Do not drive a car or operate dangerous machinery until you know how this medicine will affect you. As your body adjusts to tripelennamine the drowsiness and dizziness should decrease. Contact your doctor if they are troublesome.

Other, less common effects of tripelennamine are blurred vision, difficult or painful urination, headache, loss of appetite, nervousness, restlessness or trouble sleeping (especially in children), skin rash, unusual increase in sweating and unusually fast heartbeat. These effects usually decrease as your body adjusts to the medication. However, if they are persistent or severe, contact your doctor. He may want to adjust your dose or change your medication.

Precautions

Tripelennamine can make certain medical conditions worse. Be sure to tell your doctor if you have an enlarged prostate, heart disease, high blood pressure, glaucoma, an overactive thyroid, a stomach ulcer or urinary tract blockage.

Tell your doctor what prescription or nonprescription drugs you are taking, including barbiturates, medicine for seizures, narcotics, other medicine for allergy, prescription medicine for pain, sedatives, tranquilizers, medicine to help you sleep and medicine for depression. These drugs when taken with tripelennamine can increase the chance of or the severity of side effects.

If you do not know the names of the drugs you are taking or what they were prescribed for, bring them in their labeled containers to your doctor or pharmacist.

Do not drink alcoholic beverages while you are taking tripelennamine because alcohol can increase the severity of drowsiness and dizziness. Do not start to take any of the drugs listed above until you first check with your doctor.

Tripelennamine should be taken exactly as directed by your doctor. Do not take more of it and do not take it more often than instructed.

Before having surgery with a general anesthetic, including dental surgery, tell the doctor or dentist in charge that you are taking tripelennamine.

Tripelennamine should not be taken by women who are pregnant or breast-feeding. Tell your doctor if you are breast-feeding or if you are pregnant. This information will help him select the treatment best for you and your baby.

Dosage and Storage

Your doctor will determine how often you should take tripelennamine and how much you should take at each dose. Carefully follow the instructions on your prescription label and ask your doctor or pharmacist to explain any part of the instructions you do not understand.

Tripelennamine comes liquid, regular tablets and extended-release tablets.

If you are taking the extended-release tablets, be sure to swallow them whole. Do not break, crush or chew them before swallowing. To get an accurate dose of the liquid, use a specially marked measuring spoon. Take this medicine with milk or solid food if it upsets your stomach.

If you forget to take a dose, take it as soon as you remember. Then take the remaining doses for that day at evenly spaced intervals. If you remember a dose when it is almost time for another, omit the missed dose entirely and take only the regularly scheduled dose. *Do not take a double dose to make up for the missed one.*

Keep this medicine in the container it came in, and keep it out of the reach of children. Do not allow anyone else to take your tripelennamine.

Triprolidine
(trye proe' li deen)

Brand name: Actidil
Brand names of products containing triprolidine: Actifed, Acti-Prem
Triprolidine is an antihistamine used to prevent or relieve the symptoms of hay fever, bee stings, poison ivy and poison oak. Triprolidine causes less drowsiness than some other antihistamines and therefore is particularly good for daytime use.

UNDESIRED EFFECTS
Triprolidine often causes dry mouth and throat, which can be relieved by chewing gum, sucking hard candies or drinking fluids. Triprolidine also can upset your stomach or give you stomach pain. To prevent this, take triprolidine with milk or solid food. If stomach upsets continue or are severe, contact your doctor.

Although it causes less drowsiness than some other antihistamines, triprolidine can make some people drowsy or dizzy. Do not drive a car or operate dangerous machinery until you know how this drug will affect you.

Other effects of triprolidine that are less common are blurred vision, difficult or painful urination, headache, loss of appetite, nervousness, restlessness or difficulty sleeping (especially in children), skin rash, unusual sweating and unusually fast heartbeat. When these effects occur, they tend to disappear after you take the medicine for a few days. Contact your doctor if these effects are persistent or severe. He may want to adjust your dose or change your medication.

PRECAUTIONS
Before you start to take triprolidine, tell your doctor if you have heart trouble, high blood pressure, an enlarged prostate, glaucoma, an overactive thyroid, a stomach ulcer or urinary tract blockage. This drug may make these medical conditions worse.

Tell your doctor what prescription or nonprescription drugs you are taking, particularly barbiturates, medicine for seizures, narcotics, other medicine for allergy, prescription medicine for pain, sedatives, tranquilizers, medicine to help you sleep and medicine for depression. If you do not know the names of the drugs or what they were prescribed for, bring them in their labeled containers to your doctor or pharmacist.

Do not drink alcoholic beverages while you are taking triprolidine, and do not start to take any of the drugs listed above until you first check with your doctor. All these drugs can increase the chance of and the severity of drowsiness.

Triprolidine should be taken exactly as prescribed by your doctor. Do not take more of it and do not take it more often than directed.

Before having surgery with a general anesthetic, including dental surgery, tell the doctor or dentist that you are taking triprolidine.

Triprolidine should not be taken by women who are breast-feeding and probably should not be used by pregnant women, since it is not known whether triprolidine is safe for the unborn child.

DOSAGE AND STORAGE

Your doctor will determine how often you should take triprolidine and how much you should take at each dose. Carefully follow the instructions on your prescription label and ask your doctor or pharmacist to explain any part of the instructions you do not understand.

Triprolidine comes in liquid and tablets. Measure a dose of liquid medicine with a specially marked spoon to assure an accurate dose. Take this medicine with milk or solid food if it upsets your stomach.

If you forget to take a dose, take it as soon as you remember and take the remaining doses for that day at evenly spaced intervals. If you remember a missed dose when it is time to take another, omit the missed dose entirely and take only the regularly scheduled dose. *Do not take a double dose to make up for the missed dose.*

Keep triprolidine in the container it came in. Keep this medicine out of the reach of children, and do not allow anyone else to take your triprolidine.

MEDICATIONS FOR COLDS

DECONGESTANTS

Decongestant medications are used to relieve stuffy or runny nose caused by colds. Decongestants are available as oral tablets, as capsules, in liquid form and as nasal sprays and drops.

If you are using nose drops, follow these instructions:
1. Blow your nose gently.
2. Wash your hands thoroughly with soap and water.
3. Check the dropper tip for chips or cracks.
4. The nose drops must be kept clean. Avoid touching the dropper against the nose or anything else.
5. Draw the medicine into the dropper.
6. Lie on a flat surface, such as a bed, hang your head over the edge and tilt your head back as far as is comfortable.

7. Place the prescribed number of drops into the nose.
8. To allow the medication to spread in the nose, remain in this position for a few minutes.
9. Replace the dropper in the bottle right away.
10. Wash your hands to remove any medicine.

If you are using nose spray, follow these instructions:
1. Blow your nose gently.
2. Wash your hands thoroughly with soap and water.
3. Hold your head erect and spray once or twice into each nostril. Sniff the medicine into your nose as you spray.
4. Wait three to five minutes for the medicine to work.
5. Blow your nose again and repeat the spraying, if needed.
6. Rinse the tip of the spray bottle with hot water.
7. Wipe the tip dry with a clean tissue and replace the cap.
8. Wash your hands to remove any medicine.

Isopropamide
(eye so proe′ pa mide)

Brand name: Darbid
Brand names of products containing isopropamide: CPI, Tuss-Aid, Vernate and others
Isopropamide is a drying agent used with an antihistamine and a nasal decongestant to relieve sneezing, running nose and other symptoms of nasal congestion. Its drying effect lasts up to 12 hours.

UNDESIRED EFFECTS
Dry mouth is one of the most common side effects of isopropamide. To relieve this effect, chew gum or suck on hard candy. When you first start to take a product containing isopropamide it can cause blurred vision. This effect tends to decrease or disappear as your body adjusts to the medicine. However, contact your doctor if this effect persists or is severe.
If you experience difficulty with or pain on urination, contact your doctor.

PRECAUTIONS
Before you start to take any product containing isopropamide, tell your doctor if you have glaucoma, an enlarged prostate, obstruction of the stomach or small intestine or obstruction of the neck of the bladder.
Tell your doctor what other prescription or nonprescription drugs you are taking. If you do not know the names of the drugs or what they were prescribed for, bring them in their labeled containers to your doctor or pharmacist.

DOSAGE AND STORAGE
Carefully follow the instructions on your prescription label and ask your doctor or pharmacist to explain any part of the instructions you do not understand.
If you miss a dose of isopropamide, take only the next regularly scheduled

dose at the time it is due. *Do not take a double dose to make up for the missed dose.*

Keep isopropamide in the container it came in, and keep it out of the reach of children. Do not allow anyone else to take your isopropamide.

Oxymetazoline
(ox i met az′ oh leen)

Brand names: Afrin, Duration, St. Joseph's Spray

Oxymetazoline shrinks swollen blood vessels in the nose, reducing congestion and making it easier to breathe. Oxymetazoline is sprayed or dropped into the nose for temporary relief of congestion caused by colds or allergies.

UNDESIRED EFFECTS

When oxymetazoline is used for short periods of time in recommended doses, side effects are rare.

When sprayed or dropped into the nose, oxymetazoline may cause sneezing or temporary burning, dryness or stinging of the inside of the nose.

If oxymetazoline is used for too long a period or is used too often, it may be absorbed into the body and cause more serious side effects. If you develop headache or lightheadedness, an increase in runny or stuffy nose, pounding heartbeat or trouble in sleeping, stop using this medicine and contact your doctor.

PRECAUTIONS

Before you start taking oxymetazoline, tell your doctor or pharmacist if you have ever had an unusual reaction to nasal decongestants. You are more likely to have a reaction to oxymetazoline if you have ever had one after use of another nasal decongestant.

You should not use oxymetazoline if you have blood vessel disease, diabetes, high blood pressure or an overactive thyroid unless the doctor specifically tells you to. Before you use this medicine tell your doctor or pharmacist if you have any of these medical problems.

Tell your doctor or pharmacist what other prescription or nonprescription drugs you are taking, particularly whether you are now taking or have taken in the past two weeks any monoamine oxidase inhibitors such as isocarboxazid, pargyline, phenelzine and tranylcypromine. If you do not know the names of the drugs you are taking or what they were prescribed for, bring them in their labeled containers to your doctor or pharmacist.

Use oxymetazoline only as directed. Do not use more of it, do not use it more often and do not use it longer than three days without first checking with your doctor; otherwise, your runny or stuffy nose may get worse and you may increase the chance of side effects.

DOSAGE AND STORAGE

Carefully follow the instructions on the package label and ask your doctor or pharmacist to explain any part of the instructions you do not understand.

Oxymetazoline comes in nose drops or spray. See pages 224–25 for instructions on using the drops or spray.

If you miss a dose of oxymetazoline, take only the next regularly scheduled dose at the time it is due. Do not take the missed dose and *do not take a double dose*. If you have any questions about this, check with your doctor or pharmacist.

Keep oxymetazoline in the container it came in, and keep it out of the reach of children. Do not allow anyone else to use your oxymetazoline so your infection will not spread.

Phenylephrine
(fen ill ef' rin)

Brand names: Alcon-Efrin, Coricidin, Neo-Synephrine, Rhinall, Sinarest, Vacon

Phenylephrine applied to the inside of the nose relieves nasal congestion caused by hay fever, other allergies, colds and sinus problems. Application of this medicine inside the nose also may help open inflamed ears.

Although there are oral products (tablets, capsules and liquids) combining phenylephrine with antihistamines and other decongestants, these combinations do not appear to be more effective than phenylephrine alone. This medicine is available without a prescription, but your doctor may recommend the proper use or dose of this drug for your particular condition.

UNDESIRED EFFECTS
When phenylephrine is applied, it can cause a temporary burning, stinging or dryness in the nose.

If large amounts of this medicine are used or if an excess amount of the drops is swallowed, they can be absorbed into the body and cause more serious side effects. Stop using phenylephrine and contact your doctor if you experience headache or dizziness, an increase in runny or stuffy nose, pounding or unusually fast heartbeat, trembling, trouble in sleeping or unusual nervousness.

PRECAUTIONS
Do not use phenylephrine if you have ever had any unusual reaction to nasal decongestants; if you have, you are much more likely to have a reaction to this medicine. If you have any questions about this, check with your doctor or pharmacist.

People with blood vessel disease, diabetes, heart disease, high blood pressure or an overactive thyroid should not use phenylephrine. Before you start to use this medicine, tell your doctor or pharmacist if you have any of these medical problems.

Tell your doctor or pharmacist what other prescription or nonprescription drugs you are taking, particularly medicine for depression and monoamine oxidase inhibitors (isocarboxazid, pargyline, phenelzine and tranylcypromine). If you do not know the names of the drugs or what they were prescribed for, bring them in their labeled containers to your doctor or pharmacist.

This medicine should be used only as directed. Do not use more of it, do not use it more often and do not use it for more than three days without first checking with your doctor. If you do, your nasal stuffiness may get worse and you will increase the chance of side effects.

DOSAGE AND STORAGE

Carefully follow the instructions on the prescription label or container and ask your doctor or pharmacist to explain any part of the instructions you do not understand.

Phenylephrine comes in drops, spray and jelly, all of which are applied to the inside of the nose. See pages 224–25 for instructions on using nasal drops and spray.

To use the nasal jelly, first blow your nose. Then place a dab of jelly about the size of a pea in your nose with your finger. Sniff the jelly well back into your nose. Wipe the tip of the tube with a clean, damp tissue and replace the cap immediately.

If you forget to use a dose, use only the regularly scheduled dose at the next regular time. Do not use the missed dose and *do not use a double dose.*

Keep phenylephrine in the container it came in, and keep it out of the reach of children. Do not spread infection by allowing another person to use your phenylephrine.

Phenylpropanolamine
(fen ill proe pa nole' a meen)

Brand names: Propadrine, Rhindecon and others

Some brand names of products containing phenylpropanolamine: Anatuss, Anorexin, Appedrine, Bayer Cold Tablets, Bayer Cough Syrup, Brocon, Codimal, Comtrex, Congespirin, Control Capsules, Coricidin, Coryban-D, Daycare, Decon-aid, Decon-tuss, Dexatrim, Dextrotussin, Dimetane, Dimetapp, Dorcol, Entex, 4-Way Cold Tablets, Fiogesic, Histabid, Histalet, Histatapp, Hycomine, Kronohist, Naldecon, Napril, Milcol, Nolamine, Norel Plus, Novahistine, Ornacol, Ornade, Ornex, Polyhistine, Probacon, Prolamine, Puretapp, Rhinex, Robitussin, Ru-Tuss, S-T Forte, SineAid, Sinubid, Sinulin, Triaminic, Triaminacol, Tuss-Ornade, Vicks Formula 44D and others

Phenylpropanolamine shrinks swollen blood vessels to reduce swelling in the nose and air passages. It is taken by mouth to relieve the discomfort caused by colds, hay fever and other allergies. This drug comes alone or in products combining phenylpropanolamine with other drugs. Phenylpropanolamine is available without a prescription but your doctor may recommend the proper dose for your particular condition.

UNDESIRED EFFECTS

Phenylpropanolamine can cause nervousness, restlessness, trouble in sleeping and dizziness. These effects tend to decrease as your body adjusts to the medicine. If they are severe or persistent, contact your doctor.

Less frequently this medicine will cause more serious reactions. Stop taking phenylpropanolamine and contact your doctor if you experience headache, tightness in the chest, irregular heartbeats or unusually fast heartbeats.

Phenylpropanolamine makes some people drowsy. Do not drive a car or operate dangerous machinery until you know how this drug will affect you.

PRECAUTIONS

Before you start taking phenylpropanolamine, tell your doctor or pharmacist if you have ever had an unusual reaction to medicines similar to phenylpropanolamine such as amphetamines, ephedrine, epinephrine, isoproterenol, metaproterenol, norepinephrine, phenylephrine, pseudoephedrine and terbutaline.

Certain medical problems may become worse if you take phenylpropanolamine. People with diabetes, an enlarged prostate, glaucoma, heart or blood vessel disease, high blood pressure or an overactive thyroid should not use phenylpropanolamine.

Phenylpropanolamine can affect the way your body responds to certain other medications, including other drugs similar to phenylpropanolamine (see the list above), amphetamines, many medicines for high blood pressure, digitalis (heart medicine) and medicine for depression. Tell your doctor what other prescription or nonprescription drugs you are taking. He also will need to know if you are taking monoamine oxidase inhibitors (isocarboxazid, pargyline, phenelzine and tranylcypromine) or if you have taken them within the past three weeks. If you do not know the names of the drugs you are taking or what they were prescribed for, bring them in their labeled containers to your doctor or pharmacist.

Avoid using alcohol, pills to help you sleep and narcotics while you are taking phenylpropanolamine. These will increase the drowsiness caused by phenylpropanolamine.

Be sure to take this medication exactly as your doctor has prescribed it. Do not take more. If you think you need more to relieve your symptoms, check with your doctor.

If you are pregnant or think you may be, tell your doctor before you start to take phenylpropanolamine.

DOSAGE AND STORAGE

Carefully follow the instructions on the package label and ask your doctor or pharmacist to explain any part of the instructions you do not understand.

Phenylpropanolamine comes in capsules, tablets and liquid. If you are taking the extended-release capsules, be sure to swallow them whole. Do not crack, break or chew them.

To ensure an accurate dose of liquid, measure your dose with a specially marked spoon.

If you forget to take a dose, take it as soon as you remember. However, if you remember a missed dose at the time you are scheduled to take another, take only one dose. *Do not take a double dose to make up for the missed one.*

Keep phenylpropanolamine in the container it came in, and keep it out of the reach of children. Do not allow anyone else to take your phenylpropanolamine which was prescribed for your particular condition.

Pseudoephedrine

(soo doe a fed' rin)

Brand names: Cenafed, D-Feda, Novafed, Sudafed

Some brand names of products containing pseudoephedrine: Actifed, Acti-Prem, Afrinol, Chlorafed, Chlor-Trimeton, Codimal, CoTylenol, D-Feda, Deconamine, Dimacol, Disophrol, Drixoral, Emprazil, Fedahist, Fedazril, Histalet, Historal, Isoclor, Lo-Tussin, Nasalspan, Novafed, Nucofed, Polaramine, Poly-Histine, Pseudobid, Pseudo-Hist, Rhinosyn, Robitussin, Rondec, Ryna, Triprolidine, Tussend

Pseudoephedrine shrinks swollen blood vessels in the nose, lungs and ears. It is used to relieve the congestion and discomfort caused by colds, allergies and certain types of ear problems. Several cold and cough preparations containing pseudoephedrine are available with or without a doctor's prescription.

UNDESIRED EFFECTS

When you start to take pseudoephedrine, it may make you nervous or restless or give you trouble sleeping. These effects tend to decrease or disappear as you continue to take it and as your body adjusts to the medicine. If they are persistent or severe, contact your doctor.

Less frequently, pseudoephedrine can cause difficult or painful urination, dizziness or lightheadedness, headache, nausea or vomiting, trembling, troubled breathing, an unusual increase in sweating, unusual paleness, unusually fast or pounding heartbeat or weakness. Try taking a smaller amount of the medicine each day. If these effects continue, stop taking the medicine and contact your doctor.

Very large doses of pseudoephedrine can result in hallucinations, irregular heartbeat or unusually slow heartbeat and shortness of breath. If you experience any of these effects, stop taking the medicine and contact your doctor.

PRECAUTIONS

Before you start taking pseudoephedrine, tell your doctor if you have ever had any unusual reaction to medicines similar to pseudoephedrine, such as amphetamines, ephedrine, epinephrine, isoproterenol, metaproterenol, norepinephrine, phenylephrine, phenylpropanolamine or terbutaline. If you have had a reaction to any of these medicines, you may have a reaction to pseudoephedrine.

Certain medical problems may become worse if you take pseudoephedrine. Tell your doctor if you have diabetes, an enlarged prostate, glaucoma, heart or blood vessel disease, high blood pressure or an overactive thyroid. Because many nonprescription remedies for coughs, colds and hay fever contain pseudoephedrine, ask your pharmacist about the ingredients of such remedies before you buy them. You should not take pseudoephedrine if you have any of the medical conditions named above unless your doctor specifically says you may.

Pseudoephedrine can affect the way your body responds to certain other medications, including amphetamines, many medicines for high blood pressure, digitalis glycosides (heart medicine) and medicine for depression. Tell your doctor or pharmacist what other prescription or nonprescription medications you are taking. If you do not know the names of the drugs or what they were prescribed for, bring them in their labeled containers to your doctor or pharmacist.

Tell your doctor if you are breast-feeding. Pseudoephedrine is passed through the milk and can have an undesired effect on the baby.

Excessive consumption of coffee or tea may increase the restlessness or insomnia that pseudoephedrine can cause. You may want to reduce the amount of these beverages you drink while you are taking this drug.

Contact your doctor if any new symptoms or health problems develop while you are taking pseudoephedrine or if your symptoms do not improve within five days.

DOSAGE AND STORAGE

Your doctor will determine how often you should take pseudoephedrine and how much you should take at each dose. Carefully follow the instructions on your prescription label and ask your doctor or pharmacist to explain any part of the instructions you do not understand.

Pseudoephedrine comes in capsules, syrup and tablets. Usually it begins to work within 15 minutes to a half hour after it is taken and takes full effect in about an hour.

If you are taking the extended-release capsule or the extended-release tablet, swallow it whole. Do not crush, break or chew it before swallowing it. If the capsule is too large to swallow, you may mix its contents with jam or jelly and swallow without chewing.

To help prevent trouble in sleeping, take the last dose of pseudoephedrine several hours before bedtime. If you have any questions about this dosage procedure, ask your doctor or pharmacist.

If you forget to take a dose of pseudoephedrine, take the next dose at the regularly scheduled time. Do not take the missed dose and *do not take a double dose*.

Keep this medicine in the container it came in. Keep pseudoephedrine out of the reach of children, and do not allow anyone else to take your pseudoephedrine.

MEDICATIONS FOR COUGHS

EXPECTORANTS

Expectorants are used to help thin the mucus in the air passages. This makes it easier to cough up the mucus and clear the air passages. It also will help if you drink a lot of water while you are using expectorants. In severe cases, a vaporizer may be used to help thin the mucus.

Guaifenesin
(gwye fen i sen)

Brand names: Guaiatuss, 2G, Robitussin Syrup and others

Names of products containing guaifenesin: Actifed C Expectorant, Adatuss, Anatuss, Asbron-G, Brondecon, Bronkolixir, Chlor-Trimeton Expectorant, Conar Expectorant, Coricidin Cough Syrup, Coryban-D Cough Syrup, Co-Xan, Dimacol, Dimetane Expectorant, Donatussin Syrup, Dorcol, Emfaseem, Entex, Entuss, Fedahist Expectorant, Guistrey, Histalet X, Isoclor Expectorant, Lo-Tussin, Lufyllin, Mudrane, Nasalspan, Neothylline-GG, Nilcol, Novahistine Expectorant, P-V-Tussin, Polarmine Expectorant, Pseudo-Hist Expectorant, Quibron Elixir, Rhinex-DM, Rhinspec, Robitussin A-C (and others), Romex, Ryna-Cx, S-T Forte, Slo-Phyllin-GG, Sorbutuss, Synphylate-GG, Tedral Expectorant, Triaminic, Tussend Cough Syrup, Unproco, Verequad, Vicks Cough Syrup and others

Guaifenesin, also known as glyceryl guaiacolate, thins the mucus in air passages and makes it easier to cough it up. Guaifenesin relieves coughs of colds, tuberculosis and whooping cough. Guaifenesin is combined with decongestants, antihistamines, narcotics and bronchodilators to treat coughs.

UNDESIRED EFFECTS

When taken in larger amounts than those required for effective expectorant action, guaifenesin may cause vomiting. However, at usual doses upset stomach as an effect of taking this medicine is rare.

PRECAUTIONS

Many of the combination products containing guaifenesin are available without a prescription. Discuss with your pharmacist the other drugs in these products to be sure you do not take something you should not, such as phenylpropanolamine if you have high blood pressure, or isopropamide if you have glaucoma.

DOSAGE AND STORAGE

If your doctor has prescribed guaifenesin, carefully follow the instructions on the prescription label. If you purchase this medicine without a prescription, follow the directions included in the package or on the label. Do not take more and do not take it more often than recommended.

If you forget to take a dose of this medicine, take it as soon as you remember and then take the remaining doses for that day at evenly spaced intervals. If you remember a missed dose at the time you are to take another, take only the scheduled dose. Do not take the missed dose and *do not take a double dose*.

Keep guaifenesin in the container it came in, and keep it out of the reach of children.

Terpin Hydrate
(ter′ pin hye′ drate)

Brand names of products containing terpin hydrate: Terpin Hydrate and Codeine Elixir, Tussaminic Tablets

Terpin hydrate, in the form of an elixir with or without codeine, is used to relieve coughs. However, five milliliters of the elixir (the usual dose) contains only about one-fourth of the effective dose of terpin hydrate. The high alcohol content of the elixir (more than 40 percent) makes it unwise to give doses larger than five milliliters. Therefore, the elixir usually contains codeine, a narcotic that acts on the cough center of the brain to lessen coughing (see **codeine**, page 233, for side effects).

Undesired Effects
Although side effects are rare, terpin hydrate can cause nausea, and the alcohol in the product can cause drowsiness.

Precautions
Terpin hydrate cough medicines contain more than 40 percent alcohol. Avoid alcoholic beverages while you are taking terpin hydrate.

Dosage and Storage
Carefully follow the instructions on your prescription label or package label if you are taking a nonprescription product.

If you forget to take a dose, take it as soon as you remember it. However, if it is almost time for you to take the next dose, take only the regularly scheduled dose.

Keep this medication in the container it came in, and keep it out of the reach of children.

COUGH SUPPRESSANTS

Cough suppressants act on a portion of the brain that stimulates the cough reflex. These medications are best used to stop a dry, hacking cough that irritates the throat and may prevent sleep. It is best not to use this type of medication if a lot of mucus is being coughed up.

Codeine
(koe' deen)

Brand names of some of the many products containing codeine: Actifed-C, Ambenyl Expectorant, Cerose, Cetro-Cirose, Cheracol, Colrex Compound, Copavin, Cosanyl Cough Syrup, Cotussis, Dimetane Expectorant DC, Ephedrol, Histadyl EC Syrup, Isoclor Expectorant, Mercodol, Novahistine DH. Omnituss, Phenergan Expectorant with Codeine, Pediacof, Pyrroxate with Codeine, Robitussin A-C, Tolu-Sed, Tussar, Tussi-Organidin

Codeine is a narcotic which acts on the cough center in the brain to decrease coughing. It is used alone or combined with other cough medicines, expectorants, decongestants and antihistamines to relieve cough and colds symptoms. In higher doses it also is used to relieve pain.

Undesired Effects

When you first start to take codeine, you may become nauseated. If you lie down for a while, this effect usually will go away. Codeine also can cause vomiting or constipation. Drink plenty of fluids and if these effects continue or are severe, contact your doctor.

While you are taking codeine you may be dizzy or lightheaded or may faint when you get up from a lying or sitting position. If you get up slowly, this problem will be less bothersome. However, if it continues in spite of your precautions, contact your doctor.

A more serious problem is the effect codeine can have on the central nervous system (brain and spinal cord). If you experience shortness of breath, have difficulty breathing or notice that your heartbeat is unusually slow, contact your doctor. In children, a central nervous system problem can have the opposite effect and cause unusual excitement. Contact your doctor if your child behaves in this way after taking codeine.

Codeine makes some people drowsy or less alert than usual. Do not drive a car or operate dangerous machinery until you know what effect this medicine will have on you.

Precautions

Codeine can make certain medical conditions worse. Be sure to tell your doctor if you have colitis; emphysema, asthma or chronic lung disease; an enlarged prostate or problems with urination; gallbladder disease or gallstones; kidney or liver disease; disease of underactive adrenal glands (Addison's disease); an underactive thyroid; or an unusually slow or irregular heartbeat.

Other medicines that slow down function of the central nervous system should not be taken with codeine. Tell your doctor what other prescription or nonprescription drugs you are taking, including antihistamines, medicine for allergy or colds, barbiturates, other narcotics, prescription medicine for pain, sedatives, tranquilizers, medicine to help you sleep, medicine for seizures and medicine for depression. Also tell your doctor if you are taking prescription medicine for stomach cramps or spasms and if you are now taking or have taken monoamine oxidase (MAO) inhibitors for depression in the past two weeks.

If you do not know the names of the drugs you are taking or what they were prescribed for, bring them in their labeled containers to your doctor or pharmacist. Contact your doctor or pharmacist before you start to take any of the above drugs while you are taking codeine.

You should not consume alcohol while you are taking codeine because of the possibility of side effects. If you have any questions about this, check with your doctor or pharmacist.

Do not take codeine if you have ever had problems with it in the past.

Before having any kind of surgery with general anesthesia, including dental surgery, tell the doctor or dentist that you are taking codeine.

To help your doctor select the best treatment for you and your baby, tell him if you are pregnant or are breast-feeding a baby. Codeine can be passed from mother to baby and have undesired effects.

DOSAGE AND STORAGE

Your doctor will determine how often you should take codeine or a product containing codeine and how much you should take at each dose. Carefully follow the instructions on your prescription label and ask your doctor or pharmacist to explain any part of the instructions you do not understand.

Codeine and products containing codeine come in tablets, capsules and in liquid form. Many times codeine is prescribed to be taken as needed for coughing. However, if you have been told to take this medicine, do not take more of it or take it more often or for a longer period than your doctor has instructed. Products containing codeine can be habit-forming.

If you forget to take a dose, take the missed dose as soon as you remember, unless you remember it when you are scheduled to take another dose. Then take only the regularly scheduled dose. Omit the missed dose completely and *do not take a double dose*.

Keep codeine in the container it came in, and keep it out of the reach of children. Do not allow anyone else to take your codeine.

Dextromethorphan
(dex troe meth ore' fan)

Brand names of some of the many products containing dextromethorphan: Albatussin, Anatuss, Bayer Cough Syrup, Chloraseptic DM, Codimal DN, Comtrex, Coricidin, Coryban-D, CoTylenol, Daycare, Dextrotussin, Dimacol, Dorcol, Guaifensin-Dextromethorphan Syrup, Histalet, Nilcol, Nyquil, Ornacol, Phenergan, Quelidrine, Rhinex-DM, Robitussin-DM, Romex, Rondec-DM, Sorbutuss, Triaminic-DM, Triaminicol, Tusquelin, Tussaminic, Tussar DM, TussiOrganidin, Unproco, Vicks 44 and 44D and others

Dextromethorphan, like codeine, acts on the cough center in the brain to stop coughing. Dextromethorphan's effect on the cough reflex is about equal to that of codeine, but dextromethorphan has fewer side effects than codeine. Dextromethorphan is a common ingredient in cough preparations available without a prescription.

UNDESIRED EFFECTS

Although side effects are rare after you take dextromethorphan, it can cause nausea and drowsiness. These effects tend to decrease or disappear as your body becomes adjusted to the medicine. However, if they continue or are severe, contact your doctor or pharmacist.

PRECAUTIONS

Before you start to take products containing dextromethorphan, tell your doctor or pharmacist what prescription or nonprescription drugs you are taking.

DOSAGE AND STORAGE

If your doctor has prescribed a cough preparation containing dextromethorphan, carefully follow his instructions on how often to take the cough preparation and how much to take at each dose. If you have selected a cough preparation that does not require a prescription, carefully follow the directions on the bottle. Do not take more of this medicine, take it more often or take it longer than instructed.

If you forget to take a dose, take it as soon as you remember. However, if it is almost time for you to take another dose, omit the missed dose entirely and take only the regularly scheduled dose.

Keep this medicine in the container it came in, and keep it out of the reach of children.

Hydrocodone
(high dro co' dohn)

Brand names: Codone, Dicodid

Brand names of products containing hydrocodone: Adatuss, Citra-Forte, Codimal DH, Duradyne DHC, Entuss, Hycodan, Hycomine, Hycotuss, Norcet, P-V-Tussin, Pseudo-Hist, S-T Forte, Triaminic, Tussend, Tussionex, Vicodin

Hydrocodone is a narcotic that acts on the cough center in the brain to stop coughing. The ability of hydrocodone to stop coughing is slightly greater than that of codeine. Hydrocodone also dries the nose and throat.

This drug is used alone or with other cough suppressants, expectorants, antihistamines, decongestants and pain medicine to relieve the symptoms of colds and allergies.

UNDESIRED EFFECTS

Although side effects are uncommon with usual doses, hydrocodone can cause nausea and constipation. Drink plenty of fluids and contact your doctor if these effects continue over a period of time or are severe.

Rarely, hydrocodone will cause difficulty in breathing. If you have this problem, stop taking the medicine and contact your doctor.

Hydrocodone makes some people drowsy and dizzy. Do not drive a car or operate dangerous machinery until you know how this drug will affect you.

PRECAUTIONS

Before you start to take hydrocodone, tell your doctor if you have ever had any problem with this drug in the past or if you have asthma, emphysema, an underactive thyroid, an enlarged prostate, adrenal disease (Addison's disease) or kidney or liver disease.

Certain other medications should not be taken with hydrocodone. These include other narcotics, barbiturates, sedatives, tranquilizers, medicine to help you sleep and medicine for depression. Tell your doctor what prescription or nonprescription drugs you are taking. If you do not know the names of the drugs or what they were prescribed for, bring them in their labeled containers to your doctor or pharmacist.

Do not start to take any of the drugs listed above without first checking with your doctor.

Do not drink alcoholic beverages while you are taking hydrocodone. Alcohol can increase the chance and severity of side effects.

Before you have surgery with a general anesthetic, including dental surgery, tell the doctor or dentist that you are taking hydrocodone.

Do not take hydrocodone any longer than your doctor has told you to take it. Do not take any more of it nor take it more often than your doctor has instructed. To do so could cause problems because hydrocodone is habit-forming.

To help your doctor select the treatment best for you and your baby, tell him if you are pregnant or are breast-feeding a baby. Safe use of this drug in pregnancy has not been established and hydrocodone is passed to a nursing baby through the milk.

DOSAGE AND STORAGE

Your doctor will determine how often you should take hydrocodone and how much you should take at each dose. Carefully follow the instructions on your prescription label and ask your doctor or pharmacist to explain any part you do not understand.

Hydrocodone alone is available in tablets, and the combination products are available in liquid, tablets and capsules.

If you forget to take a dose, take it as soon as you remember. However, if you remember a missed dose when it is almost time for you to take another dose, omit the missed dose entirely and take only the regularly scheduled dose. *Do not take a double dose.*

Keep this medicine in the container it came in, and keep it out of the reach of children. Do not allow anyone else to take your hydrocodone.

ARTHRITIS

DRUGS USED TO TREAT ARTHRITIS

Arthritis

Arthritis is an inflammation of the joints. The joints become painful, red, tender, swollen and stiff. There are many different types of arthritis, but the most common ones are osteoarthritis and rheumatoid arthritis.

Osteoarthritis occurs later in life and usually is characterized by painful and knobby swelling of the fingers. Rheumatoid arthritis starts in middle age, usually involves many joints and causes you to feel stiff all over.

A type of arthritis that involves primarily the back and joints of the lower back is ankylosing spondylitis.

Gout is also a type of arthritis that occurs mostly in men and that usually is sudden in onset. Pain and swelling occur in the affected joint—frequently the big toe, ankle or knee.

Usually, a salicylate—commonly aspirin—is the first drug you will take for arthritis. If a salicylate does not help, your doctor may prescribe one of the nonsteroidal anti-inflammatory drugs discussed on the following pages. A steroid—a cortisonelike drug—may be injected into a painful arthritic joint. Rarely, use of a steroid by mouth, on a continuing basis, is justified. (See page 402 for the names of additional drugs to treat gout.)

Any of these drugs may relieve the *symptoms* of arthritis and slow down the progression of the disease. However, the basic course of the disease usually is not changed and arthritis is not cured.

SALICYLATE

Aspirin
(as' pir in)

Aspirin reduces the pain and also the arthritic swelling in the joints.
(See **aspirin**, page 415, for more information.)

If you take aspirin for arthritis, you need to take large doses—probably 12 to 16 tablets of five grains or 300 milligrams each—every day. Your doctor should still see you every so often, even though you are not taking a prescription drug.

Other salicylates besides aspirin that may be taken for arthritis are:

choline salicylate (brand names: Arthropan, Actasal)

magnesium salicylate (brand name: Magan)

salicylamide (brand names: Amid-Sal, Salrin)

sodium salicylate

There are also many products containing combinations of salicylates, many available without a prescription. Some common brand names are: Duragesic, Pabalate, Parbocyl, Persistin, Sal-Eze, Stanback and Zarumin.

NONSTEROIDAL ANTI-INFLAMMATORY DRUGS

Fenoprofen
(fen oh proe' fen)

Brand name: Nalfon

Fenoprofen is used to relieve the pain, redness, tenderness, swelling and stiffness of certain types of arthritis. The drug also is used to relieve mild to moderate pain such as that following surgery or major dental work.

UNDESIRED EFFECTS

The most common side effects of fenoprofen are stomach upsets such as indigestion, nausea, vomiting, stomach pain and diarrhea. To prevent stomach upsets after taking fenoprofen, take it with milk, meals, a snack or an antacid. If these effects continue or are severe, contact your doctor.

Fenoprofen makes some people drowsy, dizzy or less alert. Do not drive a car or operate dangerous machinery until you know how this medicine will affect you.

Other effects, which may go away as you continue to take fenoprofen and as your body adjusts to it, include constipation, headache, loss of appetite, blurred vision, dry mouth, nervousness, trembling, trouble sleeping, increased sweating and fast or pounding heartbeat. Contact your doctor if these effects continue or are bothersome.

More serious side effects can occur, which may require medical attention. Contact your doctor if you have a ringing or buzzing in your ears; skin rash; hives; itching; bloody or tarry stools; partial loss of hearing; vision problems; swelling of the hands, feet, ankles or lower legs; shortness of breath or difficult breathing, wheezing or tightness in the chest; or unusual tiredness or weakness.

PRECAUTIONS

You should not take fenoprofen if you have ever had a bad reaction to it or if you have ever had an unusual reaction to aspirin or other salicylates, ibuprofen, indomethacin, meclofenamate, mefenamic acid, naproxen, oxyphenbutazone, phenylbutazone, sulindac, tolmetin or zomepirac. If you have questions about this, check with your doctor.

Because fenoprofen can make certain medical conditions worse, tell your doctor if you have bleeding problems, heart disease, diverticulitis, kidney disease, a stomach ulcer or other stomach problems.

Tell your doctor what prescription or nonprescription drugs you are taking, including anticoagulants (blood thinners), medicine for diabetes, any other medicine for arthritis, phenytoin and sulfa medicines. If you do not know the names of the drugs or why they were prescribed, bring them in their labeled containers to your doctor or pharmacist.

It may take a few days for you to feel better after you take fenoprofen and you may have to take it for two to three weeks before you feel the full effects.

Take fenoprofen exactly as prescribed. Do not take more of it, take it more often or take it for a longer period than ordered by your doctor. If you think you need more to relieve your symptoms, contact your doctor.

Laboratory tests such as blood tests or kidney and liver function tests may be required while you are taking fenoprofen. If you experience problems with your vision or hearing after you start to take this drug, you should tell your doctor, have your eyes examined and have a test for your hearing. *Be sure to keep all appointments with your doctor and at the laboratory.*

Do not drink alcoholic beverages while you are taking fenoprofen. Do not take aspirin regularly unless you have permission from your doctor. Alcohol or aspirin can increase the chance of stomach upset.

Before you have surgery with a general anesthetic, including dental surgery, tell the doctor or dentist that you are taking fenoprofen.

Because it is not known whether this medicine may be safely used in pregnant women or nursing mothers, tell your doctor if you are pregnant or breast-feeding.

DOSAGE AND STORAGE

Your doctor will determine how often you should take fenoprofen and how much you should take at each dose. Carefully follow the instructions on your prescription label and ask your doctor or pharmacist to explain any part of the instructions you do not understand.

Fenoprofen comes in capsules and tablets. If this medicine upsets your stomach, take it with solid food, milk or an antacid.

If you forget to take a dose of this medicine, take it as soon as you remember. If you do not remember a missed dose until it is almost time for you to take the next one, omit the missed dose entirely and take only the regularly scheduled dose. *Do not take a double dose to make up for the missed one.*

Keep fenoprofen in the container it came in, and keep it out of the reach of children. Do not allow anyone else to take your fenoprofen.

Ibuprofen

(eye byoo′ proe fen)

Brand name: Motrin

Ibuprofen is used to relieve the pain, redness, tenderness, swelling and stiffness of certain types of arthritis. Ibuprofen also is used to relieve other types of mild to moderate pain.

UNDESIRED EFFECTS

The most common side effects are stomach upsets such as bloating or gas, heartburn or indigestion, nausea or vomiting, stomach cramps or stomach pain, and diarrhea. To prevent these problems, take this medicine with meals, a snack, milk or an antacid. If these problems continue, contact your doctor.

Ibuprofen makes some people dizzy. Do not drive a car or operate dangerous machinery until you know how this medicine will affect you.

Other effects, which may go away as you continue to take ibuprofen, are constipation, decreased appetite, headache and nervousness.

More serious side effects, which do not occur often, will require medical attention if they do occur. Contact your doctor if you have skin rash; hives; itching; ringing or buzzing in the ears; swelling of the feet, ankles or lower legs; unusual weight gain; bloody or tarry stools; blurred or partial loss of vision; change in color in your vision; mental depression; difficult or painful urination; shortness of breath or difficult breathing, wheezing or tightness in the chest; or sore throat or fever.

PRECAUTIONS

You should not take ibuprofen if you have ever had a bad reaction to it in the past or have ever had an unusual reaction to aspirin or other salicylates, fenoprofen, indomethacin, meclofenamate, mefenamic acid, naproxen, oxyphenbutazone, phenylbutazone, sulindac, tolmetin or zomepirac. If you have questions about this, check with your doctor.

Before you start to take ibuprofen, tell your doctor if you have bleeding problems, heart disease, kidney disease, diverticulitis, a stomach ulcer or other stomach problems. Ibuprofen may make these conditions worse.

Tell your doctor what prescription or nonprescription drugs you are taking, especially anticoagulants (blood thinners), medicine for diabetes, any other medicine for arthritis, phenytoin and sulfa drugs. If you do not know the names of the drugs or why they were prescribed, bring them in their labeled containers to your doctor or pharmacist.

For ibuprofen to relieve your symptoms, it must be taken regularly and exactly as prescribed by your doctor. It may take two to three weeks before you feel the full effect of this medicine. Do not take more of it than your doctor has ordered. If you feel you need more to relieve your symptoms, contact your doctor.

Your doctor may order laboratory tests such as blood counts or tests for liver function, or ask you to have your eyes examined.

Do not drink alcoholic beverages while you are taking ibuprofen. Do not take aspirin regularly while you are taking ibuprofen unless you have your doctor's permission. Alcohol or aspirin can increase the chance of stomach upset.

Before you have any surgery with a general anesthetic, including dental surgery, tell the doctor or dentist that you are taking ibuprofen.

It is not known whether this drug is safe for pregnant women or nursing mothers. Be sure to tell your doctor if you are pregnant or breast-feeding.

DOSAGE AND STORAGE

Your doctor will determine how often you should take ibuprofen and how much you should take at each dose. Carefully follow the instructions on your prescription label and ask your doctor or pharmacist to explain any part of the instructions you do not understand.

Ibuprofen comes in tablets. If they upset your stomach, they may be taken with solid food, milk or an antacid.

If you forget to take a dose of ibuprofen, take the missed dose as soon as you remember it. If you remember the missed dose at the time you are scheduled to take the next dose, omit it completely and take only the regularly scheduled dose. *Do not take a double dose.*

Keep ibuprofen in the container it came in, and keep it out of the reach of children. Do not allow anyone else to take your ibuprofen.

Indomethacin

(in doe meth' a sin)

Brand name: Indocin

Indomethacin is used to relieve the pain, redness, tenderness, swelling and stiffness of certain types of arthritis and other joint diseases, including gout attacks. Because of its possible side effects, indomethacin usually is only used when aspirin or other drugs are not helpful.

UNDESIRED EFFECTS

Headache is the most common effect of indomethacin and may occur within an hour after you take it. If you get severe headache, contact your doctor. It may be necessary to reduce the amount of indomethacin you are taking.

Indomethacin can cause stomach upsets such as indigestion, heartburn, nausea, vomiting, stomach pain or diarrhea. To lessen stomach upset, take this medicine with meals, a snack or milk. If this does not lessen your stomach upset, ask your doctor if you may take indomethacin with an antacid.

Indomethacin makes some people drowsy, dizzy or lightheaded. Do not drive a car or operate dangerous machinery until you know how this medicine will affect you.

Other effects, which may go away as you continue to take it and as your body adjusts to indomethacin, are constipation and unusual tiredness and weakness. Contact your doctor if these effects continue or are severe.

Serious and possibly fatal effects can occur. Stop taking indomethacin and contact your doctor if you have ringing or buzzing in the ears; bloody or tarry stools; blurred vision; hearing problems; mood or mental changes; shortness of breath; wheezing; difficult breathing; tightness in the chest; skin rash or hives; sore throat; fever; swelling of the ankles, feet or lower legs; unusual bleeding or bruising; unusual weight gain; or yellowing of the eyes and skin.

PRECAUTIONS

You should not take indomethacin if you have ever had a bad reaction to it or if you have ever had an unusual reaction to aspirin or other salicylates, fenoprofen, ibuprofen, meclofenamate, mefenamic acid, naproxen, oxyphenbutazone, phenylbutazone, sulindac, tolmetin or zomepirac. If you have questions about this, check with your doctor.

Because indomethacin can make certain medical conditions worse, tell your doctor if you have bleeding problems, colitis, diverticulitis, epilepsy, kidney or liver disease, mental illness, Parkinson's disease, a stomach ulcer or other stomach problems.

Tell your doctor what prescription or nonprescription drugs you are taking, including anticoagulants (blood thinners), medicine for diabetes, diuretics, medicine for high blood pressure, lithium, probenecid, any other medicine for arthritis, phenytoin and sulfa medicines. If you do not know the names of the drugs or why they were prescribed, bring them in their labeled containers to your doctor or pharmacist.

When you take indomethacin for arthritis, you may have to take it for several weeks before you begin to feel better. It could be a month before you feel the full effects of this medicine.

Take indomethacin exactly as prescribed by your doctor. Do not take more of it, take it more often or take it for a longer period than ordered by your doctor. Do not take indomethacin for any problem other than the one for which it was prescribed.

You may be required to have tests of your urine and blood or laboratory tests for your liver function while you are taking this drug. You also may need eye examinations or tests for your hearing if you have vision or hearing problems after you begin to take indomethacin. *Be sure to keep all appointments with your doctor and at the laboratory.*

Do not drink alcoholic beverages or take aspirin regularly while you are taking indomethacin. Alcohol or aspirin can make stomach upsets worse.

Before you have any kind of surgery with a general anesthestic, including dental surgery, tell the doctor or dentist that you are taking indomethacin.

Because indomethacin can harm an unborn child or a nursing baby, tell your doctor if you are pregnant or breast-feeding.

DOSAGE AND STORAGE

Your doctor will determine how often you should take indomethacin and how much you should take at each dose. Carefully follow the instructions on your prescription label and ask your doctor or pharmacist to explain any part of the instructions you do not understand.

Indomethacin comes in capsules. Take them with meals, a snack or milk to lessen stomach upset.

If you forget to take a dose of this medicine, take it as soon as you remember. If you remember a missed dose when it is almost time for you to take another, omit the missed dose completely and take only the regularly scheduled dose. *Do not take a double dose to make up for the missed one.*

Keep indomethacin in the container it came in, and keep it out of the reach of children. Do not allow anyone else to take your indomethacin.

Naproxen
(na prox' en)

Brand names: Anaprox, Naprosyn

Naproxen is used to relieve the pain, redness, tenderness, swelling and stiffness of certain types of arthritis. Naproxen also is used to relieve menstrual cramps and mild to moderate pain such as that following surgery or major dental work.

Undesired Effects

The most common side effects of naproxen are stomach upsets such as heartburn or indigestion, stomach pain, nausea and vomiting; diarrhea also is a common side effect. To lessen these upsets, take naproxen with meals, a snack, milk or an antacid.

Naproxen makes some people dizzy, lightheaded or drowsy. Do not drive a car or operate dangerous machinery until you know how this medicine will affect you.

Other side effects are constipation, soreness of the mouth, headache, pounding heartbeat and sweating. These effects may go away as you continue to take naproxen and as your body adjusts to it. However, if they continue or are severe, contact your doctor.

More serious side effects, which do not occur often, will need medical attention if they do occur. Contact your doctor if you have bloody or tarry stools; blurred vision or any other change in vision; mental depression; ringing or buzzing in the ears; any loss of hearing; skin rash or hives; swelling of the feet, ankles or lower legs; unusual weight gain; difficult or painful urination; shortness of breath or wheezing; difficulty in breathing or tightness in the chest; sore throat; fever; unusual bleeding or bruising; or yellowing of the skin and eyes.

Precautions

You should not take naproxen if you have ever had a bad reaction to it or if you have had an unusual reaction to aspirin or other salicylates, fenoprofen, ibuprofen, indomethacin, meclofenamate, mefenamic acid, oxyphenbutazone, phenylbutazone, sulindac, tolmetin or zomepirac. If you have any questions about this, check with your doctor.

Before you start to take naproxen, tell your doctor if you have bleeding problems, heart disease, kidney disease, a stomach ulcer or other stomach problems. Naproxen may make these conditions worse.

Tell your doctor what prescription or nonprescription drugs you are taking, including anticoagulants (blood thinners), medicine for diabetes, any other medicine for arthritis, phenytoin, probenecid and sulfa medicines. If you do not know the names of the drugs or why they were prescribed, bring them in their labeled containers to your doctor or pharmacist.

For this medicine to help you, it must be taken regularly and exactly as prescribed by your doctor. You may have to take it for several weeks before you begin to feel better and for a month before you feel the full effects.

Your doctor probably will order laboratory tests such as blood tests and tests for liver or kidney function to check on how you are reacting to this drug. You may need to have an eye examination or a hearing test if you experience vision or hearing problems after you start to take naproxen. *Be sure to keep all appointments with your doctor and at the laboratory.*

Do not drink alcoholic beverages or take aspirin regularly while you are taking naproxen. Alcohol or aspirin can make stomach upsets worse.

Before you have any surgery with a general anesthetic, including dental surgery, tell the doctor or dentist that you are taking naproxen.

Because naproxen can harm an unborn child or a nursing baby, be sure to tell your doctor if you are pregnant or are breast-feeding.

DOSAGE AND STORAGE

Your doctor will determine how often you should take naproxen and how much you should take at each dose. Carefully follow the instructions on your prescription label and ask your doctor or pharmacist to explain any part of the instructions you do not understand.

Naproxen comes in tablets. Take them with solid food, milk or an antacid to lessen the chance of stomach upset.

If you forget to take a dose, take it as soon as you remember. If you remember a missed dose when it is almost time for you to take another one, omit the missed dose completely and take only the regularly scheduled one. *Do not take a double dose to make up for the missed one.*

Keep naproxen in the container it came in, and keep it out of the reach of children. Do not allow anyone else to take your naproxen.

Oxyphenbutazone
(ox i fen byoo′ ta zone)

Brand names: Oxalid, Tandearil

Oxyphenbutazone is used for short-term relief of pain, redness, tenderness, swelling and stiffness of certain types of arthritis and other joint diseases, including gout attacks. Because of the possible side effects and potentially very serious blood problems caused by oxyphenbutazone, it usually is only used when all other drugs have not been helpful.

UNDESIRED EFFECTS

Many people have undesired effects from this drug severe enough that they cannot take it. Oxyphenbutazone frequently causes nausea, vomiting, indigestion, stomach pain or diarrhea. Taking this medicine immediately before or immediately after meals, with a full glass of milk or with an antacid, should help prevent the stomach problems. If stomach upsets continue in spite of these precautions, contact your doctor.

Oxyphenbutazone causes some people to become drowsy, confused or less alert. Do not drive a car or operate dangerous machinery until you know how this medicine will affect you.

If you gain weight, have swelling of the feet and ankles or have difficulty breathing after you have been taking oxyphenbutazone, check with your doctor. Using less salt in your diet may help relieve these problems.

More serious problems, such as intestinal bleeding, kidney or liver problems, allergic reactions and eye problems, may occur rarely. Stop taking oxyphenbutazone and contact your doctor immediately if you have any loss of hearing, bloody or black tarry stools, indigestion or stomach pain, bloody or cloudy urine, difficult or painful urination, difficult breathing, wheezing, eye pain or any change in vision, skin rash or hives or yellowing of the eyes and skin.

Serious blood problems can occur many days or weeks after you stop taking oxyphenbutazone, although these effects are rare. During this period, contact your doctor immediately if you have sore throat, fever, chills, sores or white spots in the mouth, unusual bleeding or bruising, or unusual tiredness or weakness.

PRECAUTIONS

Do not take oxyphenbutazone if you have ever had a bad reaction to it or if you have ever had an unusual reaction to aspirin or other salicylates, fenoprofen, ibuprofen, indomethacin, meclofenamate, mefenamic acid, naproxen, phenylbutazone, sulfinpyrazone, sulindac, tolmetin or zomepirac. Be sure to tell your doctor about any such reaction.

Because oxyphenbutazone can make some medical conditions worse, tell your doctor if you have or ever had asthma; diseases of the blood, heart, liver, kidneys, pancreas, salivary glands or thyroid glands; high blood pressure; a stomach ulcer or other stomach problems; or diseases characterized by muscle pain or pain in the temples.

Tell your doctor what prescription or nonprescription drugs you are taking, especially anticoagulants (blood thinners), medicine for diabetes, isoniazid, digitoxin, any other medicine for arthritis, phenytoin, tetracyclines, iron medications and sulfa medicines. If you do not know the names of the drugs or why they were prescribed, bring them in their labeled containers to your doctor or pharmacist.

If you take oxyphenbutazone for a week and still have the symptoms for which it was prescribed, contact your doctor. Take oxyphenbutazone exactly as prescribed. Do not take more of it, take it more often or take it for a longer period than ordered by your doctor. Do not take oxyphenbutazone for any problem other than that for which it was prescribed.

Certain laboratory tests should be done before you begin to take oxyphenbutazone, including blood tests and tests for your kidney, liver and thyroid function. These tests should be repeated every few weeks so your doctor can check on how you are reacting to this drug. *Be sure to keep all appointments with your doctor and at the laboratory.*

Do not drink alcoholic beverages while you are taking oxyphenbutazone. Do not take aspirin regularly while you are taking oxyphenbutazone unless you first check with your doctor about how much to take. Alcohol or aspirin can make stomach upset more likely to occur.

Before you have surgery with a general anesthetic, including dental surgery, tell your doctor or dentist that you are taking oxyphenbutazone.

To help your doctor select the treatment best for you and your baby, tell your doctor if you are pregnant or breast-feeding.

DOSAGE AND STORAGE

Your doctor will determine how often you should take oxyphenbutazone and how much you should take at each dose. Carefully follow the instructions on your prescription label and ask your doctor or pharmacist to explain any part of the instructions you do not understand.

Oxyphenbutazone comes in tablets. They should be taken immediately before or immediately after meals, with a full eight-ounce glass of milk, or with an antacid to lessen the possibility of stomach upset.

If you forget to take a dose of this medicine, take it as soon as you remember. Then take any remaining doses for that day at evenly spaced intervals. If you remember a missed dose when it is almost time for you to take another one, omit the missed dose completely and take only the regularly scheduled one. *Do not take a double dose to make up for the missed one.*

Keep oxyphenbutazone in the container it came in, and keep it out of the reach of children. Do not allow anyone else to take your oxyphenbutazone.

Phenylbutazone
(fen ill byoo' ta zone)

Brand names: Azolid, Butagen, Butazolidin, Butazone

Phenylbutazone is used for short-term relief of pain, redness, tenderness, swelling and stiffness of certain types of arthritis and other joint diseases, including gout attacks. Because of the possible side effects and potentially very serious blood problems caused by phenylbutazone, it usually is only used when all other drugs have not been helpful.

UNDESIRED EFFECTS

Many people have undesired effects from phenylbutazone severe enough that they cannot take it. Common side effects of phenylbutazone are nausea, vomiting, indigestion, heartburn, stomach pain and diarrhea. You can help prevent the stomach problems by taking this medicine immediately before or immediately after meals, with a glass of milk or with an antacid. Contact your doctor if these effects continue despite these precautions.

Some people become drowsy, confused or less alert when they take phenylbutazone. Do not drive a car or operate dangerous machinery until you know how this medicine will affect you.

Phenylbutazone may cause weight gain, swelling of your feet and ankles or difficult breathing. Check with your doctor if such problems occur. Using less salt in your diet may help prevent these problems.

More serious problems, such as intestinal bleeding, kidney or liver problems, allergic reactions and eye problems, may occur. Stop taking the drug and contact your doctor immediately if you have any loss of hearing; bloody or black, tarry stools; indigestion or stomach pain; bloody or cloudy urine; difficult or painful urination; difficulty in breathing; wheezing; eye pain or any change in vision; skin rash or hives; swelling of the neck or throat; or yellowing of the eyes and skin.

Serious blood problems can occur many days or weeks after you stop taking phenylbutazone, although these effects are rare. During this period, contact your doctor immediately if you have sore throat, fever, chills, sores or white spots in your mouth, unusual bleeding or bruising, or unusual tiredness or weakness.

PRECAUTIONS

Do not take phenylbutazone if you have ever had a bad reaction to it or if you have ever had an unusual reaction to aspirin or other salicylates, fenoprofen, ibuprofen, indomethacin, meclofenamate, mefenamic acid, naproxen, oxyphenbutazone, sulfinpyrazone, sulindac, tolmetin or zomepirac. Be sure to tell your doctor about any such reaction.

Before you start to take phenylbutazone, tell your doctor if you have or ever had asthma; diseases of the blood, heart, liver, kidneys, pancreas, salivary glands or thyroid glands; high blood pressure; a stomach ulcer or other stomach problems; or diseases characterized by muscle pain or pain in the temples. Phenylbutazone may make these conditions worse.

Tell your doctor what prescription or nonprescription drugs you are taking, especially anticoagulants (blood thinners), medicine for diabetes, isoniazid, digitoxin, any other medicine for arthritis, phenytoin, tetracyclines, iron medications and sulfa medicines. If you do not know the names of the drugs or why they were prescribed, bring them in their labeled containers to your doctor or pharmacist.

If you take phenylbutazone for a week and still have the symptoms for which it was prescribed, contact your doctor. Take phenylbutazone exactly as prescribed. Do not take more of it, take it more often or take it for a longer period of time than ordered by your doctor. Do not take phenylbutazone for any problem other than that for which it was prescribed.

You should have certain laboratory tests before you begin to take phenylbutazone, including blood tests and tests for your kidney, liver and thyroid function. These tests should be repeated every few weeks so your doctor can check on how you are reacting to this drug. *Be sure to keep all appointments with your doctor and at the laboratory.*

Do not drink alcoholic beverages while you are taking phenylbutazone. Do not take aspirin regularly while you are taking phenylbutazone unless you first check with your doctor to find out how much to take. Alcohol or aspirin can make stomach upset more likely to occur.

Before you have surgery with a general anesthetic, including dental surgery, tell your doctor or dentist that you are taking phenylbutazone.

Because phenylbutazone may affect your baby, tell your doctor if you are pregnant or breast-feeding.

DOSAGE AND STORAGE

Your doctor will determine how often you should take phenylbutazone and how much you should take at each dose. Carefully follow the instructions on your prescription label and ask your doctor or pharmacist to explain any part of the instructions you do not understand.

Phenylbutazone comes in capsules and tablets. They should be taken immediately before or immediately after meals, with a full eight-ounce glass of milk or with an antacid to lessen the possibility of stomach upset.

If you forget to take a dose of this medicine, take it as soon as you remember. Then take any remaining doses for the day at evenly spaced intervals. If you remember a missed dose when it is almost time for you to take another, omit the missed dose entirely and take only the regularly scheduled dose. *Do not take a double dose to make up for the missed dose.*

Keep phenylbutazone in the container it came in, and keep it out of the reach of children. Do not allow anyone else to take your phenylbutazone.

Tolmetin
(tole' met in)

Brand name: Tolectin

Tolmetin is used to relieve the pain, redness, tenderness, stiffness and swelling of certain types of arthritis.

UNDESIRED EFFECTS

The most common side effects of tolmetin are stomach upsets such as indigestion, heartburn, nausea, vomiting and stomach pain; diarrhea also is a side effect. To prevent or lessen stomach upset, take this medicine with a meal or snack, milk or an antacid other than sodium bicarbonate (baking soda). If stomach upsets continue, contact your doctor.

Tolmetin may cause some people to become dizzy, lightheaded or drowsy. Do not drive a car or operate dangerous machinery until you know how this medicine will affect you.

Other effects, which may disappear as you continue to take this drug and as your body adjusts to it, include headache, constipation and nervousness. Contact your doctor if these effects continue to bother you.

More serious effects, which do not occur often, will require medical attention if they do occur. Contact your doctor if you have a ringing or buzzing in the ears; skin rash or hives; swelling of the feet, ankles or lower legs; unusual weight gain; bloody or tarry stools; shortness of breath; difficulty breathing; wheezing; tightness in the chest; sore throat; or fever.

PRECAUTIONS

Do not take tolmetin if you have ever had a bad reaction to it or if you have ever had an unusual reaction to aspirin or other salicylates, fenoprofen, ibuprofen, indomethacin, meclofenamate, mefenamic acid, naproxen, oxyphenbutazone, phenylbutazone, sulindac or zomepirac. Be sure to tell your doctor about any such reaction.

Because tolmetin can make certain medical problems worse, tell your doctor if you have bleeding problems, heart disease, kidney disease, a stomach ulcer or other stomach problems.

Tell your doctor what prescription or nonprescription drugs you are taking, especially anticoagulants (blood thinners), medicine for diabetes, any other medicine for arthritis, phenytoin, sulfa medicines and sodium bicarbonate (baking soda). If you do not know the names of the drugs or why they were prescribed, bring them in their labeled containers to your doctor or pharmacist.

Tolmetin will help you only if you take it regularly as prescribed by your doctor. You should begin to feel better within a week after you start to take tolmetin.

Your doctor probably will order laboratory tests for your kidney and liver function as well as blood tests while you are taking this drug. If you have blurred vision or other problems with your eyes after you start to take tolmetin, you also will need an eye examination. *Be sure to keep all appointments with your doctor and at the laboratory*.

Do not drink alcoholic beverages or take aspirin regularly while you are taking tolmetin. Alcohol or aspirin can add to stomach upset. If you have questions about this, check with your doctor or pharmacist.

Before you have any surgery with a general anesthetic, including dental surgery, tell the doctor or dentist that you are taking tolmetin.

Although harm to an unborn child or a nursing baby has not been reported after taking tolmetin, tell your doctor if you are pregnant or breast-feeding before you start to take tolmetin.

DOSAGE AND STORAGE

Your doctor will determine how often you should take tolmetin and how much you should take at each dose. Carefully follow the instructions on your prescription label and ask your doctor or pharmacist to explain any part of the instructions you do not understand.

Tolmetin comes in capsules and tablets. Take the drug with milk or solid food or with an antacid (not sodium bicarbonate) if it upsets your stomach.

If you forget to take a dose of tolmetin, take it as soon as you remember. If you remember a missed dose when it is almost time for you to take another, omit the missed dose entirely and take only the regularly scheduled dose. *Do not take a double dose to make up for a missed dose*.

Keep tolmetin in the container it came in, and keep it out of the reach of children. Do not allow anyone else to take your tolmetin.

STEROIDS
Dexamethasone
(dex a meth' a sone)

Brand names: Decadron, Deronil, Dexameth, Dexone, Hexadrol, SK-Dexamethasone

UNDESIRED EFFECTS (See **corticosteroids**, page 201.)

PRECAUTIONS (See **corticosteroids**, page 201.)
If you are taking the oral form of dexamethasone, do not drink alcoholic beverages. Alcohol can worsen stomach upset caused by taking dexamethasone.

If dexamethasone is injected into one of your joints, you should be careful not to put too much stress or strain on that joint. Ask your doctor how much you are allowed to move the joint while it is healing. If redness or swelling occurs at the place of the injection, contact your doctor.

DOSAGE AND STORAGE

Your doctor will determine how often you should take dexamethasone. Carefully follow the instructions on your prescription label and ask your doctor or pharmacist to explain any part of the instructions you do not understand.

If you are to take dexamethasone once a day, take it in the morning with breakfast. If you are to take this medicine more than once a day, take it at regular intervals between the time you get up in the morning and the time you go to bed at night. For example, if your doctor tells you to take it three times a day, take it at 7:00 a.m., 3:00 p.m. and 11:00 p.m.

Dexamethasone comes in liquid form and in tablets. Take this medicine with meals or a snack to decrease stomach upset.

If you forget to take a dose of dexamethasone when you are on a once-a-day schedule, take the missed dose as soon as you remember it that day. If you do not remember a missed dose until the next day, take only your regularly scheduled dose. *Do not take a double dose to make up for the missed dose.*

If you are taking dexamethasone more than once a day and forget to take a dose, take it as soon as you remember. Take any remaining doses for that day at evenly spaced intervals. If you do not remember a missed dose until it is time for you to take another, you may take both doses at one time.

Keep dexamethasone in the container it came in. If you have arthritis, you may ask your pharmacist to put this medicine in a bottle without a childproof cap.

Keep dexamethasone out of the reach of children. Do not allow anyone else to take your dexamethasone.

Hydrocortisone
(hye droe kor′ ti sone)

Brand names: Cortef, Hydrocortone, Panhydrosone

UNDESIRED EFFECTS (See **corticosteroids**, page 201.)

PRECAUTIONS (See **corticosteroids**, page 201.)

If you are taking the oral form of hydrocortisone, do not drink alcoholic beverages. Alcohol can worsen the stomach upset caused by taking hydrocortisone.

If hydrocortisone is injected into one of your joints, you should be careful not to put too much stress or strain on that joint. Ask your doctor how much you are allowed to move the joint while it is healing. If redness or swelling occurs at the place of the injection, contact your doctor.

DOSAGE AND STORAGE

Your doctor will determine how often you should take hydrocortisone. Carefully follow the instructions on your prescription label and ask your doctor or pharmacist to explain any part of the instructions you do not understand.

If you are to take hydrocortisone once a day, take it in the morning with breakfast.

If you are to take this medicine more than once a day, take it at regular intervals between the time you get up in the morning and the time you go to bed at night. For example, if your doctor tells you to take it three times a day, take it at 7:00 a.m., 3:00 p.m. and 11:00 p.m.

Hydrocortisone comes in liquid form and in tablets. Take this medicine with meals or a snack to decrease stomach upset. Shake the liquid well before each dose.

If you forget to take a dose when you are on a once-a-day schedule, take the missed dose as soon as you remember it. If you do not remember a missed dose until it is time for you to take another, omit the missed dose entirely and take only the regularly scheduled dose.

If you are taking hydrocortisone more than once a day and forget to take a dose, take the missed dose as soon as you remember it. Take any remaining doses for that day at evenly spaced intervals. If you remember a missed dose when it is time for you to take another, you may take both doses at one time.

Keep hydrocortisone in the container it came in, and keep it out of the reach of children. If you have arthritis, you may ask your pharmacist to put this medicine in a bottle without a childproof cap, but be sure to keep it out of the reach of children.

Do not allow anyone else to take your hydrocortisone.

Prednisone

(pred' ni sone)

Brand names: Delta-Dome, Deltasone, Fernisone, Meticorten, Orasone, Pan-Sone, Paracort, Pred-5, Prednicen-M, Ropred, Servisone, SK-Prednisone, Sterapred

UNDESIRED EFFECTS (See **corticosteroids**, page 201.)

PRECAUTIONS (See **corticosteroids**, page 201.)

Do not drink alcoholic beverages while you are taking this medicine. Alcohol with prednisone can cause severe stomach upset.

DOSAGE AND STORAGE

Your doctor will determine how often you should take prednisone. Carefully follow the instructions on your prescription label and ask your doctor or pharmacist to explain any part of the instructions you do not understand.

If you are to take prednisone every other day, take it at breakfast the first day. Do not take it at all on the second day. Then take it at breakfast the third day.

If you are to take prednisone once a day, take it in the morning with breakfast.

If you are to take this medicine more than once a day, take it at regular intervals between the time you get up in the morning and the time you go to bed at night. For example, if your doctor tells you to take it three times a day, take it at 7:00 a.m., 3:00 p.m. and 11:00 p.m.

Prednisone comes in tablets. Take them with meals or a snack to decrease stomach upset.

If you forget to take a dose of prednisone, do one of the following, depending on your dosage schedule:

Schedule of every other day—If you remember a missed dose the morning of the day you should have taken it, take the missed dose as soon as you remember it. If you remember a missed dose on the afternoon of the day you should have taken it, start a new schedule. Take the missed dose the next morning (day one), do not take a dose the morning of day two and take the next dose the morning of day three.

Schedule of once a day—Take the missed dose as soon as you remember it. If you do not remember a missed dose until it is time for you to take another, omit the missed dose entirely and take only the regularly scheduled dose.

Schedule of more than once a day—Take the missed dose as soon as you remember it and take any remaining doses for that day at evenly spaced intervals. If you remember a missed dose when it is time for you to take another, you may take both doses at one time.

Keep prednisone in the container it came in. If you have arthritis, you may ask your pharmacist to put this medicine in a bottle without a childproof cap, but be sure to keep it out of the reach of children.

Do not allow anyone else to take your prednisone.

Triamcinolone
(trye am sin' oh lone)

Brand names: Aristocort, Aristo-Pak, Kenacort, Rocinolone, SK-Triamcinolone, Spencort

UNDESIRED EFFECTS (See **corticosteroids**, page 201.)

PRECAUTIONS (See **corticosteroids**, page 201.)
If you are taking an oral form of triamcinolone, do not drink alcoholic beverages. Alcohol can add to the stomach upset triamcinolone causes.

If triamcinolone is injected into one of your joints, you should be careful not to put too much stress or strain on that joint. Ask your doctor how much you are allowed to move this joint while it is healing. If redness or swelling occurs at the place of the injection, contact your doctor.

DOSAGE AND STORAGE
Your doctor will determine how often you should take triamcinolone. Carefully follow the instructions on your prescription label and ask your doctor or pharmacist to explain any part of the instructions you do not understand.

If you are to take triamcinolone every other day, take it at breakfast the first day. Do not take it at all the second day. Then take it at breakfast the third day.

If you are to take triamcinolone once a day, take it in the morning with breakfast.

If you are to take this medicine more than once a day, take it at regular intervals between the time you get up in the morning and the time you go to bed at night. For example, if your doctor tells you to take it three times a day, take it at 7:00 a.m., 3:00 p.m. and 11:00 p.m.

Triamcinolone comes in tablets and in liquid form. Take this medicine with meals or a snack to lessen stomach upset.

If you forget to take a dose of triamcinolone, do one of the following, depending on your dosage schedule:

Schedule of every other day—If you remember a missed dose the morning of the day you should have taken it, take the missed dose as soon as you remember it. If you remember a missed dose in the afternoon of the day you should have taken it, start a new schedule. Take the missed dose the next morning (day one), do not take it at all on day two and take the next dose the morning of day three.

Schedule of once a day—Take the missed dose as soon as you remember it. If you do not remember a missed dose until it is time for you to take another, omit the missed dose entirely and take only the regularly scheduled dose.

Schedule of more than once a day—Take the missed dose as soon as you remember it and take any remaining doses for that day at evenly spaced intervals. If you remember a missed dose when it is time for you to take another, you may take both doses at one time.

Keep triamcinolone in the container it came in, and keep it out of the reach of children. If you have arthritis, you may ask your pharmacist to put this medicine in a bottle without a childproof cap, but be sure to keep it out of the reach of children.

Do not allow anyone else to take your triamcinolone.

STOMACH AND INTESTINAL PROBLEMS

DRUGS FOR STOMACH
AND INTESTINAL PROBLEMS

Indigestion and Heartburn

"Indigestion" is a term used to describe a variety of complaints, including nausea, upper abdominal or stomach pain, gas and a sense of fullness in the abdomen that occurs during or after eating. Indigestion can be caused by disease in the gastrointestinal tract (stomach and intestines) or by many diseases originating someplace else in the body. Indigestion also can be caused by overeating, eating too fast, or eating foods that are highly seasoned or "rich" or that you are not accustomed to eating. Eating during emotional upsets or severe mental stress also can cause indigestion.

"Heartburn" is a popular term for a sensation of burning in the stomach or the esophagus, the tube connecting the mouth and the stomach. Heartburn can occur when partially digested food is retained in the lower esophagus. Heartburn is common with ulcers and gallbladder disease.

Although indigestion and heartburn can be caused by improper diet, overeating or tension, you should request a physical examination by a doctor if you have indigestion or heartburn persistently.

Antacids are widely used to relieve the symptoms of indigestion and heartburn. Antacids also are commonly prescribed to treat gastric and duodenal ulcers.

All antacids work by neutralizing the acid produced by the stomach. Neutralization of this acid helps relieve the pain and promotes healing of damaged tissue. Although all antacids work in the same way, their strengths vary because of their different capacities to neutralize acid.

When antacids are used as part of the treatment for an ulcer, it is extremely important that you take them on a regular schedule as prescribed. It is also important that you carefully follow your doctor's instructions on diet limitations. A number of drugs aggravate ulcers, and you should check with your doctor or pharmacist before using other drugs, including nonprescription drugs, while you are under treatment for an ulcer.

ANTACIDS
Aluminum Hydroxide and Magnesium Hydroxide
(a loo' min um hye drox' ide) (mag nee' zhum hye drox' ide)

Brand names: Alka-Med, Aludrox, Alumid, Alurex, Creamalin, Delcid, Kolantyl, Kudrox, Maalox, Magmalin, Magnagel, Maxamag, Neosorb Plus, Neutralox, Rolox, Rulox, Spenox, Trialka, WinGel; (with simethicone added) Antar, Di-Gel, Gelusil, Mylanta, Silain-Gel, Simeco, Simethox

Aluminum hydroxide and magnesium hydroxide are antacids that are used together to treat ulcers and to relieve heartburn, stomach gas and upset stomach.

UNDESIRED EFFECTS
This combination medicine can cause nausea, vomiting, diarrhea or constipation. If you experience any of these effects, contact your doctor.

Taking this medicine in large doses or over a long period of time may remove too much phosphorus from the body. Signs of this problem are loss of appetite, muscle weakness and unusual tiredness. Contact your doctor if you experience these symptoms.

PRECAUTIONS
Before you start to take aluminum hydroxide and magnesium hydroxide, tell your doctor or pharmacist if you have kidney disease. Some antacids may make this condition worse.

This medicine may affect the way your body responds to certain other drugs. Tell your doctor or pharmacist what prescription or nonprescription drugs you are now taking, including digoxin, arthritis medicine, ferrous sulfate, isoniazid, buffered aspirin, anticoagulants (blood thinners), pseudoephedrine (decongestant), tetracycline and tranquilizers.

If you are taking aluminum hydroxide and magnesium hydroxide for an ulcer, carefully follow the diet prescribed by your doctor.

Contact your doctor if you have taken aluminum hydroxide and magnesium hydroxide for one week and the pain has not improved or has become worse. You should not take the maximum dose for more than two weeks unless your doctor tells you to do so.

DOSAGE AND STORAGE
If this medicine was prescribed by your doctor, he has determined how often you should take it and how much you should take at each dose. Carefully follow the instructions on your prescription label. If you buy this medicine without a prescription, carefully follow the directions on the label. Ask your doctor or pharmacist to explain any part of the directions you do not understand.

This medicine comes in tablets and in liquid form. The tablets should be chewed thoroughly before they are swallowed. The liquid should be shaken well before you take it.

If you forget to take a dose of this medicine, take it as soon as you remember. Take the remaining doses for that day at the regularly scheduled times.

Keep this medicine in the container it came in. Keep it tightly closed and store the container at room temperature. Keep this medicine out of the reach of children.

Calcium Carbonate
(kal′ see um kar′ bone ate)

Brand names: Alka-2, Amitone, Calcilac, Calglycine, Dicarbosil, El-Da-Mint, Equilet, Gustalac, Mallamint, P.H., Spentacid, Titralac, Titracid, Trialka, Tums

Calcium carbonate is an antacid that neutralizes stomach acid. Calcium carbonate is used as a part of total therapy for certain types of stomach ulcers and to relieve indigestion, heartburn and sour stomach.

UNDESIRED EFFECTS

Calcium carbonate can cause constipation, belching and gas. You can expect a chalky taste with this medicine.

If you take calcium carbonate in large doses or for a long period of time, or if you drink large amounts of milk while taking this medicine regularly, too much calcium can build up in your body. This could upset your body chemistry and lead to kidney stones. Signs of this problem are nausea, vomiting, loss of appetite, weakness, headache and dizziness. Contact your doctor if you experience these effects.

Contact your doctor if you have severe stomach pain or heartburn a few hours after taking this medicine.

PRECAUTIONS

You should not take calcium carbonate if you have a history of kidney stones. If you do, ask your doctor or pharmacist to recommend a different antacid for you.

Before you start to take calcium carbonate, tell your doctor or pharmacist what prescription or nonprescription drugs you are taking, including tetracyclines, digoxin (heart medicine), indomethacin (arthritis medicine), ferrous sulfate, buffered aspirin and anticoagulants (blood thinners). If you do not know the names of the drugs or why they were prescribed, bring them in their labeled containers to your doctor or pharmacist.

You should not take the maximum dose of calcium carbonate for more than two weeks unless your doctor tells you to do so. If you are taking calcium carbonate over a long period of time, your doctor will want to check your response to this medicine at regular visits. *Be sure to keep all of your appointments with your doctor.*

DOSAGE AND STORAGE

If your doctor has prescribed calcium carbonate, he has determined how often you should take it and how much you should take at each dose. Carefully follow the instructions on your prescription label and ask your doctor or pharmacist to explain any part of the instructions you do not understand. If you buy calcium carbonate without a prescription, carefully follow the instructions on the label.

Calcium carbonate comes in tablets and in liquid form. The tablets should be chewed completely.

If you forget to take a dose of this medicine, take it as soon as you remember. Then take the remaining doses for that day on your regular dosage schedule.

Keep calcium carbonate in the container it came in, and keep it out of the reach of children.

Sodium Bicarbonate

(do' dee um bye car' bone ate)

Other name: baking soda

Brand names of some products containing sodium bicarbonate: Alka-Seltzer, Bell-Ans Citrocarbonate, Bisodol Powder, Soda Mint and others

Sodium bicarbonate is an antacid used to relieve occasional acid indigestion, heartburn and sour stomach.

UNDESIRED EFFECTS

The most common side effects of sodium bicarbonate are passing gas and swelling of the abdomen.

Sodium bicarbonate, taken in large amounts or regularly over a long period of time, can cause high blood pressure and seriously upset your body chemistry. If you drink large amounts of milk while taking this medicine regularly, too much calcium may build up in your body. Contact your doctor if you have nausea, vomiting, headache, mental confusion or loss of appetite.

PRECAUTIONS

If you have high blood pressure, heart failure, kidney disease, swelling of the legs and feet or cirrhosis of the liver, you should not take sodium bicarbonate. It can make these conditions worse. Do not use sodium bicarbonate if you are on a salt-free or sodium-free diet. If you have any questions about this, check with your doctor or pharmacist.

Sodium bicarbonate can affect the way certain medications act in your body. You should not take sodium bicarbonate if you are already taking anticoagulants (blood thinners), digoxin, indomethacin, naproxen or other medicines for arthritis, ferrous sulfate, amphetamines, buffered aspirin or quinidine (medicine for irregular heartbeat). If you do not know the names of the drugs you are taking or why they were prescribed, bring them in their labeled containers to your doctor or pharmacist.

Do not use sodium bicarbonate over a long period of time, or regularly for more than two weeks. Too much sodium in your body can cause problems. If you have questions about this, check with your doctor or pharmacist.

If you are allergic to aspirin, be sure to check the package label of combination products to avoid those that contain aspirin (for example, some types of Alka-Seltzer contain aspirin).

DOSAGE AND STORAGE

If your doctor has prescribed sodium bicarbonate, carefully follow his instructions on how often to take it and how much to take at each dose. If you buy sodium bicarbonate without a prescription, follow the directions on the container and ask your pharmacist to explain any part of the directions you do not understand.

Sodium bicarbonate comes in a powder to be dissolved in a full eight-ounce glass of water. Stir the medicine and water well before you drink it.

Keep this medicine in the container it came in, and keep it out of the reach of children.

ANTIGAS DRUG
Simethicone
(sye meth′ eye cone)

Brand names: Gas-X, Mylicon

Names of preparations containing simethicone: Di-Gel, Gelusil, Maalox Plus, Mylanta, Phazyme, Riopam Plus, Silain-Gel and others

Simethicone is an antiflatulent that acts on gas bubbles in the intestinal tract to make it possible for gas to be released by belching or by passing gas. Simethicone is used for gas pain after surgery and for many conditions in which gas in the intestines may be a problem.

UNDESIRED EFFECTS
At the present time, there are no known side effects after taking simethicone. However, if you do have undesired effects after taking simethicone, contact your doctor.

PRECAUTIONS
Do not use simethicone for infant colic. Safe use of simethicone for infants and children has not been established.

DOSAGE AND STORAGE
If your doctor has prescribed this medicine, he has determined how often you should take it and how much you should take at each dose. Carefully follow the instructions on your prescription label and ask your doctor or pharmacist to explain any part of the instructions you do not understand. If you buy simethicone without a prescription, carefully follow the label instructions on how often to take this medicine and how much to take at each dose.

Simethicone comes in tablets and in liquid form. The tablets should be thoroughly chewed before they are swallowed. Shake the liquid well before each use. Measure the proper dose with the dropper included with the container. Be sure you know how to use the dropper. Ask your pharmacist to explain the use of the dropper if you have any questions about this.

Keep simethicone in the container it came in, and keep it out of the reach of children.

CONSTIPATION

Laxatives may be the most widely misused class of drugs. Excessive use of laxatives stems from the popular belief that "regularity" (one bowel movement per day) is absolutely essential for good health. This idea is heavily promoted through advertisements by manufacturers of various laxative products.

In fact, normal frequency of bowel movements can vary from three times per day to three times per week, depending on the individual. The normal frequency for each person is determined by his or her physiology, diet and lifestyle. Laxatives are needed only when you become constipated compared to your regular bowel-movement habits.

Laxatives frequently are used to prepare a person for X rays or other diagnostic tests. When used for this purpose, your doctor will give you specific instructions on how to use the laxative.

There are several different types of laxatives available. The bulk-producing laxatives increase the size of the stool. The increase in size stimulates bowel contractions to produce a bowel movement. The lubricant laxatives coat the stool with oil to prevent them from becoming hard and difficult to pass. Castor oil and glycerin suppositories stimulate the bowel directly to produce a bowel movement.

Before using any laxative it is important to tell your doctor or pharmacist what drugs you are taking and whether you have any other medical condition, particularly if you have had recent surgery. You should not use any laxative product for more than one week unless directed to by your doctor. Prolonged use of laxatives can be habit-forming and may lead to loss of important nutrients and damage to the bowel.

LAXATIVES
Bulk-forming Laxatives

Drug name	Brand names
methylcellulose	Cellothyl
(meth ill sell′ yoo lows)	Cologel
	Hydrolose
malt soup extract	Maltsupex
	Syllamalt (combined with psyllium)
psyllium (sil′ ee yum)	Effersyllium
	Konsyl
	L.A. Formula
	Laxamead
	Metamucil

Drug name	*Brand names*
psyllium (cont.)	Modane
	Mucillium
	Mucilose
	Regacillium
	Serutan
	Siblin
	Syllact

Bulk-forming laxatives act in a way similar to that of high-fiber-content foods in the diet. They absorb water in the intestines and add bulk to the bowel contents. The bulk stimulates muscular contractions in the bowel and helps the bowel to empty. Bulk-forming laxatives begin to work in 12 to 24 hours, but you may not notice their full laxative effect until a day or two after you start taking them. Although there are several different bulk laxatives, all work in the same basic way.

These medicines are the preferred drugs for constipation during pregnancy or after childbirth. They are also used after surgery and for patients with conditions (such as heart attack, high blood pressure, blood vessel disease, anal or rectal disease and hernia) in which straining to move the bowels might cause a problem.

UNDESIRED EFFECTS
Side effects with bulk-forming laxatives are rare. If these effects occur, contact your doctor.

Bulk-forming laxatives can cause blockage of the esophagus or the bowel if they are taken without enough liquid. To prevent this problem, always take these medicines with a full eight-ounce glass of water and be sure to prepare them according to instructions.

PRECAUTIONS
Do not take a bulk-forming laxative if you have abdominal pain, bloating, nausea or vomiting. These may be symptoms of appendicitis or other abdominal problems. Contact your doctor if you have these symptoms.

Do not take bulk-forming laxatives if you have intestinal ulceration, blockage of the bowel or difficulty swallowing. If you need a laxative, check with your doctor or pharmacist about one you may use without problems. Tell your doctor if you have high blood pressure, diabetes or kidney or heart problems.

If you are taking antacids, antibiotics, anticoagulants (blood thinners), aspirin, birth-control pills, heart medicine, nitrofurantoin (antibacterial medicine for urinary tract infections), pain medicine or other laxatives, do not start to use bulk-forming laxatives before first checking with your doctor or pharmacist.

Take only as much of bulk-forming laxatives as directed by your doctor or by the instructions on the package. Do not take them for a longer time than directed. If you take a bulk-forming laxative regularly for a week and still are constipated, contact your doctor.

DOSAGE AND STORAGE

If a bulk-forming laxative has been prescribed for you, your doctor has determined how often you should take it and how much to take at each dose. Carefully follow the instructions on your prescription label and ask your doctor or pharmacist to explain any part of the instructions you do not understand.

If you buy a bulk-forming laxative without a prescription, be sure to follow the directions on the package carefully. Check with your pharmacist if you have any questions about how often to take this medicine or how much to take.

Bulk-forming laxatives come in powders, flakes, granules, tablets and liquid form and should be dissolved or diluted according to the directions on the package. All forms should be taken with a full eight-ounce glass of water. *Be sure to drink plenty of fluids while taking any laxatives.*

If you forget to take a dose of this medicine, take it as soon as you remember and take any remaining doses for that day at evenly spaced intervals. If you remember a missed dose when it is almost time for you to take another, omit the missed dose entirely and take only the regularly scheduled dose. *Do not take a double dose to make up for the missed dose.*

Keep bulk-forming laxatives in the containers they came in. Keep them out of the reach of children.

Castor Oil
(kas′ tore)

Brand names: Alphamul, Emulsoil, Neoloid

Castor oil acts on the intestines to speed up the emptying action of the bowel. The result usually is a violent emptying of bowel contents. Though once a commonly used laxative for simple constipation, castor oil now is used almost exclusively to clean the bowel before surgery, or before X-ray or scope examination of the bowel.

UNDESIRED EFFECTS

Following a dose of castor oil, you may experience intestinal discomfort, nausea, mild cramps, bowel pain or fainting.

Long-term use of castor oil may make it impossible for you to have a bowel movement without using this laxative. You may lose weight because your food is not nourishing your body as it should. Minerals that the body needs may be removed if you take castor oil too often. This can cause vomiting and muscle weakness. Contact your doctor if you have any of these problems.

If you or a child accidentally take too much castor oil, contact your doctor or a poison control center immediately. Signs of overdose are unusually rapid breathing, abdominal pain, diarrhea, nausea or vomiting.

PRECAUTIONS

Do not take castor oil if you have abdominal pain, bloating, nausea or vomiting. These may be signs of appendicitis and you should contact your doctor instead. Pregnant women, women who are menstruating and people who have bowel obstruction should not use castor oil. If you have any questions about this, check with your doctor or pharmacist. Tell your doctor if you are breast-feeding or have high blood pressure, diabetes, or kidney, heart or intestinal problems.

Tell your doctor what prescription or nonprescription drugs you are taking, especially antacids, antibiotics, anticoagulants (blood thinners), birth-control pills, medicine for your heart or other laxatives. If you do not know the names of the drugs you are taking or why they were prescribed, bring them in their labeled containers to your doctor or pharmacist.

Castor oil should be used only for infrequent bouts of constipation. Frequent or continued use can cause laxative dependence because castor oil is habit-forming. If you have used castor oil regularly for a week and still are constipated, contact your doctor.

DOSAGE AND STORAGE

Castor oil is available as an emulsion, usually flavored to mask its disagreeable taste. Shake the emulsion well before using. Carefully follow the instructions on the package for the proper dose and check with your pharmacist if you have any questions about how much to take.

Mix castor oil with one-half glass (four ounces) or a full eight-ounce glass of water, milk, fruit juice or a soft drink. *Be sure to drink plenty of fluids while taking any laxative.*

Keep castor oil in the container it came in, and keep it out of the reach of children.

Glycerin Suppositories

(gliss' ehr in supp pos' i tor eez)

Glycerin draws water from the bowel itself into the bowel contents with the result that the bowel is emptied. It is given as a rectal suppository and is particularly useful for constipation in infants and children.

UNDESIRED EFFECTS

Glycerin suppositories have few side effects when used infrequently and for a short period of time. This medicine may cause rectal discomfort, irritation, burning, bowel pain, cramps or straining without producing a bowel movement. If these effects are bothersome, contact your doctor.

If glycerin suppositories cause a bloody discharge from the rectum, contact your doctor.

Overuse of this medicine may cause continuing diarrhea, which leads to a loss of vitamins and minerals and a potentially dangerous decrease in body water. Stop using glycerin suppositories and contact your doctor if continuing diarrhea is a problem.

PRECAUTIONS

Do not use glycerin suppositories if you have abdominal pain, bloating, nausea or vomiting. These may be symptoms of appendicitis or some other problem. Instead, contact your doctor.

Do not use more of this medicine than directed by your doctor or than indicated on the package label. Do not use it for a long period of time. If you have used glycerin suppositories regularly for a week and still are constipated, contact your doctor.

DOSAGE AND STORAGE
If your doctor has prescribed glycerin suppositories, he has determined how often you should use them. Carefully follow the instructions on your prescription label and ask your doctor or pharmacist to explain any part of the instructions you do not understand.

If you buy these suppositories without a prescription, carefully follow the instructions for use on the package. Check with your pharmacist if you have questions about the instructions.

To use the suppositories, remove the foil wrapper and moisten the tip of the suppository with water. Then lie on your side, bring your top knee to your chest and insert the suppository well into the rectum with your finger. A bowel movement usually will occur within 15 to 30 minutes.

Be sure to drink enough fluids while taking any laxative. Keep glycerin suppositories in the container they came in and store them away from heat and direct sunlight. Keep them out of the reach of children. Do not allow anyone else to use your glycerin suppositories.

Mineral Oil

Brand names: Agoral Plain, Kondremul Plain Emulsion, Fleet Mineral Oil Enema, Neo-Cultol, Nujol, Petrogalar Plain, Saf-Tip Oil Enema

Brand names of some products containing mineral oil: Agoral and Agoral Raspberry (with phenolphthalein), Haley's M-O (with milk of magnesia), Kondremul with Cascara Emulsion, Kondremul with Phenolphthalein, Petrogalar and Cascara, Petrogalar and Phenolphthalein, Petro-Syllium (with psyllium)

Mineral oils puts an oily film over the lining of the bowel to prevent water from leaving the stool. This action keeps the stool soft and aids in emptying the bowel.

Mineral oil often is prescribed after surgery and for people with conditions (such as heart attack, high blood pressure, blood vessel disease, anal or rectal disease and hernia) in which straining to move the bowels might cause problems.

UNDESIRED EFFECTS
When properly used (infrequently and for short periods of time), mineral oil has few side effects. Seepage from the rectum is a common problem. This seepage can stain the clothing, cause irritation and anal itching and increase infection in bleeding hemorrhoids or rectal fissures and prevent their healing. Usually this leakage can be avoided by taking a smaller dose or by dividing the dose into several smaller ones and taking them at intervals.

Taking mineral oil over a long period of time can result in your body being unable to absorb and use vitamins A, D, E and K. It also can cause loss of essential minerals and other important nutrients, continuing diarrhea and a potentially dangerous loss of water from the body.

When mineral oil is taken in large doses over an extended period of time, it can be absorbed into the body and cause tumors in the lymph nodes, liver and spleen.

PRECAUTIONS

Do not take mineral oil if you have abdominal pain, bloating, nausea or vomiting. These may be symptoms of appendicitis or other abdominal problems and you should contact your doctor. Do not take mineral oil if you have stomach or esophagus disease, difficulty in swallowing or hiatal hernia. If you have any questions about this, check with your doctor or pharmacist. Tell your doctor if you have high blood pressure, diabetes or kidney or heart problems.

Mineral oil may make certain medicines less effective. Tell your doctor what prescription or nonprescription drugs you are taking, especially antacids, antibiotics, anticoagulants (blood thinners), birth-control pills, heart medicine, other laxatives and vitamins A, D, E or K. If you do not know the names of the drugs you are taking or why they were prescribed, bring them in their labeled containers to your doctor or pharmacist.

Check with your doctor before giving oral mineral oil to children under six years of age or to very elderly or very sick persons. There is a chance they may inhale some of the oil, which can cause inflammation of the lungs.

Do not take mineral oil any longer than directed by your doctor or the instructions on the package. If you take oral mineral oil for a week and still are constipated, contact your doctor.

If you are pregnant, do not use mineral oil. Regular use of this medicine can cause blood problems in the baby. If you have questions about this, check with your doctor.

DOSAGE AND STORAGE

If mineral oil has been prescribed for you, your doctor has determined how often you should take it and how much you should take at each dose. Carefully follow the instructions on your prescription label and ask your doctor or pharmacist to explain any part of the instructions you do not understand.

If you buy mineral oil without a prescription, carefully follow the instructions on the package as to the proper use of this medicine. Check with your pharmacist if you have questions about this.

Mineral oil comes as plain oil and as an oil emulsion to be taken by mouth, and as an enema to be given rectally.

The oral forms should be taken on an empty stomach to prevent interference with absorption of vitamins from your food. The laxative will begin to work in six to eight hours. Be sure you know how to use the enema form. If you do not understand the directions on the package, ask your pharmacist to explain them.

Be sure to drink enough fluids while taking any laxative. Keep mineral oil in the container it came in, and keep it out of the reach of children.

STOOL SOFTENER
Docusate
(dock' you sate)

Brand names: Afko-Lube, Bu-Lax, Colace, Colax, Coloctyl, Comfolax, Dilax, Dioeze, Diomedicone, Diosuccin, Disonate, Doctate, Doxinate, Doss, D.S.S., Kasof, Laxinate, Modane, Molatoc, Regul-Aids, Regutol, Revak, Sofner, Surfak

Docusate softens stools and makes them easier to pass. It often is given to women during pregnancy and after childbirth, and to patients after surgery. It also is used to ease bowel movements for people who should avoid straining (people with heart conditions, hernia or hemorrhoids).

UNDESIRED EFFECTS
Side effects with docusate are rare. Occasionally this medicine will cause mild stomach cramps, diarrhea, loose stools or throat irritation. Contact your doctor if these effects bother you.

PRECAUTIONS
Stool softeners may affect the absorption of many oral drugs. *Do not take mineral oil while you are taking this medicine.* Docusate increases the absorption of mineral oil into the body, which can cause liver or spleen problems. Tell your doctor what prescription or nonprescription drugs you are taking, including aspirin and other laxatives.

Tell your doctor if you have abdominal pain, bloating, nausea or vomiting (signs of appendicitis or intestinal disease), high blood pressure, diabetes, or kidney or heart problems. Do not take docusate longer than your doctor has told you to. If your stools still are hard after this period, ask your doctor or pharmacist whether you should change your diet or do some kind of exercise to relieve your problem.

DOSAGE AND STORAGE
If docusate has been prescribed for you, your doctor has determined how often you should take it and how much you should take at each dose. If you buy this medication without a prescription, carefully follow the directions for use on the package. If you have any questions about the proper use of this medicine or do not understand the directions on your prescription label, ask your doctor or pharmacist for an explanation.

Docusate comes in capsules, tablets and liquid form. All three forms should be taken with a full eight-ounce glass of water. You may take the liquid by adding it to milk or fruit juice.

If you forget to take a dose, take it as soon as you remember. If you do not remember a missed dose until it is almost time for you to take another, omit the missed dose completely and take only the regularly scheduled dose. *Do not take two doses at one time. Be sure to drink plenty of fluids while taking any laxatives.*

Keep this medicine in the container it came in, and keep it out of the reach of children. Do not allow anyone else to take your docusate.

DIARRHEA

Diarrhea is the frequent passage of loose stools. Because individual bowel habits vary widely, diarrhea is defined as an increase of passage of loose stools over an individual's normal pattern.

Diarrhea can be an acute, short-term condition or a chronic problem. In either case, diarrhea is a symptom of some GI disorder. The causes of acute diarrhea include infection (bacterial or viral), food poisoning, adverse drug effects and dietary imbalances.

Persistent or recurrent diarrhea may be a signal of more serious disease, particularly if other symptoms are present. Individuals who experience weight loss, weakness or loss of appetite should contact a physician to determine the underlying cause of their diarrhea.

The biggest dangers associated with diarrhea are dehydration and loss of electrolytes. These are particularly dangerous in infants and small children because their supply of water and electrolytes can be depleted very quickly. A child under three years experiencing disorder should always be seen by a doctor so the cause and severity can be evaluated. The doctor may wish to prescribe a special fluid and electrolyte solution.

ANTIDIARRHEALS
Diphenoxylate and Atropine
(dye fen ox' i late) (a' troe peen)

Brand names: Colonil, Lomotil

Diphenoxylate and atropine relax the intestinal tract. This combination of medications is used to treat certain types of severe diarrhea.

UNDESIRED EFFECTS

This medicine can cause thirst and dry mouth. To relieve these effects, drink a lot of fluids and chew gum or suck hard candies.

Some people get dizzy or drowsy when they take diphenoxylate and atropine. Do not drive a car or operate dangerous machinery until you know how this medicine will affect you.

Other side effects, which may disappear as your body adjusts to the medicine, are blurred vision, depression, fever, flushing, headache, numbness of the hands or feet, rapid heartbeat, skin rash or itching, swelling of the gums or an unusual decrease in urination. Contact your doctor if you have these effects and they continue or get worse.

More serious side effects will require medical attention. Contact your doctor if you have bloating, constipation, loss of appetite, nausea and vomiting, or stomach pain.

Taking too much diphenoxylate and atropine can be dangerous. Signs of an overdose are fainting, pinpoint pupils, shallow breathing and unusual excitement. If you have these symptoms, contact your doctor or poison control center immediately.

When you stop taking this medicine, your body may need time to adjust to it. During the adjustment period, contact your doctor if you have muscle cramps, nausea and vomiting, shaking or trembling, stomach cramps or unusual sweating.

PRECAUTIONS

Before you start to take diphenoxylate and atropine, tell your doctor if you have Addison's disease, alcoholism, colitis, difficult urination, emphysema, asthma, bronchitis or other chronic lung disease, an enlarged prostate, gallbladder disease or gallstones, glaucoma, heart disease, hiatal hernia, high blood pressure, kidney disease, liver disease, myasthenia gravis, or an overactive or underactive thyroid. This medicine may make these conditions worse.

Tell your doctor what prescription or nonprescription drugs you are taking, particularly amantadine, haloperidol, medicine for your heart, medicine for ulcers, antihistamines, medicine for allergies or colds, barbiturates, narcotics, prescription medicine for pain, sedatives, tranquilizers, medicine to help you sleep, medicine for seizures, medicine for depression and MAO inhibitors (even if you stopped taking them within the past two weeks).

If you do not know the names of the drugs or what they were prescribed for, bring them in their labeled containers to your doctor or pharmacist.

Do not drink alcoholic beverages while you are taking diphenoxylate and atropine. Do not start to take any of the drugs listed above unless you first check with your doctor or pharmacist. All of these can increase the chance of and severity of side effects.

Take diphenoxylate and atropine exactly as prescribed by your doctor. Do not take more of it, do not take it more often and do not take it for a longer period of time than your doctor has ordered. Too much of this medicine can be habit-forming, or can cause an overdose in a child.

If your diarrhea does not stop a few days after you start taking diphenoxylate and atropine or if you develop a fever, contact your doctor.

Check with your doctor if you want to stop taking this medicine. He may want you gradually to reduce the amount you are taking before you stop completely.

Keep in touch with your doctor while you are taking this medicine. Before you have any kind of surgery, including dental surgery, tell the doctor or dentist in charge that you are taking diphenoxylate and atropine.

To help your doctor choose the best treatment for you and your baby, be sure to tell him if you are pregnant or are nursing a baby. The effects of these drugs on an unborn child and a breast-fed baby are not known.

DOSAGE AND STORAGE

Your doctor will determine how often you should take this medicine and how much you should take at each dose. The effectiveness of diphenoxylate and atropine starts 45 to 60 minutes after it is taken and continues for three to four hours. This medicine often is prescribed to be taken after loose bowel movements occur. Carefully follow the instructions on your prescription label and ask your doctor or pharmacist to explain any part of the instructions you do not understand.

Diphenoxylate and atropine comes in tablets for adults and in liquid form for children. The liquid comes in a container with a special dropper to measure the exact dose. Be sure you know how to use the dropper properly. If you have any questions, check with your doctor or pharmacist. Be sure to shake the liquid well before each use.

If you forget to take a dose of this medicine and you still have diarrhea, take the dose as soon as you remember it and take any remaining doses for that day at evenly spaced intervals. If you do not have diarrhea, omit the missed dose completely and take only the next regularly scheduled dose. *Do not take a double dose to make up for the missed dose.*

Keep this medicine in the container it came in. Keep it out of the reach of children. An overdose is especially dangerous for children. Do not allow anyone else to take your diphenoxylate and atropine.

Paregoric
(par eh gore′ ik)

Brand names of preparations containing paregoric: Donnagel-PG, Infantol Pink, Kenpectin-P, Mul-Sed, Parepectolin

Paregoric is a mixture of opium, anise oil, benzoic acid, camphor, glycerin and alcohol. Paregoric relaxes the intestines to relieve diarrhea. Paregoric is available alone or in combination with kaolin, pectin and bismuth (substances also used to treat diarrhea).

UNDESIRED EFFECTS

Occasionally, paregoric will cause nausea and stomach upset. If this occurs you may take paregoric with food or milk. If stomach upsets continue or are severe, contact your doctor. Paregoric makes some people drowsy. Do not drive a car or operate dangerous machinery until you know how it will affect you.

When paregoric is taken in low doses for a short period of time, it rarely is habit-forming. However, if you take this medicine over a long period of time (for example, as treatment of diarrhea resulting from chronic inflammation of the bowel), your body may need time to adjust when you stop taking it. During this adjustment period, contact your doctor if you have convulsions or seizures, hallucinations (seeing, hearing or feeling things that are not there), increased dreaming, muscle twitching, nausea or vomiting, nightmares, trembling, trouble sleeping or unusual nervousness or restlessness.

Taking too much paregoric can be dangerous. If you accidentally take too much, contact your doctor immediately or go to the nearest hospital emergency room. Signs of an overdose are constipation, unusually slow heartbeat, shortness of breath or difficulty breathing.

PRECAUTIONS

Because paregoric can make some medical conditions worse, tell your doctor if you have emphysema, asthma, any other chronic lung disease, an enlarged prostate, liver disease, or a history of drug abuse or dependence.

Tell your doctor what prescription or nonprescription drugs you are taking, including antihistamines, medicine for allergies or colds, barbiturates, narcotics, sedatives, tranquilizers, medicine to help you sleep, prescription medicine for pain, medicine for seizures, medicine for depression and MAO inhibitors (even if you stopped taking them within the past two weeks). If you do not know the names of the drugs or what they were prescribed for, bring them in their labeled containers to your doctor or pharmacist.

Do not drink alcoholic beverages while you are taking paregoric. Do not start to take any of the drugs listed above without first checking with your doctor or pharmacist. All of these can increase the chance of and/or severity of side effects.

Take paregoric exactly as your doctor has prescribed it. Do not take more of it, do not take it more often and do not take it for a longer period of time than your doctor has ordered. If you take this medicine for a long period of time, do not stop taking it unless you first check with your doctor. He may want you gradually to reduce the amount you take before you stop completely.

To help your doctor select the best treatment for you and your baby, tell him if you are pregnant or are nursing a baby.

DOSAGE AND STORAGE

Your doctor will determine how often you should take paregoric and how much you should take at each dose. Paregoric usually is prescribed to be taken after each loose bowel movement. Carefully follow the instructions on your prescription label and ask your doctor or pharmacist to explain any part of the instructions you do not understand.

Paregoric comes in liquid form. Use a specially marked measuring spoon to be sure you get an accurate dose.

If you are taking paregoric on a regular dosage schedule and forget to take a dose, do one of the following: (1) If you still have diarrhea, take the missed dose as soon as you remember it and take any remaining doses for that day at evenly spaced intervals. (2) If you do not have diarrhea any longer, omit the missed dose entirely and take only the regularly scheduled dose. *Do not take a double dose to make up for the missed one.*

Keep paregoric in the container it came in, and store it away from heat and direct sunlight. Keep this medicine out of the reach of children. Do not allow anyone else to take your paregoric.

Nausea and Vomiting

Nausea and vomiting are symptoms common to a wide variety of illnesses. Some of the common causes of vomiting are:
- Infections, including the "flu" and various types of gastroenteritis
- Food poisoning
- Disturbances of the inner ear
- Motion sickness
- Radiation therapy
- Drugs; nausea and vomiting may be side effects or symptoms of an overdose
- Serious illness; appendicitis, migraine headache, hormonal imbalance and many other diseases may cause nausea and vomiting

If you experience vomiting for more than two days or if you notice blood in the vomit or have stomach or abdominal pain, you should contact your doctor. Sometimes blood may look like coffee grounds rather than bright red. Therefore, if you notice material that looks like coffee grounds in your vomit, you should contact your doctor.

An infant who is vomiting should be seen by a doctor if simple causes (for example, overfeeding) are not obvious.

ANTI-EMETICS
Hydroxyzine

Hydroxyzine is also used to treat nausea and vomiting. (See the section on **hydroxyzine**, page 316.)

Meclizine
(mek' li zeen)

Brand names: Antivert, Bonine, Eldezine, Roclizine, Vertrol, Wehvert

Meclizine is an antihistamine that is not used to treat allergies. It is particularly useful in preventing the nausea, vomiting and dizziness caused by motion sickness. It also is used to treat the dizziness caused by certain ear conditions such as Meniere's disease.

UNDESIRED EFFECTS

One of the most common effects of meclizine is dry mouth. To relieve this dryness, drink fluids, chew gum or suck hard candy or ice chips.

Like other antihistamines, meclizine may make you drowsy or less alert than normal. Do not operate dangerous machinery or drive a car until you know how this medicine will affect you.

Occasionally or rarely, meclizine will cause blurred vision, difficult or painful urination, headache, loss of appeite, nervousness or trouble sleeping, skin rash, unusually fast heartbeat or upset stomach. If you experience these effects, contact your doctor.

PRECAUTIONS

Before you start to take meclizine, tell your doctor if you have an enlarged prostate, a stomach ulcer, urinary tract blockage or glaucoma. This medicine can make these conditions worse.

Tell your doctor what prescription or nonprescription drugs you are taking, including barbiturates, medicine for seizures, narcotics, other antihistamines, medicine for allergies and colds, prescription medicine for pain, sedatives, tranquilizers and medicine to help you sleep. If you do not know the names of the drugs or what they were prescribed for, bring them in their labeled containers to your doctor or pharmacist.

Do not drink alcoholic beverages while you are taking meclizine. Do not start to take any of the drugs listed above without first checking with your doctor or pharmacist. All of these can increase the drowsiness caused by meclizine.

Take meclizine exactly as directed. Do not take more of it and do not take it more often than your doctor has ordered.

If you are taking large amounts of aspirin (for arthritis or other conditions), be sure your doctor knows this before you start taking meclizine on a regular basis. Meclizine may cover up symptoms that may develop after taking too much aspirin, such as ringing in the ears.

Meclizine should not be taken by children under the age of 12 because its safe use for those in this age group has not been established. Meclizine should not be taken by nursing mothers because it may dry up their milk.

Before you start to take meclizine, tell your doctor if you are pregnant or plan to become pregnant while taking this medicine. It is not known whether this medicine may have bad effects on an unborn child.

DOSAGE AND STORAGE

When meclizine is used for motion sickness, you should take this medicine one hour before you start to travel. If you are taking meclizine for the dizziness caused by an ear condition, your doctor has determined how often you should take this medicine and how much to take at each dose. Carefully follow the instructions on your prescription label and ask your doctor or pharmacist to explain any part of the instructions you do not understand.

Meclizine comes in regular tablets and chewable tablets. The chewable tablets may be chewed or swallowed whole.

If you forget to take a dose of meclizine, take it as soon as you remember. Then take any remaining doses for that day at evenly spaced intervals. *Do not take more than one dose at a time.*

Keep meclizine in the container it came in, and keep it out of the reach of children. Do not allow anyone else to take your meclizine.

Prochlorperazine

Prochlorperazine is also used to treat nausea and vomiting. (See the section on **hydroxyzine**, page 316.)

Trimethobenzamide
(trye meth oh ben′ za mide)

Brand name: Tigan

Trimethobenzamide acts on the portion of the brain that controls the vomiting center. Trimethobenzamide is used to control nausea and vomiting caused by radiation therapy and certain types of diseases.

UNDESIRED EFFECTS

Trimethobenzamide may cause some people to become drowsy, dizzy or lightheaded. Do not drive a car or operate dangerous machinery until you know how this medicine will affect you.

Other effects, which may disappear as your body adjusts to this medicine, are blurred vision, diarrhea, headache and muscle cramps. If these effects continue or bother you, contact your doctor.

More serious side effects are Reye's syndrome, blood problems and liver problems, which will need medical attention if they occur. Contact your doctor if you have back pain, mental depression, seizures, severe or continuing vomiting, shakiness or tremors, sore throat and fever, an unusual feeling of tiredness or yellowing of the eyes and skin.

PRECAUTIONS

If you are allergic to benzocaine or other local anesthetics, you should not use the suppository form of this medicine, which contains benzocaine. If you have any questions about this, check with your doctor or pharmacist.

Tell your doctor what prescription or nonprescription drugs you are taking, including antihistamines, medicine for allergies or colds, barbiturates, narcotics, phenothiazines, prescription medicine for pain, sedatives, tranquilizers, medicine to help you sleep and medicine for seizures. If you do not know the names of the drugs or what they were prescribed for, bring them in their labeled containers to your doctor or pharmacist.

Do not drink alcoholic beverages while you are taking trimethobenzamide. Do not start to take any of the drugs listed above without checking first with your doctor. All of these can increase the chance of and/or severity of side effects.

Because trimethobenzamide is used only to relieve or prevent nausea and vomiting, take it exactly as prescribed by your doctor. Do not take more of it and do not take it more often than your doctor has ordered.

Do not give this medicine to a child unless you have your doctor's permission. If you are using trimethobenzamide to control a child's nausea and vomiting, be especially careful not to give more than prescribed. Side effects may be more serious in children.

Before you start to take trimethobenzamide, tell your doctor if you are pregnant or are nursing a baby. Safe use of this drug in pregnant women and breast-feeding mothers has not been established.

DOSAGE AND STORAGE

Your doctor will determine how often you should take trimethobenzamide and how much to take at each dose. Carefully follow the instructions on your prescription label and ask your doctor or pharmacist to explain any part of the instructions you do not understand.

Trimethobenzamide comes in capsules to be taken orally and in rectal suppositories. To use the suppositories, first remove the foil wrapper and dip the tip of the suppository into water. Then lie on your side, draw your top knee up to your chest and insert the suppository well into your rectum and hold it in place for a few minutes. Try not to have a bowel movement for at least one hour after inserting the suppository.

If the suppository is too soft to insert, leave on the wrapper and refrigerate the suppository for 30 minutes or run cold water over it.

If you forget to take a dose of trimethobenzamide, take it as soon as you remember. Then take any remaining doses for that day at evenly spaced intervals. *Do not take a double dose to make up for a missed one.*

Keep trimethobenzamide in the container it came in, and keep it out of the reach of children. Do not allow anyone else to take your trimethobenzamide.

Ulcerlike Pain

An ulcer is an area of the stomach or duodenum (intestine) that has lost its normal lining. As a result, that portion is exposed to acid and enzymes that digest food. The breakdown of the stomach lining may be caused by excess formation of acid or enzymes. It also may result from a decreased resistance to acid in the lining.

The factors that are related to ulcer development include:

- Smoking—smokers have a higher rate of stomach and intestinal ulcers than other people do, but the exact reason is not known.
- Heredity—close relatives of individuals with stomach or intestinal ulcers have an increased risk of developing ulcers.
- Drugs—a number of medications will cause ulcers, particularly when used in large doses or over a long period of time. Aspirin is a well-known cause of ulcers; other drugs that cause ulcers include steroids and anti-inflammatory agents used to treat arthritis.
- Stress—stress caused by surgery, extensive burns, infection and other types of disease may induce ulcers.

Treatment of ulcers almost always includes antacid therapy. In addition, medications that reduce the amount of acid produced also are used. Although strict, bland diets were previously considered essential, recent studies have shown that spicy foods do not have an ill effect on ulcer patients. It may be helpful to eat smaller meals more frequently in order to keep some food in the stomach at all times. This prevents stomach acids from coming in direct contact with the stomach lining.

ANTISPASMODICS
Belladonna Alkaloids and Phenobarbital
(bell a don'a al' ka loyds) (fee noe bar'bi tal)

Brand name: Donnatal

This combination of drugs helps to relieve cramping pain of the stomach, intestines and bladder. This medicine often is prescribed as part of a total treatment of ulcers.

UNDESIRED EFFECTS

One of the most common side effects of this medicine is dryness of the mouth, nose and throat. To relieve the dryness, chew gum, suck hard candy or ice chips, or drink plenty of fluids.

This medicine makes some people drowsy, dizzy or less alert than normal.

Do not drive a car or operate dangerous machinery until you know how this medicine will affect you.

Belladonna alkaloids often will make you sweat less and increase the chance of a heatstroke. Avoid situations in which you might become overheated (for example, exercise, hot weather or sauna baths) while you are taking this medicine.

Other effects, which may disappear as you continue to take this medication and your body adjusts to it, are constipation, flushing of the skin, headache, mental confusion, rapid heartbeat, blurred vision, clumsiness, decreased sexual ability, difficulty urinating, nausea and vomiting, nervousness and reduced sense of taste. If these effects are persistent or severe, contact your doctor.

This medicine also may make your eyes more sensitive to light. Wear sunglasses to relieve this discomfort.

Rarely, this medicine will cause effects that will require medical attention. Contact your doctor if you have eye pain, hallucinations (seeing, hearing or feeling things that are not there), skin rash, slurred speech, sore throat and fever, unusual bleeding or bruising, or yellowing of the eyes or skin.

PRECAUTIONS

If you have ever had an unusual reaction to atropine, belladonna or any barbiturate, you should not take this medicine. If you have any questions about this, check with your doctor or pharmacist.

This combination of drugs can make certain medical conditions worse. Before you start to take this medicine, tell your doctor if you have difficulty urinating, glaucoma, kidney disease, liver disease, lung disease, an enlarged prostate, rapid heartbeat, spastic paralysis (in children) or brain damage (in children).

Tell your doctor what prescription or nonprescription drugs you are taking, including amantadine, antacids, anticoagulants (blood thinners), corticosteroids, digitalis, digitoxin, griseofulvin, medicine for Parkinson's disease, other medicine for intestinal or stomach cramping, medicine for ulcers, antihistamines, medicine for allergies or colds, medicine for seizures, narcotics, prescription medicine for pain, barbiturates, sedatives, tranquilizers, medicine to help you sleep, medicine for depression and MAO inhibitors (even if you stopped taking them within the past two weeks).

If you do not know the names of the drugs you are taking or what they were prescribed for, bring them in their labeled containers to your doctor or pharmacist.

Do not drink alcoholic beverages while you are taking this medicine. Do not start to take any of the drugs listed above without first checking with your doctor or pharmacist. All of these can increase the chance of and severity of side effects.

Because antacids and medicine for diarrhea can make belladonna less effective, do not take them together. They should be taken at least one hour apart. If you have questions about this, check with your doctor or pharmacist.

Take this medicine exactly as directed by your doctor. Do not take more or less of it, do not take it more often and do not take it for a longer period of time than ordered by your doctor.

Before you start to take this medicine, tell your doctor if you are pregnant or intend to become pregnant while you are using it. If you do become pregnant while taking this medicine, notify your doctor promptly.

DOSAGE AND STORAGE

Your doctor will determine how often you should take this medicine and how much you should take at each dose. Carefully follow the instructions on your prescription label and ask your doctor or pharmacist to explain any part of the instructions you do not understand.

If you forget to take a dose, take it as soon as you remember. Then take any remaining doses for that day at evenly spaced intervals.

Keep this medicine in the container it came in, and keep it out of the reach of children. Do not allow anyone else to take your belladonna alkaloids and phenobarbital.

Dicyclomine
(dye sye' kloe meen)

Brand names: Bentyl, Pasmin

Dicyclomine acts on the nerves and muscles to help relieve spasms in the stomach and intestines. Dicyclomine is used to relieve stomach cramps and cramping or spasms of the intestines caused by ulcers, colitis and other gastrointestinal problems.

UNDESIRED EFFECTS

Dicyclomine may make some people drowsy or dizzy. Do not drive a car or operate dangerous machinery until you know how this medicine will affect you.

Because dicyclomine may make you sweat less, there is an increased chance of heatstroke. Use extra care not to become overheated during exercise and during hot weather and avoid hot baths and saunas while you are taking this medicine.

Other side effects, which may go away as you continue to take dicyclomine and as your body adjusts to it, include a bloated feeling, headache, decreased sexual ability, mental confusion (especially in the elderly), nausea and vomiting, nervousness and rapid pulse. Contact your doctor if these effects continue or are severe. If you have heart trouble and this medicine changes the rate of your heartbeat, notify your doctor.

Contact your doctor if you experience constipation, difficult urination or skin rash.

PRECAUTIONS

You should not take dicyclomine if you have certain medical problems. Before you start to take this medicine, tell your doctor if you have difficulty urinating, an enlarged prostate, glaucoma, hiatal hernia, intestinal blockage, liver disease, myasthenia gravis or severe ulcerative colitis.

Tell your doctor what prescription or nonprescription drugs you are now taking, including amantadine, antacids, antihistamines, haloperidol, medicine for depression, medicine for diarrhea, medicine to help you sleep, medicine for Parkinson's disease, medicine for ulcers, sedatives or tranquilizers. If you do not know the names of the drugs or what they were prescribed for, bring them in their labeled containers to your doctor or pharmacist.

If you have taken MAO inhibitors within the past two weeks or are taking them now, tell your doctor.

Do not drink alcoholic beverages while you are taking dicyclomine. Do not start to take any of the drugs listed above unless you first check with your doctor or pharmacist. All of these can increase the chance of and severity of side effects.

Take this medicine exactly as prescribed by your doctor. Do not take more or less of it, do not take it more often and do not take it for a longer period of time than your doctor has ordered.

It is best not to take this medicine within one hour of taking antacids or medicine for diarrhea. If you have any questions about this, check with your doctor or pharmacist.

Before you start taking dicyclomine, it is wise to tell your doctor if you are pregnant or are nursing a baby, although no harm to the fetus or nursing baby has been reported as a result of using dicyclomine.

DOSAGE AND STORAGE

Your doctor will determine how often you should take dicyclomine and how much you should take at each dose. Carefully follow the instructions on your prescription label and ask your doctor or pharmacist to explain any part of the instructions you do not understand.

Dicyclomine comes in capsules, tablets and liquid form. If this medicine upsets your stomach, you may take it with solid food or milk.

If you forget to take a dose of dicyclomine, take it as soon as you remember. Take any remaining doses for that day at evenly spaced intervals. *Do not take a double dose to make up for a missed one.*

Keep dicyclomine in the container it came in, and keep it out of the reach of children. Do not allow anyone else to take your dicyclomine, and do not take it yourself for any condition other than the one for which it was prescribed.

Propantheline
(proe pan' the leen)

Brand name: Pro-Banthine

Propantheline relieves cramping pain and spasms in the stomach and intestines. Because propantheline also reduces the amount of acid formed in the stomach, it is used to treat stomach ulcers.

UNDESIRED EFFECTS

One of the most common side effects of propantheline is dryness of the mouth, nose and throat. To relieve this dryness, chew gum, suck hard candy or ice chips, or drink plenty of fluids.

This medicine makes some people drowsy, dizzy or less alert than usual. Do not drive a car or operate dangerous machinery until you know how propantheline will affect you.

Other side effects, which may disappear as your body adjusts to propantheline, include a bloated feeling, headache, rapid pulse, reduced sweating, blurred vision, decreased sexual ability, increased sensitivity of eyes to light, mental confusion (especially in elderly people), nausea and vomiting, nervousness, reduced sense of taste and tiredness. If you have any of these effects and they bother you, contact your doctor.

More serious side effects, though they do not occur often, will require medical attention if they do occur. Contact your doctor if you have constipation, difficulty in urinating, eye pain or skin rash.

PRECAUTIONS

Propantheline can make certain medical conditions worse. Before you start to take this medicine, tell your doctor if you have asthma, bronchitis, difficult urination, emphysema, an enlarged prostate, glaucoma, hiatal hernia, high blood pressure, intestinal blockage, kidney disease, liver disease, myasthenia gravis, overactive thyroid or severe ulcerative colitis.

Tell your doctor what prescription or nonprescription drugs you are taking, including amantadine, antacids, antihistamines, medicine for allergies or colds, haloperidol, medicine for your heart, medicine for diarrhea, medicine for Parkinson's disease, medicine to help you sleep, sedatives, tranquilizers and medicine for ulcers. If you do not know the names of the drugs or what they were prescribed for, bring them in their labeled containers to your doctor or pharmacist.

Do not drink alcoholic beverages while you are taking propantheline. Do not start to take any of the drugs listed above unless you first check with your doctor. All of these can increase the chance of and severity of side effects.

Propantheline may make your eyes more sensitive to light than normal. Wear sunglasses to help decrease the discomfort caused by bright light.

Because this medicine can make you sweat less, it may increase the chance of heatstroke. While you are taking propantheline, try to avoid situations in which you might become overheated (for example, strenuous exercise, being out in hot weather, saunas and steam baths).

Do not take propantheline for stomach ache due to gas, for sour stomach or for any problem other than the one for which it was prescribed.

To help your doctor select the best treatment for you and your baby, tell him if you are pregnant.

DOSAGE AND STORAGE

Your doctor will determine how often you should take propantheline and how much you should take at each dose. Carefully follow the instructions on your prescription label and ask your doctor or pharmacist to explain any part of the instructions you do not understand.

Propantheline comes in tablets, which are usually taken four times a day, before or with meals and at bedtime. Do not take propantheline within one hour of taking an antacid or medicine for diarrhea. If these medicines are taken too close together, propantheline may be less effective.

If you forget to take a dose of propantheline, take the missed dose with some food as soon as you remember to take the dose. Take any remaining doses for that day at evenly spaced intervals. *Do not take more than one dose at a time.*

Keep propantheline in the container it came in, and keep it out of the reach of children.

SLEEP DISTURBANCES

DRUGS USED TO TREAT SLEEP DISTURBANCES

Sleep Disturbances

A national health survey in 1970 showed that about one-third of the U.S. population experienced some type of sleep problem at some time. The exact nature and severity of sleep problems are difficult to evaluate because sleep needs vary from person to person.

Usually, trouble in sleeping is minor and only lasts for a few nights. Jet lag, ache and pain from minor illness and emotional upsets are common causes of such problems.

The following measures sometimes are helpful in avoiding sleep problems:
- Avoiding the consumption of large meals before bedtime
- Avoiding taking daytime naps
- Avoiding the consumption of coffee and soft drinks that contain caffeine
- Performing light exercise in the early evening
- Keeping the bedroom dark and quiet

In some cases, trouble sleeping can be severe enough to cause problems with normal daytime activities. If such problems continue for a period of weeks, you may have to consult your doctor to determine the cause of your sleeping problem. A number of medical conditions can cause insomnia. These include thyroid malfunction, diabetes, depression and respiratory problems. Your doctor will want to determine if any of these conditions are the cause of your sleeping problem.

Your doctor may prescribe a medication to help you sleep. Several different types of medications are available to help you sleep, but they all encourage sleep by depressing the central nervous system. These medications are used only for short periods of time because they can be habit-forming and can disrupt sleep patterns. It is important that you carefully follow your doctor's instructions. Do not take more of these medications or take them more often than your doctor has instructed.

All medications to help you sleep cause drowsiness that may linger into the daytime. Do not drive a car or operate dangerous machinery until you know how they will affect you.

Alcohol, tranquilizers, muscle relaxants, antihistamines, antidepressants and some medicines for pain will increase the effect of sleeping medications. Be sure to tell your doctor or pharmacist what medicines you are taking before you begin to use medications to help you sleep.

Medications to help you sleep are called sedatives or hypnotics. Generally, hypnotics are taken at bedtime to help you to fall asleep. Sedatives can be taken during the day to help calm you and make you less nervous or excitable and at bedtime to help you fall asleep.

SEDATIVES AND HYPNOTICS
Barbiturates
(bar bi' tyoo rates)

Drug	Brand names
amobarbital (am oh bar' bi tal)	Amytal
butabarbital (byoo ta bar' bi tal)	Buta-Kay, Butal, Butisol, Buticaps
pentobarbital (pen toe bar' bi tal)	Nembutal
phenobarbital (fee noe bar' bi tal)	Barbita, Barbipil, Luminal, Sherital, Solfoton
secobarbital (see koe bar' bi tal)	Seconal

Barbiturates depress the central nervous system. They are used to help people fall asleep and stay asleep through the night. They also are prescribed to help relieve anxiety and tension. Some of the barbiturates are helpful in controlling epileptic seizures and convulsions caused by certain diseases.

Many of the barbiturates listed above are included in combination products with other drugs. A commonly prescribed combination containing amobarbital and secobarbital has the brand name Tuinal.

UNDESIRED EFFECTS

The drowsiness caused by barbiturates may persist until the next day, even though you take the medicine at bedtime. Even low doses taken during the day to control seizures may cause drowsiness. Do not drive a car, operate dangerous machinery or engage in any activity that requires mental alertness until you know how barbiturates will affect you.

Less often barbiturates will cause diarrhea, headache, joint or muscle pain, nausea or vomiting and slurred speech. These effects may disappear as you continue to take the drug and as your body adjusts to it. If they continue or get worse, contact your doctor.

More serious side effects of barbiturates are allergic reactions, blood problems, liver problems and too much depression of the central nervous system. If any of these occur, they will require medical attention. Contact your doctor if you have mental confusion or depression; shortness of breath or difficulty breathing; skin rash or hives; sore throat and fever; swelling of the eyelids, face or lips; unusual bleeding or bruising; unusual excitement (more likely in children or older people); unusual tiredness or weakness; unusually slow heartbeat; wheezing or tightness in the chest; or yellowing of the eyes and skin.

When you stop taking a barbiturate, your body may need time to adjust, particularly if you have been taking it for a period of time. During this adjustment period, be alert for symptoms of withdrawal. Contact your doctor if you have convulsions or seizures, faint, have hallucinations (seeing, hearing or feeling things that are not there), increased dreaming, nightmares, trembling, difficulty sleeping, unusual restlessness or unusual weakness.

PRECAUTIONS

If you have ever had an unusual reaction to any of the barbiturates—the ones listed above or aprobarbital, hexobarbital, mephobarbital and talbutal—you should not take any barbiturate. If you have any questions about this, check with your doctor or pharmacist.

Because barbiturates can make some medical conditions worse, tell your doctor if you have asthma (or a history of this problem), emphysema, any other chronic disease, hyperactivity (in children), kidney disease, liver disease, porphyria (or a history of it) or underactive adrenal glands.

Barbiturates taken with certain other medicines can increase the chance of and/or severity of side effects. These include antihistamines, medicine for allergies or colds, narcotics, other barbiturates, prescription medicine for pain, sedatives, tranquilizers, medicine to help you sleep, medicine for seizures, medicine for depression, monamine oxidase (MAO) inhibitors (even if you stopped taking them within the past two weeks), anticoagulants (blood thinners), steroids, digitalis, digitoxin, doxycycline, griseofulvin and phenytoin.

Tell your doctor what prescription or nonprescription medicines you are taking. If you do not know the names of the drugs or what they were prescribed for, bring them in their labeled containers to your doctor or pharmacist.

Do not drink alcoholic beverages while you are taking barbiturates. Do not start to take any of the drugs listed above unless you have your doctor's permission. You can avoid serious side effects this way.

Because barbiturates can be habit-forming, take them only as directed by your doctor. Do not take more of them, do not take them more often and do not take them for a longer period of time than your doctor has ordered.

If you accidentally take too much of a barbiturate, contact your doctor immediately or go to the nearest hospital emergency room. Signs of overdosage are delirium, confusion, shortness of breath, difficult breathing, unusually slow or irregular heartbeat, deep sleep and coma. Overdosage can cause death.

Do not stop taking this medicine unless you first check with your doctor. He may want you gradually to reduce the amount you take before you stop completely. Be sure you have enough medicine to take all the doses prescribed. Check your supply before vacations and holidays when it may be difficult for you to get more.

If you will be taking a barbiturate for a long period of time, your doctor will want to check your response to the drug at regular visits. *Be sure to keep all appointments with your doctor.*

To help your doctor select the best treatment for you and your baby, be sure to tell your doctor if you are pregnant or are breast-feeding a baby. If you become pregnant while taking a barbiturate, notify your doctor at once.

DOSAGE AND STORAGE

Your doctor will determine how often you should take a barbiturate and how much you should take at each dose. When this medicine is prescribed to help control seizures and convulsions, it must be taken on a regular schedule to be effective. If you are taking a barbiturate to relieve anxiety and restlessness, your doctor may want you to take it at evenly spaced intervals during the day or, to help you sleep, at bedtime. Carefully follow the instructions on your prescription label and ask your doctor or pharmacist to explain any part of the instructions you do not understand.

Barbiturates come in extended-release capsules, tablets and liquid to be taken orally and in rectal suppositories. Do not break, crush or chew the capsules or tablets. They are to be swallowed whole.

The liquid form comes with a dropper for measuring the correct dose. Be sure you know how to use the dropper. If you have questions about this, ask your doctor or pharmacist. Each dose may be taken straight or mixed with water, milk or fruit juice. Do not use the liquid if it has become cloudy.

The rectal suppositories should be removed from the foil wrapper and the tip moistened with water. Then lie on your side, bring your top knee up to your chest and insert the suppository well into your rectum with your finger and hold it there for a few moments. Try not to have a bowel movement for at least an hour after inserting the suppository.

If you forget to take a dose of this medicine, take it as soon as you remember and take the remaining doses for that day at evenly spaced intervals. However, if you do not remember a missed dose until it is almost time for you to take another, omit the missed dose entirely and take only the regularly scheduled dose. *Do not take two doses to make up for a missed dose.*

Keep this medicine in the container it came in. Keep it out of the reach of children, because an overdose is especially dangerous in children. Do not allow anyone else to take your barbiturates.

Chloral Hydrate
(klor al hey′drate)

Brand names: Aquachloral, Cohidrate, Kessodrate, Noctec and others

Chloral hydrate is a sedative and hypnotic drug used to treat sleeplessness or insomnia. It helps people fall asleep and stay asleep through the night. Usually it begins to work in 30 to 60 minutes. It also is used to help calm or relax people who are anxious, tense or nervous.

UNDESIRED EFFECTS
The most common side effects of chloral hydrate are indigestion, nausea, stomach pain or vomiting. To lessen stomach upset, take this medicine with water, milk, fruit juice or ginger ale.

Chloral hydrate makes some people drowsy, dizzy, lightheaded, clumsy or unsteady on their feet. Do not drive a car or operate dangerous machinery until you know how this medicine will affect you. These effects tend to lessen or disappear as you continue to take chloral hydrate and as your body adjusts to it. If they continue or they bother you, contact your doctor.

More serious side effects do not occur very often but will need medical attention if they do occur. Contact your doctor if you have an allergic reaction (skin rash or hives), hallucinations (seeing, hearing or feeling things that are not there), mental confusion or unusual excitement.

After you stop taking chloral hydrate, your body may need time to adjust. For a few weeks after you stop taking this medicine be alert for withdrawal problems. Contact your doctor if you have hallucinations, mental confusion, nausea, nervousness, restlessness, stomach pain, trembling, unusual excitement or vomiting.

PRECAUTIONS

Before you start to take chloral hydrate, tell your doctor if you have heart disease, kidney disease or liver disease. This medicine may make these conditions worse.

Tell your doctor what prescription or nonprescription drugs you are taking, including antihistamines, medicine for allergies or colds, barbiturates, narcotics, other sedatives, tranquilizers, other medicine to help you sleep, prescription medicine for pain, medicine for seizures, medicine for depression, anticoagulants (blood thinners) or monamine oxidase (MAO) inhibitors (even if you stopped taking them within the past two weeks). If you do not know the names of the drugs or what they were prescribed for, bring them in their labeled containers to your doctor or pharmacist.

Do not drink alcoholic beverages while you are taking chloral hydrate. Do not start to take any of the drugs listed above without your doctor's permission. All of these can increase the chance of and/or severity of side effects.

Because this medicine can be habit-forming and is potentially dangerous taken in large amounts or continually over a long period of time, be sure to take chloral hydrate exactly as prescribed by your doctor. Do not take more of it, do not take it more often and do not take it for a longer period of time than your doctor has prescribed.

If you accidentally take too much chloral hydrate, contact your doctor immediately or go to the nearest hospital emergency room. Signs of overdose are delirium, confusion, shortness of breath, difficult breathing, unusually slow or irregular heartbeat, deep sleep and coma.

Do not stop taking chloral hydrate without first checking with your doctor. He may want you gradually to reduce the amount you are taking before you stop completely.

If you will be taking chloral hydrate over a long period of time, your doctor will want to check your response to this medicine. *Be sure to keep all appointments with your doctor.*

Before you start to take chloral hydrate, tell your doctor if you are pregnant or are breast-feeding a baby. Safe use of this drug in pregnancy and during the time a woman is breast-feeding has not been established. If you become pregnant while taking this medicine, stop taking the drug immediately.

DOSAGE AND STORAGE

Your doctor will determine how often you should take chloral hydrate and how much you should take at each dose. Carefully follow the instructions on your prescription label and ask your doctor or pharmacist to explain any part of the instructions you do not understand.

Chloral hydrate comes in capsules, tablets and liquid to be taken orally and in rectal suppositories. The capsules and tablets should be taken with a full eight-ounce glass of water, milk, fruit juice or ginger ale to lessen the chance of upset stomach. Do not take any of the oral forms with solid food.

If you are taking the liquid form of chloral hydrate, it can be mixed with one-half glass (four ounces) of water or fruit juice.

To use the suppository, remove the foil wrapper and moisten the tip of the suppository with water. Then lie on your side, bring the knee of your top leg up to your chest and insert the suppository well into the rectum and hold it there for a few moments. Try not to have a bowel movement for at least an hour after inserting the suppository. If the suppository is too soft to insert, leave the wrapper on and put the wrapped suppository in the refrigerator for 30 minutes, or run cold water over it.

Chloral hydrate is prescribed to help you sleep. If you do not feel you need help in falling asleep on a certain night, you may omit the dose that night.

Keep chloral hydrate in the container it came in, and keep it out of the reach of children. Do not allow anyone else to take your chloral hydrate.

Ethchlorvynol
(eth klor vi' nole)

Brand name: Placidyl

Ethchlorvynol is a sedative and hypnotic drug used primarily to help people fall asleep. Usually it works within an hour. It also is used to calm and relax people who are tense or nervous, especially people who cannot take other sedatives safely.

UNDESIRED EFFECTS
Frequently ethchlorvynol will cause temporary dizziness, clumsiness or unsteadiness very soon after you take a dose. Take this medicine with solid food or a glass of milk to prevent these effects.

Even when this medicine is taken at bedtime, it makes some people drowsy, dizzy or lightheaded the next day. Do not drive a car or operate dangerous machinery until you know how ethchlorvynol will affect you.

Other side effects, which may disappear as you continue to take ethchlorvynol and as your body adjusts to it, include blurred vision, indigestion, nausea or vomiting, numbness of the face, stomach pain, unusual tiredness or weakness, mental confusion and slurred speech. If these effects occur and they continue or they bother you, contact your doctor.

Though they do not happen often, more serious side effects will require medical attention if they occur. These include skin rash or hives (signs of an allergic reaction); unusual bleeding or bruising (signs of a blood problem); unusual excitement, nervousness or restlessness; darkening of the urine; itching; pale stools or yellowing of the eyes and skin (signs of liver problems). Contact your doctor if any of these effects occur. Your doctor may want to do some laboratory tests, such as blood counts or tests for your liver function.

Long-term therapy with ethchlorvynol can cause other side effects. Contact your doctor if you experience blurred or decreased vision; change in color in your vision; or numbness, tingling, pain or weakness in the hands or feet.

After you stop taking ethchlorvynol, your body may need time to adjust to this. During this adjustment period, be alert for symptoms of withdrawal problems. Contact your doctor if you have convulsions or seizures, hallucinations (seeing, hearing or feeling things that are not there), increased dreaming, muscle cramps or spasms, nausea or vomiting, nightmares, stomach cramps or pain, trembling, trouble sleeping or unusually fast heartbeat.

PRECAUTIONS

Because ethchlorvynol can make certain medical conditions worse, tell your doctor if you have kidney disease, liver disease, mental depression or porphyria.

Tell your doctor what prescription or nonprescription drugs you are taking, particularly antihistamines, medicine for allergies or colds, barbiturates, narcotics, other sedatives, tranquilizers, other medicine to help you sleep, prescription medicine for pain, medicine for seizures, medicine for depression and monoamine oxidase (MAO) inhibitors (even if you stopped taking them within the past two weeks). If you do not know the names of the drugs or what they were prescribed for, bring them in their labeled containers to your doctor or pharmacist.

Do not drink alcoholic beverages while you are taking ethchlorvynol. Do not start to take any of the drugs listed above without first checking with your doctor or pharmacist. All of these drugs can increase the chance of and/or severity of side effects.

Ethchlorvynol can be habit-forming and is potentially dangerous when taken in large amounts or continually over a long period of time. Take this medicine exactly as prescribed by your doctor. Do not take more of it, do not take it more often and do not take it for a longer period of time than your doctor has prescribed.

If you accidentally take too much ethchlorvynol, contact your doctor immediately or go to the nearest hospital emergency room. Signs of an overdose are delirium, confusion, incoordination, deep sleep or coma, unusually slow heartbeat, shortness of breath and difficult breathing.

Do not stop taking ethchlorvynol until your doctor tells you that you may. He may want you gradually to reduce the amount you are taking before you stop completely.

Be sure to tell your doctor, before you start to take this medicine, if you are pregnant or are nursing a baby. Safe use of ethchlorvynol during pregnancy and during the time a woman is breast-feeding has not been established. If you become pregnant while taking this medicine, contact your doctor at once.

DOSAGE AND STORAGE

Your doctor will determine how often you should take ethchlorvynol tablets and how much to take at each dose. Carefully follow the instructions on your prescription label and ask your doctor or pharmacist to explain any part of the instructions you do not understand.

If you are taking ethchlorvynol to help you fall asleep, do not be concerned if you forget to take a dose some night. If you do not feel that you need help to fall asleep on a certain night, you may omit the medicine for that night.

If you are taking ethchlorvynol to help calm or relax you and you forget to take a dose, take it as soon as you remember. Then take any remaining doses for that day at evenly spaced intervals. If you do not remember a missed dose until it is almost time for you to take another, omit the missed dose completely and take only the regularly scheduled dose. *Do not take a double dose to make up for a missed dose.*

Keep ethchlorvynol in the container it came in. Keep this medicine out of the reach of children. An overdose can be especially dangerous for children. Do not allow anyone else to take your ethchlorvynol.

Flurazepam
(flure az′ e pam)

Brand name: Dalmane

Flurazepam is one of the "benzodiazepine" group or family of drugs that is used as a sedative and hypnotic. (See **anxiety**, page 311, for more information on this family of drugs.) It is used to treat sleeplessness or insomnia and helps people fall asleep and then remain asleep through the night. It seems to help restore normal sleep patterns with fewer problems than other drugs used to treat sleeplessness. Usually, flurazepam begins to work in 30 to 60 minutes.

UNDESIRED EFFECTS
The most common effects of flurazepam are clumsiness or unsteadiness, dizziness or lightheadedness and daytime drowsiness or "hangover," even though the medicine is taken at night. Do not drive a car, operate machinery or do anything else that requires mental and/or physical alertness until you know how this medicine will affect you.

Less often, flurazepam will cause constipation, diarrhea, headache, heartburn, nausea or vomiting, slurred speech, stomach pain, or unusual weakness or tiredness. These effects may disappear as you continue to take flurazepam and your body adjusts to it. If they continue or bother you, contact your doctor.

Rarely, flurazepam will cause more serious side effects, requiring medical attention. Contact your doctor if you experience hallucinations (seeing, hearing or feeling things that are not there), mental confusion or depression, skin rash or itching (signs of allergic reaction), sore throat or fever (signs of blood problems), unusual excitement, nervousness or irritability, or yellowing of the skin and eyes (signs of a liver problem). If you take flurazepam for a long period of time, your doctor will probably ask you to have some laboratory tests, such as blood counts and tests for your liver and kidney function.

After you stop taking flurazepam, your body may need time to adjust to this, particularly if you have been taking large doses or have been taking flurazepam for a long period of time. For at least two weeks after you stop taking this medicine, be alert for signs of withdrawal problems. Contact your doctor if you have convulsions or seizures, mental confusion, muscle cramps, nausea or vomiting, stomach cramps, trembling, unusual irritability or sweating.

PRECAUTIONS

If you have ever had an unusual reaction to any medicine similar to flurazepam (chlordiazepoxide, clonazepam, clorazepate, diazepam, lorazepam, oxazepam or prazepam), you should not take flurazepam because you are more likely to have a bad reaction to it. If you have any questions about this, check with your doctor or pharmacist.

Before you start to take flurazepam, tell your doctor if you have emphysema, asthma, chronic bronchitis or any other chronic lung disease, kidney disease, liver disease, epilepsy, porphyria or mental depression. Flurazepam may make these conditions worse.

Tell your doctor what other prescription or nonprescription drugs you are taking, including barbiturates, narcotics, other sedatives, tranquilizers, other medicine to help you sleep, antihistamines, medicine for allergies or colds, prescription medicine for pain, medicine for seizures, medicine for depression or monoamine oxidase (MAO) inhibitors (even if you stopped taking them within the past two weeks). If you do not know the names of the drugs or what they were prescribed for, bring them in their labeled containers to your doctor or pharmacist.

Do not drink alcoholic beverages while you are taking flurazepam. Do not start to take any of the drugs listed above without first checking with your doctor or pharmacist. All of these can increase the chance of and/or severity of side effects.

Because flurazepam can be habit-forming and potentially dangerous when taken in very large amounts or continually for a long period of time, take this medicine exactly as prescribed by your doctor. Do not take more of it, do not take it more often and do not take it for a longer period of time than your doctor has prescribed.

If you accidentally take too much flurazepam, contact your doctor immediately or go to the nearest hospital emergency room. Signs of an overdose include deep sleep or coma, confusion, delirium, unusually slow heartbeat, shortness of breath and difficult breathing.

If you have been taking large doses of flurazepam for a long period of time, do not stop taking this medicine without your doctor's permission. He may want you gradually to reduce the amount you are taking before you stop completely.

Children under the age of 15 years should not take flurazepam. Safe use of this medicine in this age group has not been established.

Before you start to take flurazepam, be sure to tell your doctor if you are pregnant or are nursing a baby. The effects of flurazepam on an unborn child or a breast-fed baby are not known.

DOSAGE AND STORAGE

Your doctor will determine how much flurazepam you should take. Carefully follow the instructions on your prescription label and ask your doctor or pharmacist to explain any part of the instructions you do not understand.

Flurazepam comes in capsules, which are taken at bedtime. Because this medicine can lose its effectiveness after several weeks of regular use, take it only when you cannot sleep. You do not need to keep to a regular schedule.

You may have to take flurazepam for two or three nights before your sleeping problem improves. It will take this long for the medicine to reach its full effect.

Keep flurazepam in the container it came in, and keep it out of the reach of children. Do not allow anyone else to take your flurazepam.

Glutethimide
(gloo teth' i mide)

Brand names: Doriden, Dormtabs

Glutethimide is a sedative and hypnotic drug used to treat sleeplessness or insomnia. It helps people fall asleep and stay asleep through the night. Usually it begins to work in about 30 minutes. When glutethimide is used regularly— every day—it usually is effective only for about a week.

UNDESIRED EFFECTS

Although glutethimide is taken at bedtime, it may make some people drowsy or dizzy or "hungover" the next day. Do not drive a car or operate dangerous machinery until you know how this medicine will affect you.

Other side effects include blurred vision, clumsiness or unsteadiness, headache, mental confusion, nausea, slurred speech and vomiting. These effects may go away as you continue to take glutethimide and your body adjusts to the medicine. However, if they continue or bother you, contact your doctor.

More serious side effects do not occur often, but they may require medical attention if they do occur. These include skin rash or hives (sign of an allergic reaction), sore throat and fever, unusual bleeding or bruising, unusual tiredness or weakness (signs of blood problems) and unusual excitement. If you experience any of these effects, stop taking glutethimide and contact your doctor. He may want you to have some blood tests or other laboratory tests.

After you stop taking glutethimide, your body may need time to adjust to this. During this adjustment period, be alert for symptoms of withdrawal problems. Contact your doctor if you have convulsions or seizures, hallucinations (seeing, hearing or feeling things that are not there), increased dreaming, muscle cramps or spasms, nausea or vomiting, nightmares, stomach cramps or pain, trembling, trouble sleeping or unusually fast heartbeat.

PRECAUTIONS

Before you start to take glutethimide, tell your doctor if you have an enlarged prostate, glaucoma, an intestinal blockage, irregular heartbeat, kidney disease, porphyria, a stomach ulcer or a urinary tract blockage. This medicine may make these conditions worse.

Tell your doctor what prescription or nonprescription drugs you are taking, particularly antihistamines, medicine for allergies or colds, barbiturates, narcotics, other sedatives, tranquilizers, other medicine to help you sleep, prescription medicine for pain, medicine for seizures, medicine for depression, anticoagulants (blood thinners) and monoamine oxidase (MAO) inhibitors (even if you stopped taking them during the past two weeks). If you do not know the names of the drugs you are taking or what they were prescribed for, bring them in their labeled containers to your doctor or pharmacist.

Do not drink alcoholic beverages while you are taking glutethimide. Do not start to take any of the drugs listed above without first checking with your doctor or pharmacist. All of these can increase the chance of and/or severity of side effects.

Because glutethimide can be habit-forming and potentially dangerous if taken in large amounts or continually over a long period of time, take this medicine exactly as prescribed by your doctor. Do not take more of it, do not take it more often and do not take it for a longer period of time than prescribed by your doctor.

If you accidentally take too much glutethimide, contact your doctor immediately or go to the nearest hospital emergency room. Signs of an overdose are deep sleep, stupor or coma, confusion, delirium, unusually slow heartbeat, shortness of breath and difficult breathing. Death can occur from an overdosage of glutethimide.

If you have taken glutethimide for two weeks and still cannot sleep without the help of medications, contact your doctor. He may want to change your medicine, because glutethimide usually is not effective for longer than about one week.

Do not stop taking this medicine until your doctor tells you that you may. He may want you gradually to reduce the amount you are taking before you stop completely.

Before you start to take glutethimide, be sure to tell your doctor if you are pregnant or are nursing a baby. Safe use of this medicine during pregnancy and during the time a woman is breast-feeding has not been established. If you become pregnant while taking glutethimide, contact your doctor at once.

DOSAGE AND STORAGE

Carefully follow your doctor's instructions on your prescription label and ask your doctor or pharmacist to explain any part of the instructions you do not understand.

Glutethimide comes in tablets and capsules. It should be taken within a half hour of bedtime. You can expect to begin to feel drowsy 15 minutes after you take a dose and to fall asleep within an hour. Sound sleep will last from four to eight hours.

This medicine is prescribed to help you fall asleep. If you do not feel you need help falling asleep on a certain night, you may omit the dose of glutethimide for that night.

Keep this medication in the container it came in. Keep glutethimide out of the reach of children. An overdose is especially dangerous for children. Do not allow anyone else to take your glutethimide.

Meprobamate
(me proe ba' mate)

Brand names: Bamate, Bamo, Corpobate, Equanil, Kesso-Bamate, Mepriam, Meprospan, Miltown, SK-Bamate, Tranmep and others

Brand names of some products containing meprobamate in combination with other drugs: Deprol, Equagesic, Meprogesic, Mepro-Hex, Meprotrate, Milpath, Milprem, Miltrate, Pathibamate

Meprobamate is a sedative used to help people fall asleep, particularly those people who are anxious or tense. Usually it begins to work within two hours. It also is used to calm and relax people who are nervous, anxious or tense.

UNDESIRED EFFECTS

The most common side effects of meprobamate are clumsiness, unsteadiness and drowsiness. Even when you take this medicine at bedtime, you still may be drowsy and less alert than normal the next day. Do not drive a car or operate dangerous machinery until you know how this medicine will affect you.

Less often, meprobamate will cause blurred vision, a change in near or distant vision, diarrhea, dizziness or lightheadedness, headache, nausea or vomiting, slurred speech, or unusual weakness or tiredness. These effects may disappear as you continue to take meprobamate and as your body adjusts to it. Contact your doctor if they continue or bother you.

More serious side effects do not occur often, but they may require medical attention if they do occur. Contact your doctor if you experience skin rash, itching or hives (signs of allergic reaction); unusual excitement; mental confusion; sore throat and fever; unusual bleeding or bruising (signs of blood problems); or unusually fast, pounding or irregular heartbeat. If you take this drug for a long period of time, your doctor probably will order laboratory tests, including a blood count.

When you stop taking meprobamate, your body may need time to adjust to this. For the next few days, contact your doctor if you have convulsions or seizures, hallucinations (seeing, hearing or feeling things that are not there), increased dreaming, muscle twitching, nausea or vomiting, nightmares, trembling, difficulty sleeping, or unusual nervousness or restlessness.

PRECAUTIONS

You should not take meprobamate if you have ever had an unusual reaction to similar medicines such as carbromal, carisoprodol, mebutamate and tybamate. If you have questions about this, check with your doctor or pharmacist.

Because meprobamate can make some medical conditions worse, tell your doctor if you have epilepsy, kidney or liver disease, impaired kidney or liver function or porphyria.

Tell your doctor what prescription or nonprescription drugs you are taking, including antihistamines, medicine for allergies or colds, barbiturates, narcotics, other sedatives, tranquilizers, other medicine to help you sleep, prescription medicine for pain, medicine for seizures, medicine for depression and mono-amine oxidase (MAO) inhibitors (even if you stopped taking them within the past two weeks).

Do not drink alcoholic beverages while you are taking meprobamate. Do not start to take any of the drugs listed above unless you first check with your doctor. All of these can increase the chance of and/or severity of side effects.

Meprobamate can be habit-forming. It is important that you take it exactly as prescribed by your doctor. Do not take more of it, do not take it more often and do not take it for a longer time than directed by your doctor.

If you accidentally take too much meprobamate, contact your doctor immediately or go to the nearest hospital emergency room. Signs of overdose are slurred speech, staggering, unusually slow heartbeat, wheezing, shortness of breath or difficult breathing, deep sleep and coma.

If you take meprobamate in large doses or over a long period of time, do not stop taking it until your doctor tells you that you may. He may want you gradually to reduce the amount you take before stopping completely.

If you will be taking meprobamate for a long period of time, your doctor will want to check your response to this medicine regularly. *Be sure to keep all your appointments with your doctor.* Check with him at least every four months to be sure you need to continue taking meprobamate.

Before you start to take meprobamate, tell your doctor if you are pregnant or think you may be or if you are nursing a baby. The effects of this drug on an unborn child or on a breast-fed baby are not known.

DOSAGE AND STORAGE

Your doctor will determine how often you should take meprobamate and how much you should take at each dose. Carefully follow the instructions on your prescription label and ask your doctor or pharmacist to explain any part of the instructions you do not understand. Meprobamate comes in capsules and tablets.

If you forget to take a dose, *do not* take the missed dose when you remember it. Omit it and take the next dose at the regularly scheduled time. *Do not take a double dose.*

Keep meprobamate in the container it came in, and keep it out of the reach of children. Do not allow anyone else to take your meprobamate.

Methaqualone
(meth a' kwa lone)

Brand names: Mequin, Parest, Quaalude, Sopor

Methaqualone is a sedative and hypnotic drug used to treat sleeplessness or insomnia. It helps people fall asleep and stay asleep through the night. Usually it begins to work in about 30 minutes. It also is used to help calm or relax people who are nervous, anxious or tense, particularly those who cannot take barbiturates.

UNDESIRED EFFECTS

The most common effects of methaqualone are drowsiness and dizziness or "hangover" and headache in the daytime, although this medicine is taken at bedtime. Do not drive a car or operate dangerous machinery until you know how this medicine will affect you.

Other effects include diarrhea; indigestion or stomach upset (nausea, pain and vomiting); unusual tiredness or weakness; numbness, tingling, pain or weakness in the hands or feet; and sweating. These effects may disappear as you continue to take methaqualone and as your body adjusts to it. If they continue or bother you, contact your doctor.

More serious side effects do not occur often, but they will require medical attention if they do occur. Contact your doctor if you develop a skin rash or hives, unusual bleeding or bruising, fever or sore throat, unusual excitement, nervousness or restlessness. Your doctor may order laboratory tests for you while you are taking this drug.

After you stop taking methaqualone, your body may need time to adjust to this, and you may have symptoms of withdrawal. Contact your doctor if you have convulsion or seizures, hallucinations (seeing, hearing or feeling things that are not there), increased dreaming, muscle cramps or spasms, nausea or vomiting, nightmares, stomach cramps or pain, trembling, trouble sleeping or unusually fast heartbeat.

PRECAUTIONS

Before you start to take methaqualone, tell your doctor if you have liver disease or impaired liver function. Methaqualone can make these conditions worse.

Tell your doctor what prescription or nonprescription drugs you are taking, including antihistamines, medicine for allergies or colds, barbiturates, narcotics, other sedatives, tranquilizers, other medicine to help you sleep, prescription medicine for pain, medicine for seizures, medicine for depression and mono-amine oxidase (MAO) inhibitors (even if you stopped taking them within the past two weeks). If you do not know the names of the drugs or what they were prescribed for, bring them in their labeled containers to your doctor or pharmacist.

Do not drink alcoholic beverages while you are taking methaqualone. Do not start to take any of the drugs listed above without your doctor's permission. All of these drugs can increase the chance of and/or severity of side effects.

Take methaqualone exactly as prescribed by your doctor. This medicine can be habit-forming and is potentially dangerous when taken in large amounts or continually for a long period of time. Methaqualone should not be taken regularly for longer than three months. Do not take it more often, do not take more of it and do not take it for a longer period of time than your doctor has prescribed.

If you accidentally take too much methaqualone, contact your doctor immediately or go to the nearest hospital emergency room. Signs of an overdose are confusion, delirium, incoordination, unusually slow heartbeat, shortness of breath or difficult breathing, stupor, convulsions, deep sleep and coma. Death has occurred due to overdose of methaqualone.

If you have taken methaqualone for two weeks and still cannot sleep without medicine, contact your doctor. He may want to change your medication because methaqualone usually is not effective when taken every day for longer than several weeks.

Do not stop taking this medicine without first checking with your doctor. He may want you gradually to reduce the amount you are taking before you stop completely.

Be sure to tell your doctor if you are pregnant or are nursing a baby. Safe use of methaqualone during pregnancy and during the time a woman is breast-feeding has not been established. If you become pregnant while taking this medicine, stop taking it and contact your doctor.

DOSAGE AND STORAGE

Methaqualone comes in tablets and capsules. Your doctor will determine how often you should take this medicine and how much you should take at each dose. Carefully follow the instructions on your prescription label and ask your doctor or pharmacist to explain any part of the instructions you do not understand.

When you are taking this medicine to help you fall asleep, you do not need to be concerned if you forget a dose. If you do not feel that you need help falling asleep on a certain night, you may omit the dose for that night.

If you are taking methaqualone to help calm or relax you and you forget to take a dose, take it as soon as you remember. Then take any remaining doses for the day at evenly spaced intervals. If you remember a missed dose when it is almost time for you to take another, omit the missed dose entirely and take only the regularly scheduled dose. *Do not take a double dose to make up for a missed dose.*

Keep methaqualone in the container it came in. Keep it out of the reach of children, because an overdose is especially dangerous for children. Do not allow anyone else to take your methaqualone.

Methyprylon
(meth i prye' lon)

Brand name: Noludar

Methyprylon is a sedative and hypnotic drug used to treat sleeplessness and insomnia. It helps people fall asleep and then stay asleep through the night. Usually sleep occurs within an hour after taking a dose of methyprylon and may last for five to eight hours.

UNDESIRED EFFECTS

Even when it is taken at bedtime, methyprylon can make some people dizzy or drowsy or "hung over" the next day. Do not drive a car or operate dangerous machinery until you know how this medicine will affect you.

Other effects that may occur are headache, diarrhea, nausea or vomiting, and numbness or tingling in the arms, legs, hands or feet. As you continue to take methyprylon and your body adjusts to it, these effects tend to lessen or disappear. Contact your doctor if they continue or are severe.

More serious side effects do not occur often, but they may require medical attention if they do occur. Contact your doctor if you experience skin rash (sign of an allergic reaction), unusual excitement, ulcers or sores in the mouth or throat, or unusual bleeding or bruising (signs of blood problems). Periodically your doctor may order blood counts or other laboratory tests for you if you take methyprylon continually for a long period of time.

If you take large doses of methyprylon or take it over a long period of time, your body may need time to adjust when you stop taking it. Be alert for signs of withdrawal problems and contact your doctor if you have convulsions or seizures, hallucinations (seeing, hearing or feeling things that are not there), increased dreaming, mental confusion, nausea and vomiting, nightmares, stomach cramps, trembling, trouble sleeping, unusual restlessness or nervousness, unusual sweating or unusual weakness.

PRECAUTIONS

Because methyprylon can make certain medical conditions worse, tell your doctor if you have kidney disease, liver disease or porphyria.

Tell your doctor what prescription or nonprescription drugs you are taking, particularly antihistamines, medicine for allergies or colds, barbiturates, narcotics, other sedatives, tranquilizers, other medicine to help you sleep, prescription medicine for pain, medicine for seizures, medicine for depression and monoamine oxidase (MAO) inhibitors (even if you stopped taking them within the past two weeks). If you do not know the names of the drugs or what they were prescribed for, bring them in their labeled containers to your doctor or pharmacist.

Do not drink alcoholic beverages while you are taking methyprylon. Do not start to take any of the drugs listed above without first checking with your doctor or pharmacist. All of these can increase the chance of and/or severity of side effects.

Because methyprylon can be habit-forming, take it only as directed by your doctor. Do not take more of it, do not take it more often and do not take it for a longer period of time than your doctor has ordered.

If you accidentally take too much methyprylon, contact your doctor or go to the nearest hospital emergency room. Signs of overdosage are confusion, delirium, incoordination, difficult breathing, deep sleep and coma.

If you have been taking this medicine for a period of time, do not stop taking it without your doctor's permission. He may want you gradually to reduce the amount you are taking before you stop completely.

Before you start to take methyprylon, tell your doctor if you are pregnant or are breast-feeding a baby. He can then select the best and safest treatment for you and your baby.

DOSAGE AND STORAGE

Methyprylon comes in capsules and tablets that usually are taken at bedtime. Your doctor will determine how much you should take at each dose. Carefully follow the instructions on your prescription label and ask your doctor or pharmacist to explain any part of the instructions you do not understand.

Take this medicine only when you need it to help you sleep. If it is used every day it may not be effective after two weeks.

Keep methyprylon in the container it came in. Keep it out of the reach of children, because an overdose is especially dangerous for children. Do not allow anyone else to take your methyprylon.

Triclofos
(trye kloe' fos)

Brand name: Triclos

Triclofos is a sedative and hypnotic used to help people fall asleep and then stay asleep through the night. Usually it begins to work within an hour. Usually it is not effective after you have been taking it every day for about two weeks. It also is used to put a person to sleep when brain-wave activity is being measured in certain diagnostic tests.

UNDESIRED EFFECTS

Triclofos makes some people drowsy, dizzy, lightheaded, clumsy or unsteady on their feet. Do not drive a car or operate dangerous machinery until you know how this medicine will affect you. As you continue to take triclofos and as your body adjusts to it, these effects tend to lessen or disappear. If they continue or bother you, contact your doctor.

Other side effects include headache, stomach upset, gas, nausea and vomiting, nightmares, weakness and tiredness. Contact your doctor if these effects are severe.

More serious side effects do not occur often, but they may require medical attention if they do occur. Contact your doctor if you have an allergic reaction (skin rash or hives), mental confusion or unusual excitement.

PRECAUTIONS

Before you start to take triclofos, tell your doctor if you have kidney disease, liver disease, heart disease or irregular heartbeat. Triclofos can make these conditions worse.

Tell your doctor what prescription or nonprescription drugs you are taking, including antihistamines, medicine for allergies or colds, barbiturates, narcotics, other sedatives, tranquilizers, other medicine to help you sleep, prescription medicine for pain, medicine for seizures, medicine for depression, anticoagulants (blood thinners) or monoamine oxidase (MAO) inhibitors (even if you stopped taking them within the last two weeks). If you do not know the names of the drugs or what they were prescribed for, bring them in their labeled containers to your doctor or pharmacist.

Do not drink alcoholic beverages while you are taking triclofos. Do not start to take any of the drugs listed above without your doctor's permission. All of these can increase the chance of and/or severity of side effects.

Because triclofos can be habit-forming, be sure to take it exactly as prescribed by your doctor. Do not take more of it, do not take it more often and do not take it for a longer period of time than prescribed by your doctor.

If you accidentally take too much triclofos, contact your doctor immediately or go to the nearest hospital emergency room. Signs of overdosage are excessive drowsiness, deep sleep or coma, shortness of breath, difficult breathing and slow or irregular heartbeat.

Do not stop taking triclofos without first checking with your doctor. He may want you gradually to reduce the amount you are taking before you stop completely.

If you have taken triclofos for two or three weeks and still cannot sleep without medication, contact your doctor. He may want to change your medicine because triclofos may not be effective over a long period of time.

Except for a single dose prior to electroencephalography (measurement of brain-wave activity), triclofos should not be given to children under 12 years of age.

Before you start to take triclofos, be sure to tell your doctor if you are pregnant or are nursing a baby. Safe use of this medicine during pregnancy and during the time a woman is breast-feeding has not been established. If you become pregnant while taking this medicine, stop taking it.

DOSAGE AND STORAGE

Your doctor will determine how often you should take triclofos and how much you should take at each dose. Carefully follow the instructions on your prescription label and ask your doctor or pharmacist to explain any part of the instructions you do not understand.

Triclofos comes in tablets and in liquid form. If you are taking the liquid form, use a specially marked measuring spoon to make sure you have an accurate dose. Triclofos is prescribed to help you sleep. If you do not feel you need help falling asleep on a certain night, you may omit the dose that night.

Keep triclofos in the container it came in, and keep it out of the reach of children. Do not allow anyone else to take your triclofos.

PSYCHIATRIC
PROBLEMS

DRUGS USED TO TREAT PSYCHIATRIC PROBLEMS

Anxiety

A feeling of anxiety or fear in the face of danger is a normal reaction that is part of the body's "fight or flight" response. When the threat is real, fear is an appropriate response that is essential to survival. However, if the threat is nonexistent or trivial or if the level of anxiety greatly exceeds that indicated by the situation, the anxiety is considered inappropriate.

Anxiety may be manifested in many different ways. A large number of patients never experience feelings of anxiety but have symptoms such as chest pain, palpitations, breathlessness and fatigue. Often, anxiety is found to be the cause of these symptoms after a thorough evaluation rules out other disease.

Treatment of anxiety relies on both psychotherapy and drugs. Because the nature of the problem varies so greatly among individuals, the use of both forms of treatment are tailored to each individual.

Chlordiazepoxide
(klor dye az e pox' ide)

Brand names: A-Poxide, Libritabs, Librium, Sereen, SK-Lygen

Chlordiazepoxide is one of a group of drugs known as benzodiazepines. Chlordiazepoxide is a tranquilizer used to calm people who are anxious or tense. It may be prescribed for a wide variety of medical problems that cause anxiety. It also is used to calm people before an operation and to treat the symptoms of alcohol withdrawal.

UNDESIRED EFFECTS

During the first few days of chlordiazepoxide therapy, drowsiness, dizziness and weakness are common. Even if you take this medicine at bedtime, you may notice these effects when you get up in the morning. Do not drive a car or operate dangerous machinery until you know how this medicine will affect you.

Chlordiazepoxide may make your mouth dry. Suck hard candies or chew gum to relieve the dryness. Nausea and constipation may occur when you start to take this medicine and then decrease or disappear as your body adjusts to the medicine. If these effects continue or are severe, contact your doctor. He may want to adjust your dose.

More serious side effects include allergic reactions, blood problems, liver problems and signs that your body is not tolerating this medicine well. Contact your doctor if you have mental confusion, depression, skin rash or itching (allergic problems), trouble sleeping, unusual nervousness or irritability, un-usually slow heartbeat, shortness of breath, difficulty breathing, continuing ulcers or sores in the mouth or throat, or yellowing of the eyes or skin.

When you stop taking this medicine, you may experience withdrawal symptoms, especially if you have taken large doses for a long period of time. Contact your doctor if you notice mental confusion, muscle cramps, nausea or vomiting, stomach cramps, trembling, unusual sweating or seizures.

PRECAUTIONS
Before you start to take chlordiazepoxide, tell your doctor if you have ever had an unusual reaction to this medicine or any of the other benzodiazepines (clorazepate, clonazepam, diazepam, flurazepam, lorazepam, oxazepam, prazepam). You are more likely to have a bad reaction to chlordiazepoxide if you have had an unusual reaction to any of these other drugs.

Chlordiazepoxide can make certain medical conditions worse. Tell your doctor if you have asthma, emphysema, bronchitis or other chronic lung disease, glaucoma, kidney disease, liver disease, mental depression, myasthenia gravis, severe mental illness or hyperactivity (in children).

Tell your doctor what prescription or nonprescription drugs you are taking, including antihistamines or medicine for hay fever, other allergies or colds; barbiturates, narcotics or other sedatives; tranquilizers or sleeping medicine; prescription medicine for pain; medicine for depression or MAO inhibitors (even if you have not taken them for two weeks).

If you do not know the names of the drugs or what they were prescribed for, bring them in their labeled containers to your doctor or pharmacist.

Do not drink alcoholic beverages while you are taking chlordiazepoxide because serious effects may result. Do not start to take any of the drugs listed above without first checking with your doctor or pharmacist.

Because chlordiazepoxide can be habit-forming, you should take it exactly as directed by your doctor. Do not take more of it, do not take it more often and do not take it for a longer period of time than your doctor has ordered.

If you have been taking chlordiazepoxide in large doses or for a long period of time, do not stop taking it without your doctor's permission. To avoid withdrawal problems, your doctor may want you gradually to reduce the amount you are taking before you stop completely.

Your doctor will want to check your response to chlordiazepoxide if you are going to be taking it for a long period of time. He may want to check every four months or more often to determine whether you still need it. *Be sure to keep all appointments with your doctor.*

Chlordiazepoxide is passed from a mother to her unborn child and from a mother to a nursing baby. Be sure to tell your doctor if you are pregnant or plan to get pregnant while you are taking this medicine and if you are nursing a baby. If you become pregnant while taking this medicine, contact your doctor.

DOSAGE AND STORAGE
Chlordiazepoxide comes in capsules and tablets. Your doctor will determine how often you should take this medicine and how much you should take at each dose. Carefully follow the instructions on your prescription label and ask your doctor or pharmacist to explain any part of the instructions you do not understand.

If you forget to take a dose, *do not* take it when you remember. Omit the missed dose completely and take the next dose at the regularly scheduled time.

Keep this medicine in the container it came in. Keep chlordiazepoxide out of the reach of children. Do not allow anyone else to take your chlordiazepoxide.

Clorazepate
(klor az' e pate)

Brand name: Tranxene

Clorazepate is one of the benzodiazepine tranquilizers. Clorazepate is used to calm people who are anxious or tense. It may be prescribed for a wide variety of medical problems, including relief of the symptoms of alcohol withdrawal.

UNDESIRED EFFECTS

The most common side effect of clorazepate is drowsiness. Do not drive a car or operate dangerous machinery until you know what effect this medicine will have on you.

Less frequently, clorazepate will cause dizziness, stomach upset or nausea, nervousness, blurred vision, dry mouth, headache or mental confusion. If these effects bother you, contact your doctor.

More serious side effects will require medical attention if they occur. Contact your doctor if you experience difficulty sleeping, skin rash, tiredness, clumsiness or unsteadiness, irritability, double vision, depression or slurred speech. Your doctor may want to adjust your dosage or change your medication if you have any of these side effects.

When you stop taking clorazepate, it may take your body as long as two weeks to adjust to this. Be alert for symptoms of withdrawal and contact your doctor if you experience convulsions or seizures, mental confusion, muscle cramps, nausea or vomiting, stomach cramps, trembling, unusual irritability or unusual sweating.

PRECAUTIONS

Before you start to take clorazepate, tell your doctor if you have ever had an unusual reaction to this medicine or to any of the other benzodiazepines (chlordiazepoxide, clonazepam, diazepam, flurazepam, lorazepam, oxazepam, prazepam). You may be sensitive to this whole group of drugs.

Clorazepate may make certain medical conditions worse. Be sure to tell your doctor if you have emphysema, asthma, bronchitis or other chronic lung disease, glaucoma, kidney disease, liver disease, mental depression, myasthenia gravis or severe mental illness.

Tell your doctor what prescription or nonprescription drugs you are taking. Certain medications, when taken with clorazepate, can increase the possibility of and/or the severity of side effects. These include antihistamines or medicine for hay fever, other allergies or colds; barbiturates, narcotics and prescription medicine for pain; sedatives, tranquilizers or other medicine to help you sleep; medicine for seizures; medicine for depression; and MAO inhibitors (even if you stopped taking them within the past two weeks).

If you do not know the names of the drugs you are taking or what they were prescribed for, bring them in their labeled containers to your doctor or pharmacist.

Do not drink alcoholic beverages while you are taking clorazepate. If you do, you can experience side effects. Do not start to take any of the drugs listed above unless you have your doctor's permission. If you have any questions about this, check with your doctor or pharmacist.

Because clorazepate can be habit-forming, do not take more of this medicine than your doctor has directed and do not take it more often or for a longer period of time than he has directed.

Diazepam
(dye az' e pam)

Brand name: Valium

Diazepam is one of the group of drugs known as benzodiazepines. Diazepam acts on the brain to relieve anxiety and tension and to relax muscles. Diazepam is used to treat muscle spasm and cerebral palsy as well as to calm patients who are anxious or tense.

UNDESIRED EFFECTS

Common effects during the first few days of therapy are drowsiness, dizziness and weakness. Even if you take diazepam at bedtime, you may notice these effects when you get up the next morning. Do not drive a car or operate dangerous machinery until you know how diazepam will affect you. If fatigue continues past the first few days, contact your doctor.

If this medicine makes your mouth dry, suck hard candies or chew gum. Headache and slurring of speech may occur when you start to take diazepam and then disappear as your body adjusts to it.

More serious side effects, which will need medical treatment if they occur, include allergic reactions, blood problems, liver problems and signs that your body is not tolerating diazepam well. Contact your doctor if you have mental confusion, depression, skin rash or itching, trouble sleeping, unusual nervousness or irritability, unusually slow heartbeat, shortness of breath, difficulty breathing, continuing ulcers or sores in the mouth or throat, or yellowing of the eyes or skin.

If you have taken large doses of diazepam for a length of time you may have withdrawal symptoms when you stop taking this medicine. Contact your doctor if you experience mental confusion, muscle cramps, nausea or vomiting, stomach cramps, trembling, unusual sweating or seizures.

PRECAUTIONS

Before you start to take diazepam, tell your doctor if you have ever had an unusual reaction to this medicine or to any of the other benzodiazepines (chlordiazepoxide, clorazepate, clonazepam, flurazepam, lorazepam, oxazepam, prazepam). You are more likely to have a bad reaction to diazepam if you have reacted badly to any of these other drugs.

Tell your doctor if you have any of these medical problems: asthma, emphysema, bronchitis or other chronic lung disease, glaucoma, kidney disease, liver disease, mental depression, myasthenia gravis, severe mental illness or hyperactivity (in children). Diazepam may make these conditions worse.

Certain medication when taken with diazepam may increase the possibility or severity of side effects. Tell your doctor what prescription or nonprescription drugs you are taking, including antihistamines or medicine for hay fever, other allergies or colds; barbiturates, narcotics or other sedatives; tranquilizers or medicine to help you sleep; prescription medicine for pain; medicine for depression; or MAO inhibitors (even if you have not taken them for two weeks).

If you do not know the names of the drugs you are taking, check with your doctor or pharmacist before taking diazepam because serious side effects can result from certain combinations. Do not start to take any of the drugs listed above without checking first with your doctor or pharmacist.

Take diazepam exactly as directed by your doctor. Do not take more of it, do not take it more often and do not take it for a longer period of time than your doctor has ordered. This medicine can be habit-forming if you take it too often.

Do not stop taking diazepam without your doctor's permission, particularly if you have been taking it for a long period of time or have been taking large doses. You may suffer withdrawal symptoms if you stop this medicine abruptly. If you want to stop taking diazepam, contact your doctor.

If you will be taking diazepam for a long period of time, *keep all your appointments with your doctor* so that he can check your response to this medicine. He also will want to determine whether you need to continue to take this medicine.

Before you start to take diazepam, tell your doctor if you are pregnant, if you intend to become pregnant while taking this medicine or if you are nursing a baby. If you become pregnant while taking diazepam, contact your doctor. Diazepam is passed from a mother to her unborn baby and to a breast-fed baby through the milk and can have bad effects on the unborn baby and on the breast-fed baby.

DOSAGE AND STORAGE

Your doctor will determine how often you should take diazepam tablets and how many you should take at each dose. Carefully follow the instructions on your prescription label and ask your doctor or pharmacist to explain any part of the instructions you do not understand.

If you forget to take a dose, do not take it when you remember. Omit the missed dose completely and take the next dose at the regularly scheduled time.

Keep this medicine in the container it came in. Keep diazepam out of the reach of children. Do not allow anyone else to take your diazepam.

Hydroxyzine
(hye drox' i zeen)

Brand names: Atarax, Hy-Pam, Sedaril, Vistaril

Names of preparations containing hydroxyzine: Catarax, Enarax, Marax, Theophedrizine, Vistrax

Hydroxyzine is a tranquilizer used to calm people who are tense or anxious because of a nervous or emotional condition. Because this medicine also acts as an antihistamine, it is used to help relieve the itching of allergies and the symptoms of hay fever.

The injectable form of hydroxyzine is used to control nausea and vomiting, and to relieve anxiety before dental procedures, minor surgery and childbirth.

UNDESIRED EFFECTS

With usual doses of hydroxyzine, there are few side effects. This medicine can cause some people to be drowsy or less alert than they normally are. Do not drive a car or operate dangerous machinery until you know how this medicine will affect you. Drowsiness tends to disappear as your body adjusts to hydroxyzine.

If hydroxyzine gives you a dry mouth, chew gum or suck hard candies or bits of ice to relieve the dryness.

Large doses of this medicine can cause a skin rash or shakiness. If you experience these effects, contact your doctor.

PRECAUTIONS

Do not take hydroxyzine if you have ever had an unusual reaction to this medicine in the past.

Before you start to take hydroxyzine, tell your doctor what prescription or nonprescription drugs you are taking, including antihistamines or medicine for hay fever, other allergies or colds (check the labels of nonprescription drugs); barbiturates, narcotics or prescription medicine for pain; medicine for seizures; sedatives, tranquilizers or sleeping medicine; and medicine for depression.

If you do not know the names of the drugs you are taking or what they were prescribed for, bring them in their labeled containers to your doctor or pharmacist.

Do not drink alcoholic beverages while you are taking this medicine. Alcohol will add to the drowsiness caused by hydroxyzine. Do not start to take any of the drugs listed above unless you have permission from your doctor. They may increase the possibility of and severity of side effects.

Do not take more of this medicine and do not take it more often than directed by your doctor.

Because hydroxyzine may affect an unborn child if taken in the early part of a pregnancy, tell your doctor if you are pregnant or think you may be. Also tell your doctor if you are breast-feeding a baby.

DOSAGE AND STORAGE

Your doctor will determine how often you should take hydroxyzine and how much you should take at each dose. Carefully follow the instructions on your prescription label and ask your doctor or pharmacist to explain any part of the instructions you do not understand.

Hydroxyzine comes in capsules, tablets and liquid form. Your doctor will choose the form best for you. If you are taking hydroxyzine liquid, shake it well before using to distribute the medication evenly.

If you forget to take a dose of hydroxyzine, *do not* take the missed dose when you remember it. Take the next dose at the regularly scheduled time.

Keep hydroxyzine in the container it came in, and keep it out of the reach of children. Do not allow anyone else to take your hydroxyzine.

Oxazepam

(ox aze' e pam)

Brand name: Serax

Oxazepam is one of the benzodiazepine tranquilizers. Oxazepam is used to treat the anxiety, tension, restlessness and irritability caused by a wide variety of medical problems, including alcohol withdrawal.

UNDESIRED EFFECTS

Transient, mild drowsiness is common during the first days of therapy. Do not drive a car or operate dangerous machinery until you know how oxazepam will affect you or until the drowsiness disappears. If the drowsiness continues, contact your doctor. He may want to adjust the dose.

Unsteadiness, dizziness or headache can occur with or without drowsiness. These effects tend to decrease as you continue to take oxazepam and as your body adjusts to it. If they are persistent or severe, contact your doctor. Less often this medicine will cause blurred vision, nausea, slurred speech or unusual weakness or tiredness. Contact your doctor if these effects continue or are severe.

More serious effects, although they do not occur often, will require medical attention if they do occur. Contact your doctor if you experience mental confusion (a sign that you are not tolerating this medicine), skin rash or itching (signs of allergic reaction), trouble sleeping or unusual nervousness and irritability (signs of a reaction opposite to the desired one), unusually slow heartbeat or difficulty breathing (signs of slowed function of the central nervous system), sore throat and fever (signs of blood problems) or yellowing of the eyes or skin (signs of a liver problem).

When you stop taking oxazepam, it may take your body up to two weeks to adjust to this. Be alert for symptoms of withdrawal and contact your doctor if you experience convulsions or seizures, mental confusion, muscle cramps, nausea or vomiting, stomach cramps, trembling, unusual irritability or unusual sweating.

PRECAUTIONS

Anyone who has had an unusual reaction to any of the other benzodiazepines is more likely to react badly to oxazepam. Tell your doctor if you have ever had an unusual reaction to chlordiazepoxide, clorazepate, clonazepam, diazepam, flurazepam, lorazepam or prazepam.

Tell your doctor if you have asthma, emphysema, bronchitis or other chronic lung disease, glaucoma, kidney disease, liver disease, mental depression, myasthenia gravis, severe mental illness or hyperactivity (in children). Oxazepam can make these conditions worse.

Certain medications, when taken with oxazepam, can increase the possibility of and/or severity of side effects. Tell your doctor what prescription or nonprescription medicines you are taking, including antihistamines or medicine for hay fever, other allergies or colds; barbiturates, narcotics or other sedatives; tranquilizers or medicine to help you sleep; prescription medicine for pain; medicine for depression or MAO inhibitors (even if you have not taken them for two weeks).

If you do not know the names of the drugs you are taking or what they were prescribed for, bring them in their labeled containers to your doctor or pharmacist.

Do not drink alcoholic beverages while you are taking oxazepam because serious side effects may result. Do not start to take any of the drugs listed above unless you have permission from your doctor. If you have any questions about this, check with your doctor or pharmacist.

Take oxazepam exactly as directed by your doctor. Do not take more of it, do not take it more often and do not take it longer than your doctor has ordered. This medicine can be habit-forming if you take it too often.

Your doctor will want to check your response to oxazepam if you are going to be taking it for a long period of time. He will check at least every four months to determine if you need to continue to take this medicine. *Be sure to keep all your appointments with your doctor.*

If you have been taking oxazepam in large doses or for a long period of time, do not stop taking it without your doctor's permission. To avoid withdrawal problems, your doctor may want you gradually to reduce the amount you are taking before you stop completely.

Before you start to take oxazepam, tell your doctor if you are pregnant, if you plan to become pregnant while taking this medicine or if you are breast-feeding a baby. This drug can be passed from a mother to her unborn child and to a nursing baby through the milk. It can create problems for the baby. If you become pregnant while taking this medicine, contact your doctor.

DOSAGE AND STORAGE

Your doctor will determine how often you should take oxazepam capsules and how much of this medicine you should take at each dose. Carefully follow the instructions on your prescription label and ask your doctor or pharmacist to explain any part of the instructions you do not understand.

If you forget to take a dose, *do not* take it when you remember. Omit the missed dose completely and take only the next dose at the regularly scheduled time.

Keep oxazepam in the container it came in. Keep it out of the reach of children. Do not allow anyone else to take your oxazepam.

Depression

Grief is the normal response to loss of a loved one, illness, failure or frustration. Depression is a state of continual feelings of demoralization, unhappiness and pessimism that is not related to a specific event or situation. In bipolar depression, periods of elation alternate with depression.

Depression causes many different symptoms, depending on the exact nature and severity of the disease. Weight loss, insomnia and "agitated" behavior such as hand wringing or pacing are common. Anxiety and depression often appear together, making diagnosis of the underlying problem difficult even for professionals.

The treatment of depression may involve electroconvulsive therapy, psychotherapy or antidepressant drugs. Often these treatments are used together.

Amitriptyline
(a mee trip′ ti leen)

Brand names: Amitid, Amitril, Elavil, Endep, SK-Amitriptyline

Names of preparations containing amitriptyline: Etrafon (with perphenazine), Limbitrol (with chlordiazepoxide), Triavil (with perphenazine)

Amitriptyline is one of the group of drugs called antidepressants or mood elevators. It is used to treat mental depression and the depression that can occur with anxiety.

UNDESIRED EFFECTS

The most common side effects of amitriptyline are dry mouth (suck hard candy or chew gum to relieve the dryness), headache, increased appetite for sweets, tiredness and weakness. Less often this medicine will cause diarrhea, excessive sweating, heartburn, sleeping difficulty or vomiting. All of these effects tend to decrease and may disappear as your body adjusts to the medicine. If they continue or are severe, contact your doctor.

Amitriptyline makes some people drowsy or dizzy, particularly when they begin to take it. Do not drive a car or operate dangerous machinery until you know how this medicine will affect you.

If this medicine makes you dizzy, lightheaded or faint when you get up from a lying or sitting position, try getting up slowly. Contact your doctor if this problem continues or gets worse.

Although more serious side effects do not occur often, they will require medical attention if they do occur. Contact your doctor if you have blurred vision, constipation, irregular heartbeat, difficulty urinating, eye pain, hallucinations (seeing, hearing or feeling things that are not there), shakiness, unusually slow pulse, skin rash and itching, sore throat and fever, or yellowing of the eyes or skin.

PRECAUTIONS
If you have ever had an allergic reaction to any of the other tricyclic anti-depressants (desipramine, doxepin, notriptyline, imipramine and protriptyline), you are more likely to have a bad reaction to amitriptyline. Talk this over with your doctor.

This medicine can make some medical conditions worse. Be sure to tell your doctor if you have a history of asthma, alcoholism, difficult urination, an enlarged prostate, glaucoma, heart disease, high blood pressure, liver disease, an overactive thyroid, or stomach or bowel problems.

Tell your doctor what prescription or nonprescription drugs you are taking, particularly antihistamines, allergy medicine, barbiturates, medicine for blood pressure, cold remedies, medicine for hay fever, narcotics, other medicine for depression, medicine for pain, sedatives, medicine for seizures, medicine to help you sleep, tranquilizers and MAO inhibitors (even if you stopped taking them within the past two weeks). If you do not know the names of the drugs or what they were prescribed for, bring them in their labeled containers to your doctor or pharmacist.

Do not drink alcoholic beverages while you are taking amitriptyline. Do not start to take any of the drugs listed above without your doctor's permission. All of these can increase the possibility and/or severity of side effects.

You may have to take amitriptyline for several weeks before you begin to feel better. Do not stop taking amitriptyline unless your doctor tells you to. He may want you gradually to decrease the amount you are taking before you stop completely.

Before you have any kind of surgery (including dental surgery) or emergency treatment, tell the doctor or dentist in charge that you are taking amitriptyline.

Children under 12 years of age should not take this medicine. Safe use of amitriptyline in this age group has not been established.

Before beginning to take amitriptyline, tell your doctor if you are pregnant or are breast-feeding. If you become pregnant while taking this medicine, contact your doctor at once.

DOSAGE AND STORAGE
Your doctor will determine how often you should take amitriptyline and how much you should take at each dose. Carefully follow the instructions on your prescription label and ask your doctor or pharmacist to explain any part of the instructions you do not understand.

Amitriptyline comes in tablets. They may be taken with food to decrease the chance of an upset stomach, unless your doctor has told you to take them on an empty stomach.

If you forget to take a dose of this medicine, take it as soon as you remember it and take any remaining doses for that day at evenly spaced intervals. If you remember a missed dose when it is almost time for you to take another, take only the regularly scheduled dose. Omit the missed dose completely. *Do not take a double dose.*

Keep this medicine in the container it came in. Keep amitriptyline out of the reach of children, because an overdose can be especially dangerous to young children. Do not allow anyone else to take your amitriptyline.

Desipramine
(dess ip' ra meen)

Brand names: Norpramin, Pertofrane

Desipramine is one of the group of drugs called antidepressants or mood elevators. Desipramine is used to treat anxiety and depression, particularly when these conditions exist together.

UNDESIRED EFFECTS

Desipramine often causes dry mouth (suck hard candy or chew gum to relieve the dryness), headache, increased appetite for sweets, tiredness or weakness. Less common effects are diarrhea, excessive sweating, heartburn, difficulty sleeping and vomiting. All of these effects tend to decrease or disappear as your body adjusts to desipramine. If they continue or get worse, contact your doctor.

Some people become drowsy when they start to take desipramine. Do not drive a car or operate dangerous machinery until you know what effect this medicine will have on you.

Desipramine can make you dizzy, lightheaded or faint when you get up from a sitting or lying position. Getting up slowly may help to relieve this problem. Contact your doctor if this problem continues or gets worse.

Although more serious side effects do not occur often, they will require medical attention if they do occur. Contact your doctor if you have blurred vision, constipation, irregular heartbeat, difficulty urinating, eye pain, hallucinations (seeing, hearing or feeling things that are not there), shakiness, unusually slow pulse, skin rash and itching, sore throat and fever, or yellowing of the eyes or skin.

PRECAUTIONS

Before you start to take desipramine, tell your doctor if you have ever had an unusual reaction to any of the other tricyclic antidepressants (amitriptyline, doxepin, nortriptyline, imipramine, protriptyline). If you have had a bad reaction to any of these drugs, you may be more likely to have a bad reaction to desipramine and should not take desipramine.

Because desipramine can make certain medical conditions worse, tell your doctor if you have a history of asthma, alcoholism, difficult urination, an enlarged prostate, glaucoma, heart disease, high blood pressure, liver disease, an overactive thyroid, or stomach or bowel problems.

Tell your doctor what prescription or nonprescription drugs you are taking, including antihistamines, medicine for allergy, barbiturates, medicine for high blood pressure, remedies for colds, medicine for hay fever, narcotics, other medicine for depression, medicine for pain, tranquilizers, sedatives, medicine for seizures, medicine to help you sleep and MAO inhibitors (even if you stopped taking them within the past two weeks). If you do not know the names of the drugs you are taking or what they were prescribed for, bring them in their labeled containers to your doctor or pharmacist.

Do not drink alcoholic beverages while you are taking desipramine. Do not start to take any of the drugs listed above without your doctor's permission. All of these can increase the possibility and severity of side effects.

It may take several weeks before you notice the full effects of desipramine. Do not stop taking this medicine unless your doctor tells you that you may. He probably will want you gradually to cut down on the amount you take before you stop taking this medicine completely.

Before you have emergency treatment or any kind of surgery, including dental surgery, tell the doctor or dentist in charge that you are taking desipramine.

Children under 12 years of age should not take this medicine. Safe use of desipramine in this age group has not been established.

Before you start to take this medicine, tell your doctor if you are pregnant or are breast-feeding. If you become pregnant while taking desipramine, contact your doctor at once.

DOSAGE AND STORAGE

Your doctor will determine how often you should take desipramine and how much you should take at each dose. Carefully follow the instructions on your prescription label and ask your doctor or pharmacist to explain any part of the instructions you do not understand.

Desipramine comes in tablets and capsules. Unless your doctor instructs you otherwise, if desipramine upsets your stomach, you may take it with food.

If you forget to take a dose of desipramine, take it as soon as you remember and take any remaining doses for that day at evenly spaced intervals. If you do not remember a missed dose until it is almost time for you to take another, take only the regularly scheduled dose. Omit the missed dose completely. *Do not take a double dose to make up for a missed one.*

Keep desipramine in the container it came in. Keep this medicine out of the reach of children. An overdose of desipramine may be particularly dangerous for young children. Do not allow anyone else to take your desipramine.

Doxepin
(dox′ e pin)

Brand names: Adapin, Sinequan

Doxepin is one of the antidepressant or mood-elevating drugs. Doxepin is used to treat anxiety and depression, particularly when these conditions exist together. It also is used to treat alcoholism.

UNDESIRED EFFECTS

Drowsiness and dizziness are common side effects during the first few weeks of therapy. Do not drive a car or operate dangerous machinery until you know how doxepin will affect you. These effects tend to decrease or disappear as your body adjusts to doxepin. If they continue, contact your doctor.

Other common effects are dry mouth (suck hard candy or chew gum to relieve the dryness), headache, increased appetite for sweets, nausea, and tiredness or weakness. Less often, doxepin will cause diarrhea, excessive sweating, heartburn, sleeping difficulty or vomiting. Contact your doctor if these effects continue or are severe.

More serious side effects, which require medical attention, do not occur very often. However, you should contact your doctor if you have blurred vision, constipation, irregular heartbeat, problems urinating, eye pain, fainting, hallucinations (seeing, hearing or feeling things that are not there), shakiness, unusually slow pulse, skin rash and itching, sore throat and fever, or yellowing of the eyes or skin.

PRECAUTIONS

Before you start to take doxepin, be sure to tell your doctor if you have ever had an unusual reaction to any of the other tricyclic antidepressants (amitriptyline, desipramine, nortriptyline, imipramine, protriptyline). If you have had a bad reaction to any of these, you are more likely to have a bad reaction to doxepin.

Because doxepin can make certain medical conditions worse, tell your doctor if you have any of the following: alcoholism, a history of asthma, difficulty urinating, an enlarged prostate, glaucoma, heart disease, high blood pressure, liver disease, an overactive thyroid, or stomach or bowel problems.

Tell your doctor what prescription or nonprescription drugs you are taking, particularly medicine for allergy, antihistamines, medicine for high blood pressure, remedies for colds, medicine for hay fever, narcotics, other medicine for depression, medicine for pain, sedatives, medicine for seizures, medicine to help you sleep, tranquilizers and MAO inhibitors (even if you stopped taking them within the past two weeks). If you do not know the names of the drugs or what they were prescribed for, bring them in their labeled containers to your doctor or pharmacist.

Do not drink alcoholic beverages while you are taking doxepin. Do not start to take any of the drugs listed above without your doctor's permission. All of these can increase the chance and severity of side effects.

Take doxepin only as directed, and *keep all your appointments with your doctor* so he can determine how you are responding to this medicine.

Sometimes doxepin must be taken for several weeks before you begin to feel better. Do not stop taking this medicine unless your doctor says you may. He may want you gradually to cut down the amount you are taking before you stop taking the medicine completely.

If you need emergency treatment or surgery, including dental surgery, tell the doctor or dentist in charge that you are taking doxepin.

Children under the age of 12 years should not take doxepin. Safe use of this medicine in this age group has not been established.

Before you start to take doxepin, tell your doctor if you are pregnant or are breast-feeding. If you become pregnant while taking this medicine, contact your doctor at once.

DOSAGE AND STORAGE

Your doctor will determine how often you should take doxepin and how much you should take at each dose. Carefully follow the instructions on your prescription label and ask your doctor or pharmacist to explain any part of the instructions you do not understand.

Doxepin comes in capsules and in liquid form to be taken orally. You may take this medicine with food to decrease stomach upset, unless your doctor has told you to take it on an empty stomach.

If you are taking the liquid form, be sure you know how to measure the proper dose with the enclosed dropper. The liquid must be diluted. Just before you take this medicine, place the dose in at least half a glass of water, milk or juice. Do not mix this medicine with grape juice or carbonated beverages because they may reduce doxepin's effectiveness.

If you forget to take a dose of doxepin, take it as soon as you remember and take any remaining doses for that day at evenly spaced intervals. If you remember a missed dose when it is almost time for you to take another, omit the missed dose completely and take only the regularly scheduled dose. *Do not take a double dose to make up for a missed one.*

Keep doxepin in the container it came in. Keep this medicine out of the reach of children. Overdose is especially dangerous for young children. Do not allow anyone else to take your doxepin.

Imipramine
(im ip' ra meen)

Brand names: Imavate, Janimine, Presamine, SK-Pramine, Tofranil

Imipramine is one of the antidepressant or mood-elevating drugs. Imipramine is used to treat depression in adults and bed-wetting in children.

UNDESIRED EFFECTS

Imipramine makes some people drowsy or dizzy, especially during the first few weeks of treatment. Do not drive a car or operate dangerous machinery until you know how this drug will affect you.

If imipramine makes your mouth dry, suck hard candy or chew gum to relieve the dryness. Imipramine may cause nausea, vomiting or diarrhea. Taking this medicine with food or a light snack may help prevent stomach upset. Contact your doctor if these effects continue in spite of your precautions.

Other effects, which may occur early in treatment and then disappear as your body adjusts to the medicine, are headache, increased appetite for sweets, tiredness or weakness, excessive sweating, heartburn and difficulty sleeping. If these effects continue or bother you, contact your doctor.

Though more serious effects do not occur often, they may require medical attention if they do occur. Contact your doctor if you have blurred vision, constipation, irregular heartbeat, difficulty urinating, eye pain, fainting, hallucinations (seeing, hearing or feeling things that are not there), shakiness, unusually slow pulse, skin rash and itching, sore throat and fever, or yellowing of the eyes or skin.

The most common side effects in children taking imipramine for bed-wetting are nervousness, sleeping problems, tiredness and mild stomach upset. Although these effects usually disappear as the child continues to take the medicine, contact your doctor if they continue.

PRECAUTIONS

If you have ever had an unusual reaction to any of the other tricyclic anti-depressants (amitriptyline, desipramine, doxepin, nortriptyline and protripty-line), you are more likely to have a bad reaction to imipramine. Tell your doctor if you have had any such problem with these other drugs.

Imipramine can make certain medical conditions worse. Tell your doctor if you have a history of asthma, alcoholism, difficult urination, an enlarged prostate, glaucoma, heart disease, high blood pressure, liver disease, an overactive thyroid, or stomach or bowel problems.

Tell your doctor what prescription or nonprescription drugs you are taking, particularly medicine for allergy, antihistamines, barbiturates, medicine for high blood pressure, remedies for colds, medicine for hay fever, narcotics, other medicine for depression, medicine for pain, sedatives, medicine for seizures, medicine to help you sleep, tranquilizers and MAO inhibitors (even if you stopped taking them within the past two weeks). If you do not know the names of the drugs or what they were prescribed for, bring them in their labeled containers to your doctor or pharmacist.

Do not drink alcoholic beverages while you are taking imipramine. Do not start to take any of the drugs listed above without your doctor's permission. All of these can increase the chance of and the severity of side effects.

Take imipramine exactly as directed by your doctor and *keep all your appointments with your doctor* so he can check on your response to this medicine.

You may have to take imipramine for several weeks before you begin to feel better. Do not stop taking this medicine until your doctor says that you may. He may want you gradually to decrease the amount you are taking before you stop taking imipramine completely.

If you have to have emergency treatment or any kind of surgery, including dental surgery, be sure to tell the doctor or dentist in charge that you are taking imipramine.

Before you start to take imipramine, tell your doctor if you are pregnant or are breast-feeding. If you become pregnant while you are taking this medicine, contact your doctor at once.

DOSAGE AND STORAGE

Your doctor will determine how often you should take imipramine and how much you should take at each dose. Carefully follow the instructions on your prescription label and ask your doctor or pharmacist to explain any part of the instructions you do not understand.

Imipramine comes in tablets and capsules. If this medicine upsets your stomach, take it with food or a light snack.

If you forget to take a dose of imipramine, take it as soon as you remember and take any remaining doses for the day at evenly sapced intervals. If you remember a missed dose when it is almost time for you to take another, omit the missed dose entirely and take only the regularly scheduled dose. *Do not take a double dose to make up for a missed one.*

Keep imipramine in the container it came in. Keep this medicine out of the reach of children. An overdose of imipramine is especially dangerous for young children. Do not let anyone else take your imipramine.

Nortriptyline
(nor trip' ti leen)

Brand names: Aventyl Hydrochloride, Pamelor

Nortriptyline belongs to the group of drugs known as antidepressants or mood elevators. Nortriptyline is used to relieve mental depression and anxiety, particularly when these conditions exist together.

UNDESIRED EFFECTS

The most common side effects of nortriptyline are dry mouth (suck hard candy or chew gum to relieve the dryness), headache, increased appetite for sweets, tiredness and weakness. Less often this medicine will cause diarrhea, excessive sweating, heartburn, sleeping difficulty or vomiting. These effects tend to decrease and may disappear as your body adjusts to nortriptyline. If they continue or bother you, contact your doctor.

Some people become drowsy or dizzy when they begin to take nortriptyline. Do not drive a car or operate dangerous machinery until you know how this medicine will affect you.

Nortriptyline may make you dizzy, lightheaded or faint when you get up from a lying or sitting position. Getting up slowly may help. If this problem continues or gets worse, contact your doctor.

Although more serious side effects do not occur often, they will require medical attention if they do occur. Contact your doctor if you have blurred vision, constipation, irregular heartbeat, difficulty urinating, eye pain, hallucinations (seeing, hearing or feeling things that are not there), shakiness, unusually slow pulse, skin rash and itching, sore throat and fever, or yellowing of the eyes or skin.

PRECAUTIONS

If you have ever had an unusual reaction to any of the other tricyclic antidepressants (amitriptyline, desipramine, doxepin, imipramine and protriptyline), you are more likely to have a bad reaction to nortriptyline and should not take it. If you have any questions about this, ask your doctor.

Because nortriptyline can make some medical conditions worse, tell your doctor if you have a history of asthma, alcoholism, difficult urination, an enlarged prostate, glaucoma, heart disease, high blood pressure, liver disease, an overactive thyroid, or stomach or bowel problems.

Tell your doctor what prescription or nonprescription drugs you are taking, particularly antihistamines, medicine for allergy, barbiturates, medicine for high blood pressure, remedies for colds, medicine for hay fever, narcotics, other medicine for depression, medicine for pain, sedatives, medicine for seizures, medicine to help you sleep, tranquilizers and MAO inhibitors (even if you stopped taking them within the past two weeks). If you do not know the names of the drugs or what they were prescribed for, bring them in their labeled containers to your doctor or pharmacist.

Do not drink alcoholic beverages while you are taking nortriptyline. Do not start to take any of the drugs listed above without your doctor's permission. All of these can increase the chance of and severity of side effects.

You may have to take this medicine for a week to several weeks before you begin to feel better. Do not stop taking nortriptyline unless your doctor tells you to. He may want you gradually to decrease the amount you are taking before you stop taking nortriptyline completely.

Before you have emergency treatment or surgery, including dental surgery, tell the doctor or dentist in charge that you are taking nortriptyline.

Children under 12 years of age should not take this medicine. Safe use of nortriptyline in this age group has not been established.

Before beginning to take nortriptyline, be sure to tell your doctor if you are pregnant or are breast-feeding. If you become pregnant while taking this medicine, contact your doctor at once.

DOSAGE AND STORAGE

Your doctor will determine how often you should take nortriptyline and how much you should take at each dose. Carefully follow the instructions on your prescription label and ask your doctor or pharmacist to explain any part of the instructions you do not understand.

Nortriptyline comes in capsules and in liquid form. It may be taken with food or a light snack to decrease the chance of an upset stomach, unless your doctor has told you to take it on an empty stomach.

To make sure of an accurate dose of the liquid form, measure it in a specially marked measuring spoon. The liquid must be diluted. Just before you take this medicine, place the dose in at least half a glass of water, milk or juice. Do not mix this medicine with grape juice or carbonated beverages because they may decrease the effectiveness of nortriptyline.

If you forget to take a dose of this medicine, take it as soon as you remember it and take any remaining doses for that day at evenly spaced intervals. If you remember a missed dose when it is almost time for you to take another, take only the regularly scheduled dose. Omit the missed dose completely. *Do not take a double dose.*

Keep nortriptyline in the container it came in. Keep this medicine out of the reach of children. An overdose of nortriptyline can be especially dangerous to young children. Do not allow anyone else to take your nortriptyline.

Schizophrenia

Schizophrenia is a very serious mental illness characterized by delusions, hallucinations and changes in behavior. Often, schizophrenics have delusions about body control. They feel that they are under the control of some outside force or power and are forced to speak a certain way or perform certain actions. In many cases, expression of emotions is disturbed and inappropriate. For example, the schizophrenic may laugh while describing a sad event.

The causes of schizophrenia are controversial. Although the disease appears to be hereditary, it seems that heredity may only make a person susceptible to having schizophrenia, and other contributing factors must be present for a person to develop the disease. Environment and life experiences are major factors. Currently there are investigations under way that suggest chemical imbalances may also play a part in the development of the disease.

Treatment of schizophrenia usually involves a period of hospitalization followed by psychotherapy, drug treatment and social planning.

Chlorpromazine
(klor proe' ma zeen)

Brand name: Thorazine

Chlorpromazine is a tranquilizer used to treat patients who are anxious, tense, apprehensive or overexcited. Sometimes it is prescribed to control nausea, vomiting and severe hiccups.

UNDESIRED EFFECTS

During the first few weeks in which you are taking chlorpromazine it may make you drowsy or less alert than normal. Do not drive a car or operate dangerous machinery until you know how this medicine will affect you. The drowsiness usually will disappear after a period of time, but if it continues to trouble you, contact your doctor.

Chlorpromazine can cause dry mouth. Suck hard candy or chew gum to relieve this dryness. Other side effects, which may go away as your body adjusts to chlorpromazine, include blurred vision, constipation, decreased sweating, dizziness, nasal congestion, unusually fast heartbeat, changes in menstrual period, decreased sexual ability, difficult urination and swelling of the breasts. If these effects continue or are severe, contact your doctor.

If your doctor increases your dosage of chlorpromazine, you may experience other effects. Contact your doctor if you have muscle spasm in the neck or back; restlessness; shuffling walk; jerky movements of the head, neck, face and mouth; or trembling and shaking of the hands and fingers.

Other side effects, which may require medical attention if they occur, are fainting; fine, wormlike movements of the tongue; skin rash; eye problems; sore throat and fever; and yellowing of the eyes or skin. Contact your doctor if you have any of these effects.

Chlorpromazine may turn your urine red or brown. This effect is harmless.

PRECAUTIONS

If you have ever had an unusual reaction to any of the phenothiazines, you should not take chlorpromazine. If you have questions about this, check with your doctor or pharmacist.

Before you start to take chlorpromazine, tell your doctor if you have any of the following medical problems: alcholism, blood disease, glaucoma, heart or blood vessel disease, liver disease, lung disease, Parkinson's disease, an enlarged prostate, stomach ulcers or urination problems. Chlorpromazine may make these conditions worse.

Tell your doctor what prescription or nonprescription drugs you are taking, because certain medications can increase the possibility of and severity of side effects. These include amphetamines, medicine for seizures, medicine for asthma, epinephrine, guanethidine (medicine for high blood pressure), levodopa and medicine for ulcers. If you do not know the names of the drugs or what they were prescribed for, bring them in their labeled containers to your doctor or pharmacist.

Other medicines that can influence the effect of chlorpromazine are antihistamines or medicine for hay fever, other allergies or colds; bartiburates, narcotics or prescription medicine for pain; sedatives, tranquilizers or medicine to help you sleep; medicine for depression and MAO inhibitors (even if you stopped taking them within the past two weeks). Tell your doctor if you are taking any of these medicines.

Take chlorpromazine exactly as prescribed by your doctor. Do not take more of it or take it more often than your doctor has ordered. This is particularly important when you give this medicine to children, since they may react very strongly to its effects.

It may take several weeks before you notice the full effects of this medicine. Do not stop taking chlorpromazine without your doctor's permission. Your doctor may want you gradually to reduce the amount you take before you stop taking it completely.

Do not drink alcoholic beverages while you are taking chlorpromazine. It can make the side effects more severe. Do not start to take any other type of medicine while you are taking chlorpromazine unless you first check with your doctor or pharmacist.

Chlorpromazine often will make you sweat less than normal and your body temperature will increase. Be careful to avoid situations in which you might become overheated (such as exercise and hot weather) while you are taking this medicine.

When taking chlorpromazine, some people are more sensitive to sunlight.

Stay out of sunlight or use a sunscreen preparation until you know how this medicine will affect you. If you find that you sunburn more easily while taking chlorpromazine, contact your doctor.

Before you start to take chlorpromazine, tell your doctor if you are pregnant or think you may become pregnant while you are taking this medicine, or if you are nursing a baby. Chlorpromazine is passed to an unborn baby and to a breast-feeding baby and can have bad effects on the baby. If you become pregnant while taking chlorpromazine, contact your doctor at once.

DOSAGE AND STORAGE

Your doctor will determine how often you should take chlorpromazine and how much you should take at each dose. Carefully follow the instructions on your prescription label and ask your doctor or pharmacist to explain any part of the instructions you do not understand.

Chlorpromazine comes in extended-release capsules, tablets and liquid form to be taken orally, and in rectal suppositories. The tablets and capsules should be taken with a full eight-ounce glass of water or milk to avoid stomach irritation. The extended-release capsules should be swallowed whole. Do not break, crush or chew them before swallowing them.

If you are taking the liquid form you may take it in water, milk, a soft drink, coffee, tea, or tomato or fruit juice. Try to avoid getting this medicine on your skin or clothing. It may cause a skin rash.

To use the rectal suppository, remove the foil wrapper and dip the tip of the suppository in water. Lie on your side and bring the knee of your top leg up to your chest. Then insert the suppository well into your rectum and hold it there for a few minutes. Try to avoid having a bowel movement for at least an hour after inserting the suppository.

If the suppository is too soft to insert because it was stored in a warm place, leave the foil wrapper on and refrigerate the suppository for 30 minutes, or run cold water over it.

If you forget to take a dose of chlorpromazine, take it as soon as you remember and take any remaining doses for that day at evenly spaced intervals. If you do not remember to take a missed dose until it is almost time to take another one, omit the missed dose completely and take only the regularly scheduled dose. *Do not take a double dose.*

Keep chlorpromazine in the container it came in, and keep it out of the reach of children. Do not allow anyone else to take your chlorpromazine.

Droperidol
(droe per' i dole)

Brand name: Inapsine

Droperidol is a tranquilizer given by injection to calm people before surgery and certain diagnostic procedures and to reduce the nausea and vomiting that may follow use of an anesthetic.

UNDESIRED EFFECTS

When droperidol is injected it may make you dizzy or lightheaded or it may make your heartbeat unusually fast. These effects usually are mild and disappear after a while, but tell your doctor if you experience these effects.

Other effects include chills or shivering; facial sweating; restlessness; leg muscle cramps; stiffness of the arms and legs; jerky movements of the head, face, neck and mouth; and trembling and shaking of the hands and fingers. Contact your doctor if you have any of these effects.

PRECAUTIONS

Because droperidol can make some medical conditions worse, tell your doctor if you have heart or blood vessel disease, kidney disease, liver disease, Parkinson's disease, lung disease or low blood pressure.

Tell your doctor what prescription or nonprescription drugs you are taking, including amphetamines, medicine for seizures, medicine for high blood pressure, medicine for asthma, epinephrine, medicine for ulcers, antihistamines, medicine for allergies or colds, barbiturates, narcotics, prescription medicine for pain, sedatives, tranquilizers, medicine to help you sleep and medicine for depression. If you do not know the names of the drugs or what they were prescribed for, bring them in their labeled containers to your doctor or pharmacist.

Do not drink alcoholic beverages before you are to take droperidol and for at least a day after the injection. If you have any questions about this, check with your doctor.

Droperidol should not be given to children under the age of two years. Safe use of the drug in this age group has not been established.

Before you take droperidol, tell your doctor if you are pregnant. The safe use of this medicine in pregnant women has not been established.

Haloperidol
(ha loe per′ i dole)

Brand name: Haldol

Haloperidol is a tranquilizer used to treat emotional and mental conditions. It also is used to control nausea and vomiting; muscular tics of the face, neck, hands and shoulders; and severe behavior problems in children.

UNDESIRED EFFECTS

The most common side effects are dry mouth (suck hard candies or chew gum to relieve it), constipation and blurred vision. Less often, haloperidol will cause nausea or vomiting and decreased sexual ability. These side effects tend to decrease or disappear as your body adjusts to the medicine. If they continue or are severe, contact your doctor.

Haloperidol causes some people to become drowsy or less alert than normal. Do not drive a car or operate dangerous machinery until you know how haloperidol will affect you.

Larger doses of haloperidol can cause shuffling walk; stiffness of the arms and legs; jerky movements of the head, face, mouth and neck; or trembling and shaking of the hands and fingers. If you experience any of these effects, contact your doctor. He may want to adjust your dose or prescribe another drug that will control these effects.

Other effects, which may require medical attention if they occur, include difficult urination, dizziness, lightheadedness, fainting, wormlike movements of the tongue, skin rash, sore throat and fever and yellowing of the eyes or skin. Contact your doctor if you have any of these effects.

PRECAUTIONS
Because haloperidol can make certain medical conditions worse, tell your doctor if you have blood disease, alcoholism, epilepsy, glaucoma, heart or blood vessel disease, kidney disease, liver disease, lung disease, an overactive thyroid, Parkinson's disease, an enlarged prostate, severe mental depression, stomach ulcers or problems urinating.

Tell your doctor what prescription or nonprescription drugs you are taking, including amphetamines, medicine for seizures, medicine for high blood pressure, medicine for asthma, epinephrine, medicine for ulcers, antihistamines, medicine for allergies or colds, barbiturates, narcotics, prescription medicine for pain, sedatives, tranquilizers, medicine to help you sleep, medicine for depression and MAO inhibitors (even if you stopped taking them within the past two weeks). If you do not know the names of the drugs or what they were prescribed for, bring them in their labeled containers to your doctor or pharmacist.

Do not drink alcoholic beverages while you are taking haloperidol. Do not start to take any of the drugs listed above without your doctor's permission. All of these can increase the possibility and severity of side effects.

Take haloperidol exactly as directed by your doctor. Do not take more of it, do not take it more often and do not take it for a longer period of time than your doctor has instructed.

Do not stop taking haloperidol without your doctor's permission. He may want you gradually to cut down on the amount you take before you stop taking it completely.

To help your doctor select the best treatment for you and your baby, tell him if you are pregnant or are breast-feeding. If you become pregnant while taking haloperidol, contact your doctor at once.

DOSAGE AND STORAGE
Your doctor will determine how often you should take haloperidol and how much you should take at each dose. Carefully follow the instructions on your prescription label and ask your doctor or pharmacist to explain any part of the instructions you do not understand.

Haloperidol comes in tablets and in liquid form. If this medicine upsets your stomach, the tablets may be taken with solid food or milk.

The liquid comes in a container with a dropper to be used in measuring the proper dose. Be sure you understand how much to take and how to measure it. If you have any questions about this, check with your doctor or pharmacist.

The liquid should be taken with a four-ounce glass of milk, water, soft drink or juice. Put the medicine in the beverage just before you take it. If you get any of the beverage on the dropper, rinse it with tap water before you put it back into the container.

Try not to get any liquid haloperidol on your skin or clothing. Liquid haloperidol may cause a skin rash.

If you forget to take a dose of haloperidol, take it as soon as you remember and take any remaining doses for the day at evenly spaced intervals. If you remember a missed dose when it is almost time to take another, omit the missed dose completely and take only the regularly scheduled dose. *Do not take more than one dose at a time.*

Keep haloperidol in the container it came in, and store it away from heat and out of direct sunlight. Keep this medicine out of the reach of children. Do not allow anyone else to take your haloperidol.

Perphenazine
(per fen′ a zeen)

Brand name: Trilafon

Perphenazine is a tranquilizer used to treat patients who are anxious, tense, apprehensive or overexcited. It also is prescribed to control severe nausea and vomiting, and severe hiccups.

UNDESIRED EFFECTS

Perphenazine may make you drowsy, especially during the first few weeks you are taking it. Do not drive a car or operate dangerous machinery until you know how this medicine will affect you. If the drowsiness does not disappear or is severe, contact your doctor.

Other side effects, which tend to decrease or disappear as your body adjusts to perphenazine, include dry mouth (suck hard candy or chew gum to relieve this), blurred vision, constipation, decreased sweating, dizziness, nasal congestion, unusually fast heartbeat, changes in menstrual period, decreased sexual ability, difficult urination and swelling of the breasts. Contact your doctor if these effects continue or are severe.

An increase in dosage can cause muscle spasm in the neck or back; restlessness; shuffling walk; jerky movements of the head, neck, face and mouth; or trembling and shaking of the hands and fingers. Contact your doctor if any of these occur.

Side effects that may require medical attention include fainting, wormlike movements of the tongue, skin rash, eye problems, sore throat and fever, and yellowing of the skin or eyes. If any of these occur, contact your doctor.

This medicine may color your urine red or brown. This effect is harmless.

PRECAUTIONS

Tell your doctor if you have ever had an unusual reaction to any other phenothiazine. If you have, you will be more likely to have a bad reaction to perphenazine.

Perphenazine can make some medical problems worse. Before you start to take this medicine tell your doctor if you have blood disease, alcoholism, glaucoma, heart or blood vessel disease, liver disease, lung disease, Parkinson's disease, an enlarged prostate, stomach ulcers or urination problems.

Certain medications, when taken with perphenazine, can increase the possibility and severity of side effects. Tell your doctor what prescription or non-prescription drugs you are taking, including amphetamines, medicine for seizures, medicine for asthma, epinephrine, guanethidine (medicine for high blood pressure), levodopa, medicine for ulcers, antihistamines, medicine for allergies or colds, barbiturates, narcotics, prescription medicine for pain, sedatives, tranquilizers, medicine to help you sleep, medicine for depression and MAO inhibitors (even if you stopped taking them within the past two weeks).

If you do not know the names of the drugs or what they were prescribed for, bring them in their labeled containers to your doctor or pharmacist.

Do not drink alcoholic beverages while you are taking perphenazine. Do not start to take any of the drugs listed above without your doctor's permission. All of these can increase the severity of side effects.

Take perphenazine exactly as prescribed by your doctor. Do not take more of it and do not take it more often than ordered by your doctor. This is particularly important if you are giving perphenazine to a child. Children may react strongly to this medicine's effects.

It may take several weeks for you to notice the full effects of perphenazine. Do not stop taking it without first checking with your doctor. He may want you gradually to reduce the amount you are taking before you stop taking it completely.

Be careful to avoid situations in which you may become overheated while you are taking perphenazine. This medicine can cause you to sweat less and as a result your body temperature will increase. Strenuous exercise and hot weather can create problems in this regard.

Some people become more sensitive to sunlight when they are taking perphenazine. Limit the amount of time you spend in sunlight until you know what effect this medicine will have on you. If you find that this medicine causes you to sunburn easily, contact your doctor.

Perphenazine is passed by a mother to her unborn child or to a breast-feeding baby. Be sure to tell your doctor if you are nursing a baby, if you are pregnant or if you plan to get pregnant while you are taking perphenazine. If you become pregnant while taking this medicine, contact your doctor at once.

DOSAGE AND STORAGE
Your doctor will determine how often you should take perphenazine and how much you should take at each dose. Carefully follow the instructions on your prescription label and ask your doctor or pharmacist to explain any part of the instructions you do not understand.

Perphenazine comes in extended-release tablets, regular tablets and concentrated liquid form. The regular tablets should be taken with a full eight-ounce glass of water or milk to avoid stomach irritation. The extended-release tablets should be swallowed whole. Do not break, crush or chew them before swallowing them.

The concentrated liquid form must be diluted. Just before taking it, measure the correct dose and put it in half a glass (four ounces) of tomato or fruit juice, water, soup, coffee, tea or a soft drink. Try to avoid getting liquid perphenazine on your skin or clothing. Liquid perphenazine may cause a skin rash.

If you forget to take a dose of perphenazine, take it as soon as you remember and take any remaining doses for that day at evenly spaced intervals. If you do not remember a missed dose until it is almost time to take another one, omit the missed dose completely and take only the regularly scheduled dose. *Do not take a double dose.*

Keep this medicine in the container it came in, and keep it out of the reach of children. Do not allow anyone else to take your perphenazine.

Prochlorperazine
(pro klor peer' a zeen)

Brand name: Compazine

Prochlorperazine is a tranquilizer used to treat emotional and mental conditions. It also is prescribed to control anxiety, nausea and vomiting, and severe hiccups.

UNDESIRED EFFECTS

During the first few weeks in which you are taking prochlorperazine, it may make you drowsy or less alert than normal. Do not drive a car or operate dangerous machinery until you know how this medicine will affect you. The drowsiness should disappear. If it does not, contact your doctor.

If prochlorperazine makes your mouth dry, suck hard candies or chew gum to relieve the dryness. Other side effects include blurred vision, unusually fast heartbeat, constipation, decreased sweating, dizziness, nasal congestion, changes in menstrual period, decreased sexual ability, difficult urination and swelling of the breasts. These effects tend to decrease as your body adjusts to prochlorperazine. If they continue or are severe, contact your doctor.

Muscle spasm in the neck or back; restlessness; shuffling walk; jerky movements of the head, neck, face and mouth; and trembling and shaking of the hands and fingers can occur when the dosage of prochlorperazine is increased. Contact your doctor if you experience any of these effects.

Side effects that may require medical attention include fainting, wormlike movements of the tongue, skin rash, eye problems, sore throat and fever, and yellowing of the skin or eyes. Contact your doctor if these occur.

Prochlorperazine may change the color of your urine to red or brown. This effect is harmless.

PRECAUTIONS

If you have ever had an unusual reaction to any of the phenothiazines, you should not take prochlorperazine because you may have a bad reaction to it. If you have any questions about this, ask your doctor or pharmacist.

Before you start to take prochlorperazine, tell your doctor if you have any of the following medical conditions: blood disease, alcoholism, glaucoma, heart or blood vessel disease, liver disease, lung disease, Parkinson's disease, an enlarged prostate, stomach ulcers or urination problems. This medicine may make these conditions worse.

Certain medication can increase or decrease the effects of prochlorperazine. Tell your doctor if you are taking amphetamines, medicine for seizures, medicine for asthma, epinephrine, guanethidine (medicine for high blood pressure), levodopa, medicine for ulcers, antihistamines, medicine for allergies or colds, barbiturates, narcotics, prescription medicine for pain, sedatives, tranquilizers, medicine to help you sleep, medicine for depression and MAO inhibitors (even if you stopped taking them within the past two weeks).

If you do not know the names of the drugs you are taking or what they were prescribed for, bring them in their labeled containers to your doctor or pharmacist.

Do not drink alcoholic beverages while you are taking prochlorperazine. Do not start to take any of the drugs listed above without your doctor's permission. All of these can increase the possibility and severity of side effects.

Take this medicine exactly as prescribed by your doctor. Do not take more of it and do not take it more often than instructed. This is particularly important if you are giving prochlorperazine to a child. Children may react strongly to this medicine's effects.

You may not notice the full effects of this medicine until you have taken it for several weeks. Do not stop taking prochlorperazine without your doctor's permission. He may want you gradually to reduce the amount you are taking before you stop taking it completely.

This medicine can cause you to sweat less, and as a result your body temperature will increase. Be careful to avoid situations (such as strenuous exercise and.hot weather) in which you may become overheated while you are taking prochlorperazine.

Because prochlorperazine makes some people more sensitive to sunlight than they normally are, limit the amount of time you spend in the sunlight until you know what effect this medicine will have on you. If you find that you sunburn easily while taking prochlorperazine, contact your doctor.

Prochlorperazine should not be taken by pregnant women or by women who are breast-feeding. Be sure to tell your doctor if you are pregnant or are nursing a baby. If you become pregnant while you are taking this medicine, contact your doctor at once.

DOSAGE AND STORAGE

Your doctor will determine how often you should take prochlorperazine and how much you should take at each dose. Carefully follow the instructions on your prescription label and ask your doctor or pharmacist to explain any part of the instructions you do not understand.

Prochlorperazine comes in extended-release capsules, tablets and liquid to be taken orally and in rectal suppositories. The tablets should be taken with a full eight-ounce glass of water or milk to avoid stomach upset. The extended-release capsules should be swallowed whole. Do not break, crush or chew them before swallowing them.

If you are taking the liquid form of prochlorperazine, try to avoid getting it on your skin or clothing. Liquid prochlorperazine may cause a skin rash. The liquid may be taken in juice, water, soup, coffee, tea or a soft drink.

To use the rectal suppositories, remove the foil wrapper and dip the tip of the suppository in water. Then lie on your side, bring the knee of your top leg up to your chest and insert the suppository well into your rectum and hold it there for a few moments. Try not to have a bowel movement for at least an hour after inserting the suppository. If the suppository has been stored in a warm place and is too soft to insert easily, leave the wrapper on and refrigerate the suppository for 30 minutes or run cold water over it.

If you forget to take a dose of prochlorperazine, take it as soon as you remember and take any remaining doses for that day at evenly spaced intervals. If you do not remember a missed dose until it is almost time for another, omit the missed dose completely and take only the regularly scheduled dose. *Do not take a double dose*.

Keep this medicine in the container it came in. Keep it out of the reach of children. Do not allow anyone else to take your prochlorperazine.

Thioridazine
(the oh rid′ a zeen)

Brand name: Mellaril

Thioridazine is one of the phenothiazine tranquilizers used to treat mental depression and the depression often associated with anxiety. Thioridazine also is used to treat children with severe behavioral problems, and children who are hyperactive.

UNDESIRED EFFECTS

Some common side effects of thioridazine are dry mouth (suck hard candy or chew gum to relieve it), blurred vision, constipation, decreased sweating, dizziness, nasal congestion and unusually fast heartbeat. Less often, thioridazine can cause difficulty urinating, changes in menstrual period, decreased sexual ability or swelling of the breasts. These effects usually disappear as your body adjusts to the medicine. Let your doctor know if they continue or are severe.

Some people become drowsy or less alert than normal when they take thioridazine, particularly when they start to take it. Do not drive a car or operate dangerous machinery until you know how this medicine will affect you. Usually the drowsiness will disappear after a few weeks. Contact your doctor if it does not.

If thioridazine makes you dizzy, lightheaded or faint when you get up from a sitting or lying position, try to get up slowly; this may help. If this problem continues, contact your doctor.

More serious side effects do not occur often, but they may require medical attention if they do occur. Most often, these effects result from high doses or long-term therapy. Contact your doctor if you experience muscle spasm in the neck or back; restlessness; shuffling walk; jerky movements of the head, neck, face and mouth; trembling and shaking of the hands and fingers; fainting; wormlike movements of the tongue; skin rash; eye problems; sore throat and fever; or yellowing of the skin or eyes. Thioridazine may color your urine red or brown. This effect is harmless.

PRECAUTIONS

You should not take thioridazine if you have ever had an unusual reaction to any of the other phenothiazines. If you have any questions about this, check with your doctor or pharmacist.

Because thioridazine can make some medical problems worse, tell your doctor if you have blood disease, alcoholism, glaucoma, heart or blood vessel disease, lung disease, Parkinson's disease, an enlarged prostate, stomach ulcers or urination problems.

Tell your doctor what prescription or nonprescription drugs you are taking, including amphetamines, medicine for seizures, medicine for asthma, epinephrine, guanethidine (medicine for high blood pressure), levodopa, medicine for ulcers, antihistamines, medicine for allergies and colds, barbiturates, narcotics, prescription medicine for pain, sedatives, tranquilizers, medicine to help you sleep, medicine for depression and MAO inhibitors (even if you stopped taking them within the past two weeks).

If you do not know the names of the drugs you are taking or what they were prescribed for, bring them in their labeled containers to your doctor or pharmacist.

Do not drink alcoholic beverages while you are taking thioridazine. Do not start to take any of the drugs listed above without your doctor's permission. All of these can increase the chance of and severity of side effects.

Do not take more of this medicine or take it more often than instructed by your doctor. It is particularly important that you use thioridazine exactly as prescribed by your doctor when you are giving it to a child. Children may react strongly to this medicine's effects.

You may have to take thioridazine for several weeks before you feel its full effects. Do not stop taking it without first getting your doctor's permission. He may want you gradually to reduce the amount you are taking before you stop taking it completely.

Thioridazine can cause you to sweat less; and as a result, your body temperature will rise. Be careful to avoid situations in which you may become overheated (such as strenuous exercise, hot weather, and hot or sauna baths) while you are taking this medicine.

Thioridazine makes some people more susceptible to sunburn than they normally are. Avoid excessive exposure to sunlight, or use a sunscreen preparation until you know whether this medicine will cause you to sunburn easily.

Pregnant women and women who are breast-feeding should not take this medicine because of possible bad effects on the baby. Before you start to take thioridazine, tell your doctor if you are pregnant or are nursing a baby. If you become pregnant while taking thioridazine, contact your doctor at once.

DOSAGE AND STORAGE

Your doctor will determine how often you should take thioridazine and how much you should take at each dose. Carefully follow the instructions on your prescription label and ask your doctor or pharmacist to explain any part of the instructions you do not understand.

Thioridazine comes in tablets and in liquid form. It may be taken with food or with a full eight-ounce glass of water or milk to decrease stomach upset.

If you are taking the liquid form, use a specially marked measuring spoon to be sure you get an accurate dose. Some forms of the liquid must be diluted before you take it. Be sure that you carefully follow the instructions on your prescription label. Try to avoid getting the liquid on your skin or clothing. Liquid thioridazine may cause a skin rash.

If you forget to take a dose of thioridazine, take it as soon as you remember and take any remaining doses for that day at evenly spaced intervals. If you do not remember a missed dose until it is almost time to take another one, omit the missed dose completely and take only the regularly scheduled dose. *Do not take a double dose.*

Keep this medicine in the container it came in, and store away from heat and direct sunlight. Keep it out of the reach of children. Do not allow anyone else to take your thioridazine.

Thiothixene
(thye oh thix' een)

Brand name: Navane

Thiothixene is a tranquilizer used to treat emotional and mental conditions. It may be particularly useful in treating people with chronic mental illness who have not responded to other drugs of this type.

UNDESIRED EFFECTS

During the first few weeks in which you take thiothixene, you may be drowsy or less alert than normal. Do not drive a car or operate dangerous machinery until you know how this medicine will affect you. The drowsiness should disappear as you continue to take this medicine. If it does not, contact your doctor.

You may become dizzy, lightheaded or faint when getting up from a sitting or lying position. Getting up slowly may help, but you should contact your doctor if these problems continue or get worse.

Other side effects that may occur are dry mouth (suck hard candy or chew gum to relieve it), blurred vision, constipation, decreased sweating, nasal congestion and unusually fast heartbeat. Less often, thiothixene can cause difficulty urinating, swelling of the breasts, changes in menstrual period and decreased sexual ability. If you experience any of these effects and they bother you, contact your doctor.

If your doctor increases your dose of thiothixene, you may have muscle spasms of the neck or back; restlessness; shuffling walk; jerky movements of the head, face, mouth and neck; or trembling of the hands and fingers. Contact your doctor if these effects occur. He may want to adjust your dose or prescribe another medicine that will relieve these problems.

Other side effects may require medical attention if they occur. Contact your doctor if you experience fainting, wormlike movements of the tongue, skin rash, eye problems, sore throat and fever, or yellowing of the skin or eyes.

PRECAUTIONS

Before you start to take thiothixene, tell your doctor if you have ever had an unusual reaction to chlorprothixene or to any phenothiazine. If so, you will be more likely to have a bad reaction to thiothixene.

Because thiothixene can make some medical conditions worse, tell your doctor if you have blood disease, alcoholism, glaucoma, heart or blood vessel disease, liver disease, lung disease, Parkinson's disease, an enlarged prostate, stomach ulcers or urination problems.

Tell your doctor what prescription or nonprescription drugs you are taking, including amphetamines, medicine for seizures, medicine for asthma, epinephrine, guanethidine (medicine for high blood pressure), levodopa, medicine for ulcers, antihistamines, medicine for allergies and colds, barbiturates, narcotics, prescription medicine for pain, sedatives, tranquilizers, medicine to help you sleep, medicine for depression and MAO inhibitors (even if you stopped taking them within the past two weeks). These drugs can influence the effects of thiothixene.

If you do not know the names of the drugs you are taking or what they were prescribed for, bring them in their labeled containers to your doctor or pharmacist.

Do not drink alcoholic beverages while you are taking this medicine. Do not start to take any of the drugs listed above without your doctor's permission. All of these can increase the possibility and severity of side effects.

Take thiothixene exactly as prescribed by your doctor. Do not take more of it and do not take it more often than instructed.

You may have to take thiothixene for several weeks before you feel its full effects. Do not stop taking this medicine without your doctor's permission. He may want you gradually to cut down the amount you are taking before you stop taking it completely.

Thiothixene can cause you to sweat less; as a result, your body temperature will rise. Be careful to avoid situations in which you may become overheated (such as strenuous exercise, hot weather and sauna baths) while you are taking this medicine.

Thiothixene may make some people more sensitive to sunlight than they normally are. Limit the amount of time you spend in sunlight until you know how this medicine will affect you. If you find that you sunburn more easily while taking thiothixene, contact your doctor.

Do not take thiothixene within an hour of taking antacids or medicine for diarrhea. If these drugs are taken too close together, thiothixene may be less effective.

To help your doctor select the best and safest treatment for you and your baby, tell him if you are pregnant or if you are nursing a baby.

Thiothixene should not be given to children under 12 years of age. Its safe use in this age group has not been established.

DOSAGE AND STORAGE

Your doctor will determine how often you should take thiothixene and how much you should take at each dose. Carefully follow the instructions on your prescription label and ask your doctor or pharmacist to explain any part of the instructions you do not understand.

Thiothixene comes in capsules and concentrated liquid. The capsules should be taken with a full eight-ounce glass of water or milk to avoid stomach upset.

Thiothixene liquid comes in a container that includes a measuring dropper. If you are taking this form, be sure you understand how much to take and how to measure it with the dropper. Just before you take the liquid, measure the proper amount into a half glass (four ounces) of juice, water, soup, coffee, tea, milk or a soft drink. If any of the liquid with which you are diluting the medicine gets on the dropper, rinse the dropper with tap water before you put the dropper back in the container.

Try to avoid getting liquid thiothixene on your skin or clothing. Liquid thiothixene may cause a skin rash.

If you forget to take a dose of thiothixene, take it as soon as you remember and take any remaining doses for that day at evenly spaced intervals. If you do not remember a missed dose until it is almost time to take another one, omit the missed dose completely and take only the regularly scheduled dose. *Do not take a double dose*.

Keep thiothixene in the container it came in, and store it away from heat and out of direct sunlight. Keep it out of the reach of children. Do not allow anyone else to take your thiothixene.

Trifluoperazine
(trye floo oh peer' a zeen)

Brand name: Stelazine

Trifluoperazine is a tranquilizer used to treat emotional and mental conditions. It also is prescribed to control anxiety, nausea and vomiting and severe hiccups.

UNDESIRED EFFECTS

When you start to take trifluoperazine, you may be drowsy or less alert than normal. Do not drive a car or operate dangerous machinery until you know how this medicine will affect you. The drowsiness disappears after a few weeks. If it does not, contact your doctor.

Some common effects of this medicine are dry mouth (suck hard candy or chew gum to relieve it), blurred vision, constipation, decreased sweating, dizziness, nasal congestion and unusually fast heartbeat. Less often, trifluoperazine can cause difficulty urinating, changes in menstrual period, decreased sexual ability and swelling of the breasts. Tell your doctor if you experience these effects and they bother you.

If your doctor increases the amount of trifluoperazine you take, you may experience muscle spasm in the neck or back; restlessness; shuffling walk; jerky movements of the head, neck, face and mouth; or trembling and shaking of the hands and fingers. Contact your doctor if you have any of these problems.

Other side effects that may require medical attention are fainting, wormlike movements of the tongue, skin rash, eye problems, sore throat and fever, and yellowing of the skin or eyes. If any of these occur, contact your doctor.

You may notice a change in the color of your urine to red or brown. This effect is harmless.

PRECAUTIONS

If you have ever had an unusual reaction to any other phenothiazine, you are more likely to have a bad reaction to trifluoperazine and should not take it. If you have any questions about this, check with your doctor or pharmacist.

Before you start to take trifluoperazine, tell your doctor if you have blood disease, alcoholism, glaucoma, heart or blood vessel disease, liver disease, lung disease, Parkinson's disease, an enlarged prostate, stomach ulcers or urination problems. This medicine may make these problems worse.

Tell your doctor what prescription or nonprescription drugs you are taking, including amphetamines, medicine for seizures, medicine for asthma, epinephrine, guanethidine (medicine for high blood pressure), levodopa, medicine for ulcers, antihistamines, medicine for allergies and colds, barbiturates, narcotics, prescription medicine for pain, sedatives, tranquilizers, medicine to help you sleep, medicine for depression and MAO inhibitors (even if you stopped taking them within the past two weeks). These drugs can influence the effect of trifluoperazine.

If you do not know the names of the drugs you are taking or what they were prescribed for, bring them in their labeled containers to your doctor or pharmacist.

Do not drink alcoholic beverages while you are taking trifluoperazine. Do not start to take any of the drugs listed above without your doctor's permission. All of these can increase the possibility and severity of side effects.

Do not take more of this medicine or take it more often than instructed by your doctor. It is particularly important that trifluoperazine be taken exactly as prescribed by your doctor when you are giving it to a child. Children may react strongly to this medicine's effects.

You may have to take trifluoperazine for several weeks before you feel its full effects. Do not stop taking this medicine without first checking with your doctor. He may want you gradually to reduce the amount you are taking before you stop taking it completely.

Trifluoperazine can cause you to sweat less; as a result, your body temperature will rise. Be careful to avoid situations in which you may become overheated (such as strenuous exercise or hot weather) while you are taking this medicine.

Some people become more sensitive to sunlight while they are taking trifluoperazine. Limit the amount of time you spend in sunlight until you know how this medicine will affect you. If you find that you sunburn easily while taking trifluoperazine, contact your doctor.

Pregnant women and women who are breast-feeding should not take trifluoperazine because of possible bad effects on the baby. Before you start to take this medicine, tell your doctor if you are pregnant or are nursing a baby. If you become pregnant while taking trifluoperazine, contact your doctor at once.

DOSAGE AND STORAGE

Your doctor will determine how often you should take trifluoperazine and how much you should take at each dose. Carefully follow the instructions on your prescription label and ask your doctor or pharmacist to explain any part of the instructions you do not understand.

Trifluoperazine comes in tablets and in concentrated liquid form to be taken orally. The tablets should be taken with a full eight-ounce glass of water or milk to avoid stomach upset.

Trifluoperazine liquid comes in a container that includes a measuring dropper. If you are taking this form be sure you understand how much to take and how to measure it with the dropper. Just before you take the liquid, measure the proper amount into one-half glass (four ounces) of juice, water, soup, coffee, tea, milk or a soft drink. If any of the liquid with which you are diluting the medicine gets on the dropper, rinse the dropper with tap water before you put it back in the container.

Try to avoid getting liquid trifluoperazine on your skin or clothing. Liquid trifluoperazine may cause a skin rash.

If you forget to take a dose of trifluoperazine, take it as soon as you remember and take any remaining doses for that day at evenly spaced intervals. If you do not remember a missed dose until it is almost time to take another one, omit the missed dose completely and take only the regularly scheduled dose. *Do not take a double dose.*

Keep trifluoperazine in the container it came in, and store it away from heat and out of direct sunlight. Keep it out of the reach of children. Do not allow anyone else to take your trifluoperazine.

Lithium
(li' thee um)

Brand names: Eskalith, Lithane, Lithionate
Lithium works on the nervous system to stabilize the mood of people with manic-depressive illness.

UNDESIRED EFFECTS

When you begin to take lithium, you may have shaking of the hands and fingers, thirst, frequent urination, or brief episodes of nausea and diarrhea. Usually these effects disappear as your body adjusts to the medicine. If they do not stop, contact your doctor.

Lithium also can decrease the function of the thyroid gland. Symptoms of this problem include coldness of the fingers and toes, constipation, dry and puffy skin, headache, menstrual changes, muscle aches, sleepiness, tiredness and unusual weight gain. Contact your doctor if you experience any of these effects. He may want to prescribe a thyroid supplement for you.

The most serious side effect of this medicine is lithium poisoning. Stop taking lithium and contact your doctor if you experience nausea and vomiting, shakiness, drowsiness, mental confusion, slurred speech, ringing in the ears, weakness, blurred vision or jerking of the arms and legs. Also contact your doctor if you have pains in the lower stomach (a sign of stomach irritation) or swelling of the feet and lower legs (a sign that your body is retaining water).

PRECAUTIONS

Because lithium can make some medical conditions worse, tell your doctor if you have heart disease, kidney disease, Parkinson's disease, any kind of severe infection or thyroid disease.

Tell your doctor what prescription or nonprescription drugs you are taking, including medicine for asthma; caffeine (a common ingredient of many colas and nonprescription medicines for pain); chlorpromazine; diuretics (water pills), especially the thiazide type; haloperidol; potassium iodide; and sodium bicarbonate (baking soda). If you do not know the names of the drugs or what they were prescribed for, bring them in their labeled containers to your doctor or pharmacist.

While you are taking lithium, drink two or three quarts of water or other fluids each day and use a normal amount of salt in your food. If you are on a low-salt diet, discuss this with your doctor.

Lithium may cause some people to become drowsy or less alert than they normally are. Do not drive a car or operate machinery until you know how lithium will affect you.

Be careful to avoid situations in which you will sweat heavily (such as hot weather, strenuous exercise and hot or sauna baths). The loss of too much water and salt from your body may lead to serious side effects from taking lithium.

Do not drink large amounts of beverages that contain caffeine (such as coffee, tea or cola) while you are taking lithium. Lithium is excreted from the body in the urine, and the increased flow of urine caused by caffeine may decrease the effect of lithium.

While you are taking lithium, your doctor will want to monitor the amount of drug in your blood to make sure you do not have serious side effects. *Be sure to keep all your appointments with your doctor for checks of your blood level.*

Usually lithium must be taken for seven to 10 days before you begin to feel better. Do not take more of this medicine, do not take it more often and do not take it for a longer time than your doctor has ordered.

Do not drink alcoholic beverages or take any other drugs while you are taking lithium unless your doctor tells you that you may.

Lithium should not be given to children under 12 years of age. Safe use of lithium in this age group has not been established.

Be sure to tell your doctor if you are pregnant or think you may become pregnant while you are taking this medicine. Also tell him if you are breast-feeding. Lithium is passed from a mother to her unborn baby and from a mother to a nursing baby, and lithium may have bad effects on the baby. If you become pregnant while you are taking lithium, contact your doctor at once.

Dosage and Storage

Your doctor will determine how often you should take lithium and how much you should take at each dose. Carefully follow the instructions on your pre-scription label and ask your doctor or pharmacist to explain any part of the instructions you do not understand.

Lithium comes in tablets and capsules. If this medicine upsets your stomach, it may be taken immediately after meals or with solid food or milk. If you have any questions about this, check with your doctor or pharmacist.

If you forget to take a dose of lithium, *do not* take it when you remember. Omit the missed dose and take the next dose at the regularly scheduled time. *Do not take a double dose to make up for a missed dose.*

Keep lithium in the container it came in, and store the container out of direct sunlight. Keep this medicine out of the reach of children. Do not allow anyone else to take your lithium.

SEIZURES AND EPILEPSY

DRUGS USED TO TREAT SEIZURES AND EPILEPSY

Seizures and Epilepsy

The two most common types of epilepsy are grand mal epilepsy and petit mal epilepsy. Both types are caused by excessive electrical activity in the brain. The difference between them is primarily a matter of the degree to which the excessive activity spreads over the brain and nervous system.

In grand mal seizures, excessive activity spreads throughout the brain and even to the spinal cord. This produces a loss of consciousness and muscle rigidity, which is followed by uncontrollable rhythmic jerking movements. Usually a grand mal seizure is followed by a feeling of severe fatigue lasting up to several hours.

Petit mal seizures (also called absence seizures) are brief periods (five to 20 seconds) of loss of consciousness. During this period the individual shows a blank, staring expression and may have some minor twitching. Usually the person is unaware of the seizure and resumes previous activities as if nothing happened.

Other types of seizures include psychomotor and psychosensory seizures. These are disorders that vary quite a bit, depending on the portion of the brain involved. In some cases, several types of seizures may occur at once, and diagnosis often is difficult.

Carbamazepine
(kar ba maz' e peen)

Brand name: Tegretol

Carbamazepine is used to treat certain types of convulsions and seizures. However, since this medicine has dangerous side effects, it usually is prescribed only when other anticonvulsant drugs have been unable to control the seizures. Carbamazepine also is used to treat facial nerve pain (trigeminal neuralgia).

Undesired Effects

Carbamazepine can cause dizziness, blurred vision, drowsiness and poor coordination. Do not drive a car, operate dangerous machinery or do anything that requires you to be mentally and physically alert until you know how this medicine will affect you.

Nausea and vomiting, common side effects of carbamazepine, can be avoided if you take this medicine with meals or immediately after eating.

Serious side effects, such as blood problems, liver problems, kidney problems, and heart and blood vessel problems, can occur when you are taking carbamazepine. Contact your doctor immediately if you develop fever, sore throat, mouth ulcers, unusual bleeding or bruising, purple-colored spots on the skin, yellowing of the eyes or skin, frequent or difficult urination, swelling of the feet and legs, irregular heartbeat, or skin rash or hives.

PRECAUTIONS

If you have ever had a bad reaction to any of the tricyclic drugs (amitriptyline, desipramine, imipramine, protriptyline, nortriptyline, etc.), you should not take carbamazepine.

Because carbamazepine can make certain medical conditions worse, tell your doctor if you have a history of blood disease such as bone marrow depression, heart disease, liver disease, high blood pressure, thrombophlebitis (blood clots), kidney disease or thyroid disease.

Before you start to take carbamazepine, tell your doctor what prescription or nonprescription drugs you are taking, including barbiturates, tranquilizers, other anticonvulsant drugs, doxycycline, coumarin-type anticoagulants (blood thinners), MAO inhibitors (even if you stopped taking them in the past two weeks) and oral contraceptives. If you do not know the names of the drugs or what they were prescribed for, bring them in their labeled containers to your doctor or pharmacist.

While you are taking carbamazepine, do not take any other medicines unless your doctor specifically tells you that you may. Take carbamazepine exactly as your doctor has prescribed, and do not take more of it or take it more often than he tells you to.

Do not stop taking carbamazepine until your doctor tells you that you may. You can have problems if you abruptly stop taking this medicine. Your doctor probably will want you gradually to reduce the amount you take before you stop taking the medicine completely.

Keep in touch with your doctor while you are taking carbamazepine so he can check your response to it and adjust the amount you take. He also will want to check how this medicine is affecting you by doing complete blood counts (usually once a week when you start therapy), tests for liver function and tests of your urine. He also may want you to have your eyes checked. *Be sure to keep all your appointments for checkups.*

If you are pregnant or are nursing a baby, tell your doctor. Pregnant women and breast-feeding mothers should not take this medicine. If you become pregnant while you are taking carbamazepine, inform your doctor immediately.

DOSAGE AND STORAGE

Your doctor will determine how much carbamazepine you should take and how often you should take it. Carefully follow the instructions on your prescription label and ask your doctor or pharmacist to explain any part of the instructions you do not understand.

Carbamazepine comes in tablets, which may be taken with milk or solid food to decrease the chance of stomach upset.

If you forget to take a dose of carbamazepine, take it as soon as you remember and take any remaining doses for that day at evenly spaced intervals. If you do not remember a missed dose until it is almost time for you to take another, omit the missed dose entirely. Take only the regularly scheduled dose. *Do not take a double dose to make up for a missed dose.*

Keep carbamazepine in the container it came in, and keep it out of the reach of children. Do not allow anyone else to take your carbamazepine, which was prescribed for your particular condition.

Ethosuximide
(eth oh sux′ i mide)

Brand name: Zarontin

Ethosuximide is used to treat petit mal seizures, the form of epilepsy that makes a person lose consciousness for very short periods of time.

UNDESIRED EFFECTS

The most common side effects of ethosuximide are nausea, vomiting, stomach cramps and loss of appetite. If you take this medicine after meals, you will decrease the chance of stomach upset. These effects should disappear as you continue to take ethosuximide and as your body adjusts to it. If they do not, contact your doctor.

Ethosuximide makes some people dizzy or drowsy. Do not drive a car or operate dangerous machinery until you know how this medicine will affect you. Less often, this medicine may cause headache, tiredness or irritability. If these effects bother you, contact your doctor.

More serious side effects of ethosuximide are allergic reactions or blood problems. Contact your doctor if you develop a skin rash or itching, sore throat and fever, hiccups, unusual bruising or bleeding, or swollen lymph glands.

PRECAUTIONS

If you have ever had an unusual reaction to an anticonvulsant (seizure medicine) in the past, you should not take ethosuximide.

Because this medicine can make some medical conditions worse, tell your doctor if you have blood disease, kidney disease or liver disease.

Tell your doctor what prescription or nonprescription medicines you are taking, including medicine for mental illness or depression and any other anticonvulsant drugs. If you do not know the names of the drugs or what they were prescribed for, take them in their labeled containers to your doctor or pharmacist.

Your doctor will want to check on your response to this medicine so that he can prescribe more or less of it, depending on your need. Keep in touch with your doctor and *keep all your appointments for checkups* so that your doctor can do blood counts and other tests to be sure this medicine is not affecting you badly.

Take ethosuximide exactly as prescribed by your doctor. Do not take more of it or take it more often than he has ordered. Do not stop taking this medicine unless your doctor tells you to do so. Your doctor may want you gradually to reduce the amount you are taking before you stop taking this medicine completely.

Tell your doctor if you are pregnant or are nursing a baby. Pregnant women and women who are breast-feeding should not take ethosuximide. If you become pregnant while taking ethosuximide, contact your doctor immediately.

DOSAGE AND STORAGE

Your doctor will determine how much ethosuximide you should take and how often you should take it. Carefully follow the instructions on your prescription label and ask your doctor or pharmacist to explain any part of the instructions that you do not understand.

Ethosuximide comes in capsules and in liquid form. Your doctor will choose the form best for you.

If you forget to take a dose of this medicine, take it as soon as you remember. Take any remaining doses for the day at evenly spaced intervals. If you do not remember a missed dose until it is almost time for you to take another, omit the missed dose completely and take only the regularly scheduled dose. *Do not take a double dose.*

Keep ethosuximide in the container it came in and store the tightly closed container away from extreme heat and sunlight. Keep this medicine out of the reach of children. Do not allow anyone else to take your ethosuximide.

Methsuximide

(meth sux′ i mide)

Brand name: Celontin

Methsuximide is used to control petit mal seizures, the form of epilepsy that involves brief periods of loss of consciousness and/or jerking of the eyelids and muscles of the face and arms. Methsuximide also may be used in combination with other drugs to treat medical conditions that result in convulsions.

UNDESIRED EFFECTS

The most common side effect of methsuximide is stomach upset. Take this medicine with food or a glass of milk to avoid this problem.

Methsuximide makes some people dizzy or drowsy. Do not drive a car or operate dangerous machinery until you know how this medicine will affect you.

Some effects that may decrease or disappear as your body adjusts to methsuximide are headache, irritability, tiredness, loss of appetite, nausea and vomiting. If you experience any of these effects and they are severe or continue over a period of time, contact your doctor.

Less often, methsuximide will cause allergic reactions and, rarely, blood problems. Contact your doctor immediately if you have a skin rash or itching, sore throat and fever, swollen lymph glands, unusual bruising or bleeding, or mood changes.

PRECAUTIONS

If you have ever had an unusual reaction to another type of medicine for seizures, you should not take methsuximide. Your doctor should know if you have certain medical problems, such as blood disease, kidney disease or liver disease, before you start to take methsuximide.

Tell your doctor what prescription or nonprescription drugs you are taking, including medicine for mental illness or depression and any other anticonvulsant drugs. If you do not know the names of the drugs or what they were prescribed for, bring them in their labeled containers to your doctor or pharmacist.

While you are taking methsuximide, do not drink alcoholic beverages, because they may make the side effects worse. If you have questions about this, check with your doctor or pharmacist.

Your doctor will want to adjust the amount of methsuximide you take according to the way you respond to it. *Be sure to keep all appointments for checkups with your doctor.* Your doctor also will want to do blood counts and other tests to determine how this medicine is affecting you.

Take this medicine exactly as prescribed by your doctor. Do not stop taking it unless your doctor tells you to do so. Your doctor may want you gradually to reduce the amount you are taking before you stop taking methsuximide completely.

Be sure you have enough medicine on hand to take all the doses prescribed for you. Check your supply before vacations, holidays and other times when you might have difficulty getting more.

Tell your doctor if you are pregnant or are nursing a baby. Pregnant women and women who are breast-feeding should not take this medicine. If you become pregnant while taking methsuximide, contact your doctor immediately.

DOSAGE AND STORAGE

Your doctor will determine how much methsuximide you should take and how often you should take it. Carefully follow the instructions on your prescription label and ask your doctor or pharmacist to explain any part of the instructions you do not understand.

Methsuximide comes in capsules, which can be taken with solid food or milk to decrease the chance of stomach upset.

If you forget to take a dose of methsuximide, take it as soon as you remember it. Then take any remaining doses for the day at evenly spaced intervals. If you do not remember a missed dose until it is almost time for you to take another, omit the missed dose entirely and take only the regularly scheduled dose. *Do not take a double dose to make up for a missed dose.*

Keep methsuximide in the container it came in, and keep it out of the reach of children. Do not allow anyone else to take your methsuximide.

Phenytoin
(fen' itoe in)

Brand names: Didan-TDC, Dihycon, Dilantin, Ki-Phenyl, Diphenylan, Ekko, Kessodanten, Toin

Phenytoin is used alone or in combination with other medicines to control various types of convulsions or seizures.

UNDESIRED EFFECTS

Phenytoin can cause redness, swelling or bleeding of the gums, usually after you have been taking it for two to three months. Be sure to brush your teeth carefully and regularly, to use dental floss and to see your dentist on a regular basis for checkups. If you have any questions about how to care for your teeth and gums, check with your doctor or dentist. Contact your doctor or dentist if you develop problems as a result of taking phenytoin.

Nausea and vomiting can occur when you take phenytoin. Take this medicine with meals or immediately after eating to help prevent upset stomach.

Other effects, which require medical attention if they occur, include skin rash, blurred vision, slurred speech, difficulty walking, mental confusion, pain in the joints, unexplained fever, enlarged lymph glands, unusual bleeding or bruising, and yellowing of the eyes or skin. Contact your doctor if you experience any of these effects.

Phenytoin may color your urine pink, red or brown. This effect is harmless and should not concern you.

PRECAUTIONS

If you have ever had an unusual reaction to any other kind of anticonvulsant medicine, you should not take phenytoin. If you have questions about this, check with your doctor.

If you have high blood sugar, liver disease or alcoholism, tell your doctor. Phenytoin may make these conditions worse.

Certain medications should not be taken with phenytoin. Tell your doctor what prescription or nonprescription drugs you are taking, particularly barbiturates, chloramphenicol, coumarin-type anticoagulants (blood thinners), dexamethasone or other cortisonelike medicines, oral medicine for diabetes, disulfiram (medicine for alcoholism), doxycycline, folic acid (found in many vitamin formulas), isoniazid, medicine for mental illness, oxyphenbutazone, phenylbutazone, sulfa drugs and medicine for depression.

If you do not know the names of the drugs you are taking or what they were prescribed for, bring them in their labeled containers to your doctor or pharmacist.

Keep in touch with your doctor while you are taking phenytoin. He may want to adjust your dose or change your medication schedule, depending on your response to phenytoin.

Take phenytoin exactly as prescribed by your doctor. Do not take more of it and do not take it more often than your doctor has prescribed. If you have been taking phenytoin regularly for several weeks, do not stop taking it without your doctor's permission. He may want you gradually to reduce the amount you are taking before you stop taking it completely.

Be sure you have enough of this medicine on hand at all times so that you can take all of the doses that have been prescribed for you. Check your supply before vacations, holidays and other occasions when it may be difficult for you to get more.

Alcoholic beverages may alter the way phenytoin works. Check with your doctor before drinking alcoholic beverages while you are taking this medicine.

If you have diabetes, phenytoin may affect your blood sugar level. If you notice a change in the results of your urine sugar tests, check with your doctor.

Before you have any surgery, including dental surgery, tell the doctor or dentist in charge that you are taking phenytoin.

Be sure to tell your doctor if you are pregnant or are breast-feeding. Pregnant women and breast-feeding mothers should not take phenytoin. If you become pregnant while you are taking this medicine, contact your doctor at once.

DOSAGE AND STORAGE

Your doctor will determine how much phenytoin you should take and how often you should take it. Carefully follow the instructions on your prescription label and ask your doctor or pharmacist to explain any part of the instructions you do not understand.

Phenytoin comes in capsules, chewable tablets and liquid form. Your doctor will choose the form best for you. If you are taking the liquid form, be sure to shake it well before each use. The chewable tablets should be chewed well before they are swallowed. All forms of this medicine may be taken with milk or solid food to prevent stomach upset.

If you forget to take a dose of phenytoin, take the missed dose as soon as you remember it. Take the remaining doses for that day at regularly spaced intervals. If you remember a missed dose when it is almost time for you to take another, omit the missed dose entirely and take only the regularly scheduled dose. *Do not take two doses at one time.*

Keep phenytoin in the container it came in, and store the container at room temperature. Keep this medicine out of the reach of children. Do not allow anyone else to take your phenytoin.

Primidone
(pri′ mi done)

Brand name: Mysoline

Primidone is an anticonvulsant chemically related to phenobarbital. Primidone acts on the brain and central nervous system to control certain types of muscular convulsions or seizures. When used with other drugs it also helps control grand mal epilepsy seizures.

UNDESIRED EFFECTS

Among the most common side effects of primidone are nausea and vomiting. These effects may occur when you start to take this medicine and then disappear later as your body adjusts to the medicine. If you take primidone with meals, you may decrease the chance of stomach upset.

Primidone may make some people dizzy, drowsy or less alert than they usually are. Even when taken at bedtime, it can cause these effects the next morning. Do not drive a car or operate dangerous machinery until you know how this medicine will affect you.

Occasionally children and some older people may show signs of restlessness and excitement after taking primidone. If this occurs, contact your doctor.

More serious side effects with primidone are rare. However, contact your doctor if you experience skin rash, pain in the joints, unexplained fever, swelling of the eyelids, or wheezing or tightness in the chest.

An overdose of or intolerance to primidone can cause symptoms similar to barbiturate poisoning. Contact your doctor immediately if you have changes in vision, mental confusion, shortness of breath or difficulty breathing.

PRECAUTIONS

If you have ever had an unusual reaction to any barbiturate (such as amobarbital, butabarbital, pentobarbital, phenobarbital or secobarbital), you should not take primidone. If you have questions about this, check with your doctor or pharmacist.

To help your doctor select the best treatment for you, tell him if you have asthma, emphysema, chronic lung disease, hyperactivity (in children), kidney disease, liver disease or porphyria.

Before you start to take primidone, tell your doctor what prescription or nonprescription drugs you are taking. Some drugs that will affect the way your body responds to primidone are antihistamines, medicine for allergies and colds, narcotics, other barbiturates, other medicine for seizures, prescription medicine for pain, sedatives, tranquilizers, medicine to help you sleep, medicine for depression, MAO inhibitors (even if you stopped taking them two weeks ago), anticoagulants (blood thinners), corticosteroids (cortisonelike medicine), digitalis, digitoxin, doxycycline, griseofulvin and phenytoin.

If you do not know the names of the drugs you are taking or what they were prescribed for, bring them in their labeled containers to your doctor or pharmacist.

Do not drink alcoholic beverages while you are taking primidone. Alcohol can increase the possibility of or severity of side effects. Do not start to take any of the drugs listed above unless you first check with your doctor.

Take primidone exactly as prescribed by your doctor. Do not take more of it and do not take it more often than he has indicated. Be sure you have enough of this medicine to take all the doses prescribed. Check your supply before vacations, holidays and other occasions on which you may not be able to get more.

Do not stop taking this medicine unless your doctor tells you to do so. Your doctor probably will want you gradually to reduce the amount of primidone you are taking before you stop taking it entirely.

While you are taking this medicine keep in touch with your doctor. He will want to check your response to primidone and he may adjust your dose, depending on your needs.

Before you have any kind of surgery, including dental surgery, be sure to tell the doctor or dentist in charge that you are taking primidone.

If you are pregnant or breast-feeding a baby, be sure to tell your doctor before you begin to take primidone. If you become pregnant while you are taking this medicine, contact your doctor immediately.

DOSAGE AND STORAGE

Your doctor will determine how much primidone you should take and how often you should take it. Carefully follow the instructions on your prescription

label and ask your doctor or pharmacist to explain any part of the instructions you do not understand.

Primidone comes in tablets and in liquid form. It may be taken with meals to decrease the chance of stomach upset. The liquid should be shaken well before each use.

If you forget to take a dose of primidone, take it as soon as you remember. Take any remaining doses for that day at evenly spaced intervals. If you do not remember a missed dose until it is almost time for you to take another, omit the missed dose completely. Take only the regularly scheduled dose. *Do not take a double dose*.

Keep primidone in the container it came in, and store it at room temperature. Keep this medicine out of the reach of children. Do not allow anyone else to take your primidone.

PARKINSON'S DISEASE

DRUGS USED TO TREAT PARKINSON'S DISEASE

Parkinson's Disease

Parkinson's disease is caused by chemical imbalances in portions of the brain. The reasons for developing these imbalances are not known. Since the disease usually begins between the ages of 50 and 65, it is assumed that the aging process is partially responsible. Parkinson's disease affects both men and women of all races and does not appear to be hereditary.

The symptoms of Parkinson's disease usually begin as muscle tremors in one or both hands. This is followed by stiffness of the arms and legs, a general slowing of movements and increasing difficulty in performing routine activities. As the disease progresses further, facial muscles are affected so that facial expressions and eye blinking are decreased and speech is slowed.

Some types of medications, particularly certain tranquilizers, can cause symptoms similar to those of Parkinson's disease. Although these symptoms usually disappear within a few days after you stop taking the medication, they may last considerably longer in susceptible individuals.

Parkinson's disease is treated with a variety of medications that act to correct the chemical imbalances responsible. In addition to these medications, physical therapy often is used to keep muscles in tone and to slow progression of the disease.

Amantadine
(a man′ ta deen)

Brand name: Symmetrel

Amantadine is used to treat Parkinson's disease and symptoms similar to those of Parkinson's disease that can result from disease, injury or certain drugs. Amantadine also is used to prevent influenza caused by type A virus.

UNDESIRED EFFECTS

Amantadine can cause loss of appetite, nausea or vomiting. To decrease the chance of stomach upset, take it after meals or with food.

Amantadine makes some people dizzy, drowsy or less alert than usual. Do not drive a car or operate dangerous machinery until you know how this medicine will affect you.

Other effects that may occur are double vision, mental confusion, difficulty sleeping, tiredness and hallucinations (seeing, hearing or feeling things that are not there). Contact your doctor if any of these effects continue over a period of time or cause you a great deal of discomfort.

More serious side effects will require medical attention if they occur. Contact your doctor if you develop a skin rash, swelling of the feet and legs, a feeling of depression, difficulty in urinating or convulsions.

PRECAUTIONS

Because amantadine can make some medical conditions worse, tell your doctor if you have epilepsy or any other form of seizures, heart disease, kidney disease, liver disease, a recurring skin rash or mental illness.

Before you start to take amantadine, tell your doctor what prescription or nonprescription drugs you are taking, including benztropine, trihexyphenidyl, other medicine for Parkinson's disease, ulcer medicine, medicine for seizures, and medicine for spasms of the intestines. If you do not know the names of the drugs or what they were prescribed for, bring them in their labeled containers to your doctor or pharmacist.

Do not stop taking this medicine unless your doctor tells you that you may. If you stop taking amantadine abruptly your condition may get worse. Your doctor will want you gradually to decrease the amount you take before you stop taking this medicine entirely.

Tell your doctor if you are pregnant or are nursing a baby. Amantadine can be passed to a baby through the mother's milk. Safe use of this medicine in pregnant women has not been established.

DOSAGE AND STORAGE

Your doctor will determine how much amantadine you should take and how often you should take it. Carefully follow the instructions on your prescription label and ask your doctor or pharmacist to explain any part of the instructions you do not understand.

Amantadine comes in capsules and in liquid form. It can be taken after meals or with food to lessen stomach upset. This medicine usually is taken once or twice a day.

If you forget to take a dose of amantadine, take it as soon as you remember the missed dose. However, if you do not remember a missed dose until it is time for you to take another, take only the regularly scheduled dose. Omit the missed dose entirely. *Do not take a double dose to make up for a missed dose.*

Keep amantadine in the container it came in, and keep it out of the reach of children. Do not allow anyone else to take your amantadine.

Benztropine
(benz' troe peen)

Brand name: Cogentin

Benztropine is used alone or with other drugs to treat Parkinson's disease or "shaking palsy." Benztropine improves muscle control and allows more normal movement of the body. It is also used to control side effects resembling Parkinson's disease that some drugs used to treat mental illness may bring about.

UNDESIRED EFFECTS

One of the most common effects of benztropine is dry mouth. To relieve this, suck hard candies, chew gum or dissolve bits of ice in your mouth.

Other effects, which usually are mild when they occur, include blurred vision, nervousness, heart palpitation, loss of appetite, nausea and difficulty urinating. If you experience any of these effects and they are severe or cause you a great deal of discomfort, contact your doctor.

Benztropine will cause some people to become drowsy, dizzy or less alert than usual. Do not drive a car or operate dangerous machinery until you know how this medicine will affect you.

While you are taking benztropine your eyes may be more sensitive to light than they normally are. Wear sunglasses to help decrease the discomfort from bright light.

Because benztropine causes you to sweat less, you may easily become overheated while you are taking this medicine. To prevent heat prostration or sunstroke, be careful not to exert yourself to excess on a hot day, in a heated place or in the sunlight.

Although they do not occur often, more serious side effects will require medical attention if they do occur. Contact your doctor if you develop a skin rash or become constipated. Intestinal problems, such as constipation, can be serious if they are not corrected.

PRECAUTIONS

Because benztropine can make some medical conditions worse, tell your doctor if you have asthma, bronchitis, difficulty urinating, emphysema, an enlarged prostate, glaucoma, hiatal hernia, high blood pressure, an intestinal blockage, kidney disease, liver disease, myasthenia gravis, an overactive thyroid or ulcerative colitis.

To help your doctor select the best treatment for you, tell him what prescription or nonprescription drugs you are taking, including amantadine, antacids, antihistamines, medicine for allergy or colds, haloperidol, medicine for your heart, medicine for diarrhea, other medicine for Parkinson's disease, medicine for sleep, medicine for your nerves, sedatives, tranquilizers, medicine for ulcers and MAO inhibitors (even if you stopped taking them within the past two weeks).

If you do not know the names of the drugs you are taking or what they were prescribed for, bring them in their labeled containers to your doctor or pharmacist.

Do not drink alcoholic beverages while you are taking benztropine. Alcohol can increase the chance of and severity of side effects. Do not start to take any of the drugs listed above unless you have permission from your doctor.

Do not take this medicine within one hour of taking antacids or medicine for diarrhea. Taking these medications close together may decrease the effect of benztropine.

Before you start to take benztropine, tell your doctor if you are pregnant. The safety of this medicine in pregnant women has not been established.

DOSAGE AND STORAGE

Your doctor will determine how much benztropine you should take and how often you should take it. Carefully follow the instructions on your prescription

label and ask your doctor or pharmacist to explain any part of the instructions you do not understand.

Benztropine comes in tablets, which can be taken immediately after meals or with a snack to decrease stomach upset. Benztropine also is given by injection.

What to do if you forget to take a dose of benztropine depends on when you remember the missed dose. If your next scheduled dose is more than four hours away, take the missed dose when you remember it and then continue with your regular dosing schedule. If your next scheduled dose is less than four hours away, take the missed dose when you remember it but do not take another dose for four hours. Take any remaining doses for that day at least four hours apart. If you miss two or more doses in a row, take only one dose when you remember the missed doses. *Do not take more than one dose at a time.*

Keep benztropine in the container it came in, and keep it out of the reach of children. Do not allow anyone else to take your benztropine.

Levodopa
(lee voe doe′ pa)

Brand names: Bendopa, Bio-Dopa, Dopar, Larodopa, Sinemet (a combination of levodopa and carbidopa)

Levodopa is used to relieve the shaking, stiffness and slowness of movement that are some of the symptoms of Parkinson's disease. Levodopa is given alone or in combination with other medicines for Parkinson's disease.

Levodopa also is used to relieve the severe pain caused by some kinds of tumors.

UNDESIRED EFFECTS

Nausea, vomiting, stomach pain and loss of appetite are among the most common side effects of levodopa. Take this medicine with solid food to decrease the chance of stomach upset. Usually these effects occur when you start to take levodopa, then tend to disappear as your body adjusts to the medicine. If they continue or are severe, contact your doctor. He may want to change the amount you are taking.

Other common but mild effects include dry or watery mouth, increased shaking of the hands, inability to walk straight, difficulty falling asleep, headache, dizziness, nightmares, fatigue, depression, constipation and diarrhea. Contact your doctor if any of these effects cause you a great deal of discomfort.

Levodopa causes some people to become dizzy or drowsy. Do not drive a car or operate dangerous machinery until you know how this medication will affect you.

Levodopa may cause your urine, saliva and sweat to change color, becoming pinkish-red to almost black. This effect is not important and can be expected during treatment with this medicine.

More serious side effects can occur, and they require medical attention when they do. Contact your doctor if you experience unusual behavior; abnormal and uncontrollable movements of the mouth, tongue, face, neck, arms or legs;

difficulty urinating; dizziness when arising quickly from a sitting or lying position; or rapid heartbeat.

PRECAUTIONS

Because levodopa may make some medical conditions worse, tell your doctor if you have diabetes, emphysema, asthma, bronchitis or other chronic lung disease, glaucoma, heart or blood vessel disease, hormone problems, kidney disease, liver disease, mental illness, skin cancer or a stomach ulcer.

Before you start to take levodopa, tell your doctor what prescription or nonprescription drugs you are taking, including medicine for asthma or bronchitis (such as epinephrine, ephedrine or isoproterenol), haloperidol, medicine for appetite control, medicine for high blood pressure, methyldopa, papaverine, phenytoin, pyridoxine (vitamin B_6) and reserpine. If you do not know the names of the drugs or what they were prescribed for, bring them in their labeled containers to your doctor or pharmacist.

If you are taking any of the phenothiazine medicines (chlorpromazine, fluphenazine, perphenazine, prochlorperazine, trifluoperazine or triflupromazine) or MAO inhibitors, tell your doctor.

Vitamin B_6 has been shown to reduce the effects of levodopa. Do not take vitamin products containing vitamin B_6 or eat large amounts of food that have a lot of vitamin B_6 in them. These foods include avocado, bacon, beans, beef liver, dry skim milk, oatmeal, peas, pork, sweet potatoes, tuna fish and certain health foods. If you have questions about choosing vitamin products or about your diet, check with your doctor or pharmacist.

Take levodopa exactly as directed. Do not take more or less of it and do not take it more often than your doctor tells you to. Do not stop taking this medicine unless your doctor tells you to do so.

As your condition improves and it is easier for you to move about, be careful not to overdo physical activities. It is important that you increase your activity gradually so you can avoid falls and injuries from falling.

Before having any kind of surgery, including dental surgery, tell the doctor or dentist in charge that you are taking levodopa.

If you have diabetes, levodopa may cause inaccurate test results for sugar and ketones in your urine. Check with your doctor before changing your medicine for diabetes on the basis of tests done by the paper-strip or tablet methods.

Be sure to tell your doctor if you are pregnant or are nursing a baby. Levodopa may cause your milk to dry up, and levodopa can be passed to the baby through the milk. Safe use of levodopa in pregnant women has not been established.

DOSAGE AND STORAGE

Your doctor will determine how much levodopa you should take and how often you should take it. Carefully follow the instructions on your prescription label and ask your doctor or pharmacist to explain any part of the instructions you do not understand.

Levodopa comes in tablets and capsules and usually is taken several times a day. This medicine should be taken with solid food or a glass of milk to prevent stomach upset.

Your doctor may have you take only a small amount of levodopa when you first start treatment and then increase the amount gradually. This is done so your body can adjust to the medicine. Be sure to keep in touch with your doctor while you are taking levodopa, and carefully follow his instructions concerning the amount you should take.

Levodopa takes time to work. Some people do not obtain relief from their symptoms until they have been taking it for several months. If you have any questions about this, check with your doctor or pharmacist.

If you forget to take a dose of levodopa, take it as soon as you remember. Take any remaining doses for the day at evenly spaced intervals. *Do not take a double dose to make up for a missed dose.*

Keep levodopa in the container it came in. Store the container away from direct sunlight and excessive heat and out of the reach of children. Keep the container tightly closed.

Do not allow anyone else to take your levodopa, which was prescribed for your particular condition.

Trihexyphenidyl
(trye hex ee fen' i dill)

Brand names: Artane, Pipanol, Tremin

Trihexyphenidyl is used to treat Parkinson's disease and the palsylike side effects of certain other drugs. Trihexyphenidyl improves muscle control and relieves stiffness to allow more normal body movements.

UNDESIRED EFFECTS

Trihexyphenidyl may cause excess saliva in the mouth or stomach upset. To relieve stomach upset, take the medicine after meals or with food.

Dry mouth is a common effect of trihexyphenidyl. Chewing gum, sucking hard candy or dissolving bits of ice in your mouth will help relieve this effect.

Trihexyphenidyl causes some people to become drowsy or dizzy. Do not drive a car or operate dangerous machinery until you know how trihexyphenidyl will affect you. These effects often are mild and tend to disappear as your body adjusts to the medicine. However, if they continue or are severe, contact your doctor.

More serious side effects will require medical attention if they occur. Contact your doctor if you have difficulty urinating, constipation, blurred vision, fast heartbeat or pulse, fever, skin rash, extreme confusion or agitation.

PRECAUTIONS

To help your doctor select the best treatment for you, tell him if you have difficulty urinating, an enlarged prostate, glaucoma, high blood pressure, an intestinal blockage, kidney disease, liver disease or myasthenia gravis. Trihexyphenidyl may make these medical conditions worse.

Before you start to take trihexyphenidyl, tell your doctor what prescription or nonprescription drugs you are taking, including amatadine, antacids, antihistamines, medicines for allergies or colds, haloperidol, medicine for your heart, medicine for diarrhea, medicine to help you sleep, medicine for your nerves, other medicine for Parkinson's disease, sedatives, tranquilizers, medicine for ulcers and MAO inhibitors (even if you stopped taking them in the past two weeks).

If you do not know the names of the drugs you are taking or what they were prescribed for, bring them in their labeled containers to your doctor or pharmacist.

Take trihexyphenidyl exactly as prescribed by your doctor. He may want you to start with a small dose and increase it gradually, after he determines your response to it. *Keep all your appointments for checkups with your doctor.*

Because trihexyphenidyl may cause you to sweat less, you may easily become overheated while you are taking this medicine. To prevent heat prostration or sunstroke, be careful not to exert yourself excessively on hot days or in heated places.

Do not drink alcoholic beverages while you are taking trihexyphenidyl. Alcohol can increase the chance of and severity of side effects. If you have questions about this, check with your doctor or pharmacist. Do not start to take any of the medicines listed above unless you have your doctor's permission.

Do not take trihexyphenidyl within an hour of taking an antacid or a medicine for diarrhea. If these two medicines are taken too close together, trihexyphenidyl may be less effective.

DOSAGE AND STORAGE

Your doctor will determine how much trihexyphenidyl you should take and how often you should take it. Carefully follow the instructions on your prescription label and ask your doctor or pharmacist to explain any part of the instructions you do not understand.

Trihexyphenidyl comes in tablets and in liquid form and usually is taken three or four times a day. Both forms may be taken after meals or with food to lessen the chance of stomach upset.

If you forget to take a dose of trihexyphenidyl, take it as soon as you remember. Then take any remaining doses for that day at evenly spaced intervals. However, if you remember the missed dose when it is time for you to take another, take only the regularly scheduled dose. Omit the missed dose entirely. *Do not take a double dose to make up for a missed dose.*

Keep this medicine in the container it came in, and keep it out of the reach of children. Do not allow anyone else to take your trihexyphenidyl.

DIABETES

DRUGS USED TO TREAT DIABETES

Diabetes

Diabetes is caused by the inability of the pancreas to produce sufficient amounts of insulin for the body's needs. Insulin is required to regulate the metabolism of glucose. It has been estimated that 2 to 4 percent of the U.S. population have diabetes. It is a hereditary disease.

Diabetes varies according to the degree of insulin deficiency. The term "juvenile-onset diabetes" refers to a condition where almost no insulin is produced. In this situation, insulin injections are required to maintain normal glucose metabolism. "Adult-onset diabetes" refers to a less severe shortfall of insulin. In many cases this form of diabetes can be treated with diet or oral medications.

The symptoms vary with the severity of the disease. Individuals with severe insulin deficiency will develop marked high blood sugar, leading to dehydration and collapse unless insulin is administered.

In contrast, individuals with a milder condition may experience no symptoms, and diabetes may be diagnosed only upon results from laboratory tests.

Diabetes can cause damage to many organs throughout the body. Most commonly affected are the eyes, kidneys and skin. Damage to these results from a buildup of sugar deposits in blood vessels and impairment of circulation. In order to minimize or prevent such damage, it is essential that you take your medication regularly, as prescribed by your doctor. In addition to medications, special diets often are prescribed, and procedures to measure urine sugar are used to determine appropriate dosages.

Insulin
(in' sul in)

Brand name: Iletin

Insulin is a hormone produced in the pancreas. Insulin is necessary to move sugar from the blood into other body tissues, where it produces energy. In people with diabetes, the pancreas does not produce enough insulin for the body's needs, so that injection of additional insulin is necessary. This insulin comes from cattle and pigs. It must be injected because stomach acids would destroy it.

UNDESIRED EFFECTS

Undesired effects from insulin use usually result from using too much or too little insulin, resulting in low or high blood sugar. This can occur even though your doctor has carefully determined your needs. Your body's need for insulin can be affected by diet, exercise, drugs and other diseases.

Symptoms are as follows:

1. Low blood sugar (hypoglycemia). Giving yourself too much insulin, or strenuous exercise, can result in low blood sugar. This is often called an "insulin reaction." The symptoms of this may be weakness, tiredness, nervousness, anxiety, trembling, headache, sweating or dizziness. Drinking orange juice or eating a candy bar will stop these reactions quickly. Always carry a candy bar or some kind of sugar candy with you when you are not at home. These reactions may happen anytime but they are most common late in the afternoon or during the night. Usually they happen around the time when insulin is working hardest.

2. High blood sugar (hyperglycemia). By forgetting to use or by not using enough insulin, you may develop high blood sugar. Some of the signs of high blood sugar may be frequent urination, thirst, headache, weakness, nausea, dizziness and even loss of consciousness and coma.

Often it is difficult to tell if your level of blood sugar is too high or too low; call your doctor if you are not sure. You can keep tabs on your level of blood sugar by measuring the amount of sugar in your urine. Several methods are available to do this, such as the use of a tape, tablet or a plastic stick that changes color according to how much sugar is in the urine. If your doctor wishes you to test your urine, he will determine the best method for you to use. You will be shown how to measure, read and record the amount of your urine sugar accurately.

PRECAUTIONS

Your doctor will prescribe a diet for you to follow while you are using insulin. It is extremely important that you stick to this diet because your insulin dose is based in part on your intake of calories from food.

Tell your doctor if you are allergic to beef or pork insulin, are pregnant or have any other medical problems such as thyroid, liver or kidney disease or infection.

Many types of medications will affect your body's response to insulin. Be sure to tell your doctor what medications you are taking, including nonprescription medications. Do not begin to take any medications unless you first check with your doctor.

You should obtain either a Medic-Alert necklace or keep a card in your wallet that indicates you have diabetes. Write on the card your doctor's name, phone number and the current dose of insulin you are taking. Ask your doctor or pharmacist how you may get one of these cards.

It is a good idea to carry an extra prescription for insulin syringes with you at all times.

DOSAGE AND STORAGE

Your doctor will tell you how often and at what time of day to inject your insulin.

Insulin usually is given by subcutaneous injection. The amount of insulin you need depends on a lot of things, such as other diseases you may have, how much exercise you get and your diet, and may change with time.

There are several different types of insulin. The differences among them mostly involve how long they work to lower the sugar in the blood. For example, short-acting insulins such as regular insulin or semilente work for six to 12 hours; long-acting insulins such as ultralente work for over a day. Your doctor will determine which is the best insulin or insulin combination to control the level of sugar in your blood.

All bottles for insulin are marked with large black letters to remind you which insulin they contain. For example, Regular = R and NPH = N. It is very important that you know which one you use.

All types of insulin are measured in units. No matter what type of insulin you use, you always must know how many units of insulin you take with each injection. Although most diabetics use U-100 insulin (100 units in one milliliter), some may still be using the red-capped bottle of U-40 insulin or the green-capped bottle of U-80 insulin. If you are using these insulins, it is important that you let all your doctors and your pharmacist know this.

Different syringes must be used with U-40 insulin and with U-80 insulin. Be sure you have the right kind of syringe for your type of insulin.

Use a new syringe each time you take your insulin. Never reuse a syringe. Used needles will be dull, will hurt more and may cause an infection.

Be sure you fill the syringe to the correct number of units. If you have trouble seeing the small markings, have a friend or family member help you, and let your doctor or pharmacist know about this problem. They can provide syringes which are easier to read or special tools that help you fill the syringe more easily.

Do not inject cold insulin. Take it out of the refrigerator and allow it to reach room temperature before you administer it. Never heat the bottle of insulin to warm it up. Some doctors recommend storing the bottle you are using at room temperature.

Do not use the insulin if it looks as though it changed color or if the expiration date has passed. Roll the bottle between the palms of your hands to mix before preparing the dose. Do not shake the bottle.

It is easier to withdraw insulin from the bottle if you first inject air into the bottle. Inject the same number of units of air as insulin you will be taking. If you are taking two types of insulin at the same time—Regular and NPH for example—draw up the Regular (the clear solution) first.

You will be shown how to inject the insulin correctly. It is important that you do not use the same injection site on your body repeatedly. Change sites frequently. You can inject insulin into your stomach, thighs and arms. Clean the skin at the injection site with an alcohol pad or rubbing alcohol before injection.

You do not need a prescription to buy insulin. All you need do is ask the pharmacist for the right kind. It's best if you bring an empty bottle to the pharmacy. You may need a prescription for the syringes, depending on the state you live in. Check with your pharmacist.

Ask your doctor ahead of time what to do if you forget to take a dose of insulin at the correct time.

Unopened vials of insulin should be stored in the refrigerator; however, the vial in use may be stored at room temperature. If you are traveling, you do not need to refrigerate the insulin. It is a good idea to make sure insulin bottles are protected from bumps or other rough handling (if you are traveling, keep them wrapped in some clothes in the middle of a suitcase). Do not keep the insulin in hot parts of a car, such as glove compartment or trunk.

Chlorpropamide
(klor proe' pa mide)

Brand name: Diabinese

Chlorpropamide is used to treat adult-onset diabetes mellitus (sugar diabetes), particularly in those people whose diabetes cannot be controlled by diet alone or who cannot tolerate insulin injections.

Chlorpropamide helps to lower blood sugar by increasing the output of insulin by the pancreas. The pancreas must be capable of producing insulin before this medicine can work. Chlorpropamide is not used in the treatment of juvenile-onset diabetes (the type that requires insulin).

People who are taking chlorpropamide or any other oral medicine for diabetes may have to switch to insulin injections if they develop diabetic coma or ketoacidosis, have a severe injury or burn, develop a severe infection, need surgery or become pregnant.

UNDESIRED EFFECTS

Chlorpropamide may cause diarrhea, headache, heartburn, loss of appetite, nausea, vomiting or general stomach upset. Check with your doctor about taking less of this medicine or taking it in several small doses rather than in a single dose. Decreasing the dose or taking this medicine in several small doses may decrease these effects.

If chlorpropamide gives you a skin rash, stop taking the medicine and contact your doctor. Chlorpropamide also may make you sunburn more easily than usual. Be careful about exposing yourself to sunlight until you know how this medicine will affect you.

Rarely, chlorpropamide may cause liver or blood problems that will require medical attention. Contact your doctor if you have dark urine, itching of the skin, light-colored stools, yellowing of the eyes or skin, fatigue, fever and sore throat, or unusual bleeding or bruising.

Some people who take chlorpropamide retain more body water than usual. Symptoms of this problem are drowsiness; muscle cramps; seizures; swelling or puffiness of the face, hands or ankles; tiredness and weakness. Contact your doctor if you experience any of these effects.

Drowsiness, nervousness, headache, excessive hunger, warmth, sweating, or numbness of the finger, lips and nose may indicate your blood sugar is too low. If you experience any of these effects, drink orange juice or eat something sweet and contact your doctor immediately. If you think you are going to faint, instruct someone with you to take you to your doctor or to a hospital right away.

PRECAUTIONS
Because chlorpropamide may make some medical conditions worse, tell your doctor if you have kidney disease, liver disease, thyroid disease or a severe infection.

Before you start to take this medicine, tell your doctor what prescription or nonprescription drugs you are taking, particularly anticoagulants (blood thinners), aspirin or other salicylates, chloramphenicol, cortisonelike medicines, dextrothyroxine, epinephrine, guanethidine, insulin, MAO inhibitors, oxyphenbutazone, oxytetracycline, phenylbutazone, phenytoin (medicine for seizures), probenecid, propranolol, sulfonamides, thiazide diuretics (water pills) and thyroid medicine.

If you do not know the names of the drugs or what they were prescribed for, bring them in their labeled containers to your doctor or pharmacist.

Do not take any other medicine, including nonprescription medicine, while you are taking chlorpropamide unless you have your doctor's permission.

Before having any kind of surgery, including dental surgery, tell the doctor or dentist in charge that you are taking chlorpropamide.

Diet is extremely important in the treatment of diabetes. Chlorpropamide will work properly only if you follow your doctor's instructions concerning diet and exercise.

If you drink alcoholic beverages while taking chlorpropamide, your blood sugar may drop and you may experience the symptoms of hypoglycemia described earlier. If you have any of these symptoms, contact your doctor. It is better not to drink alcohol while you are taking chlorpropamide. If you have any questions about this, contact your doctor or pharmacist.

Skipping or delaying meals or exercising a great deal more than usual can cause your blood sugar to drop. (See symptoms of low blood sugar under **undesired effects**.) Maintaining a proper diet and exercise schedule will help you avoid this problem.

Women who are pregnant or who are nursing babies should not take chlorpropamide. During pregnancy, insulin is required to control their diabetes properly. If you become pregnant while taking chlorpropamide, contact your doctor immediately.

DOSAGE AND STORAGE
Your doctor will determine how often you should take chlorpropamide and at what time of day you should take it. Carefully follow the instructions on your prescription label and ask your doctor or pharmacist to explain any part of the instructions you do not understand.

Chlorpropamide comes in tablets and should be taken exactly as prescribed by your doctor. This medicine begins to work after the first dose, but it may be necessary for you to take chlorpropamide every day for a week or two before it is fully effective in controlling your diabetes. In addition, your doctor may need to adjust your dose to your particular needs. Keep in close touch with your doctor, particularly during the first few weeks you are taking this medicine.

Before you start to take chlorpropamide, ask your doctor what you should do if occasionally you forget to take a dose at the right time. Write down his instructions so you will be able to refer to them later if you forget to take a dose at the proper time.

Keep chlorpropamide in the container it came in, and store the container in a cool, dry place. Keep this medicine out of the reach of children. Do not allow anyone else to take your chlorpropamide.

Tolbutamide
(tole byoo' ta mide)

Brand name: Orinase

Tolbutamide is used to treat adult-onset sugar diabetes in people who cannot tolerate insulin or whose problem cannot be controlled by diet. Tolbutamide helps to lower the blood sugar by stimulating the secretion of insulin from the pancreas and will not work unless the pancreas is functioning. Tolbutamide is not used to treat juvenile-onset diabetes. People using tolbutamide or any other oral medication for diabetes may be switched to insulin injections if they develop ketoacidosis, have a severe injury or infection, need surgery or become pregnant.

UNDESIRED EFFECTS

Tolbutamide may cause diarrhea, headache, heartburn, loss of appetite, nausea, vomiting or general stomach upset. If you experience any of these effects, check with your doctor. He may want you to take less of this medicine or to take it in several smaller doses rather than in a single dose. Taking less tolbutamide or taking it in smaller doses may help to relieve these symptoms.

If tolbutamide gives you a skin rash, stop taking the medicine and contact your doctor. Tolbutamide also may make you more sensitive to sunlight than you usually are. Until you know how tolbutamide will affect you, protect yourself from sunlight.

Tolbutamide may cause liver or blood problems Although these effects are rare, they require medical attention when they occur. Contact your doctor if you have dark urine, itching of the skin, light-colored stools, yellowing of the eyes or skin, fatigue, fever and sore throat, or unusual bleeding or bruising.

Be alert for signs of low blood sugar, such as drowsiness, nervousness, headache, excessive hunger, warmth, sweating, and numbness of the fingers, lips and nose. If you experience these effects, drink orange juice or eat something sweet and contact your doctor immediately. If you think you are going to faint, instruct someone with you to take you to your doctor or to a hospital right away.

PRECAUTIONS

Before you start to take tolbutamide, tell your doctor if you have kidney disease, liver disease, thyroid disease or a severe infection. Tolbutamide can make these conditions worse or may not have the desired effect when these conditions are present.

Tell your doctor what prescription or nonprescription medicine you are taking, including anticoagulants (blood thinners), aspirin or other salicylates, chloramphenicol, cortisonelike medicines, dextrothyroxine, epinephrine, guanethidine, insulin, MAO inhibitors, oxyphenbutazone, oxytetracycline, phenylbutazone, phenytoin (medicine for seizures), probenecid, propranolol, sulfonamides, thiazide diuretics (water pills) and medicine for your thyroid. If you do not know the names of the drugs or what they were prescribed for, bring them in their labeled containers to your doctor or pharmacist.

Do not take any other medicine, including nonprescription medicine, while you are taking tolbutamide unless you have your doctor's permission.

Diet is extremely important in the treatment of diabetes. Be sure to follow your doctor's instructions concerning diet and exercise so that tolbutamide can work properly. If you skip meals, delay meals or exercise a great deal more than usual, your blood sugar may drop (see **undesired effects** for symptoms of low blood sugar).

Drinking alcoholic beverages while you are taking tolbutamide may cause a severe drop in blood sugar with the symptoms described earlier. Contact your doctor if you have any of these effects. If you have any questions about your consumption of alcohol, check with your doctor or pharmacist.

Before having any kind of surgery, including dental surgery, tell the doctor or dentist in charge that you are taking tolbutamide.

Women who are pregnant or who are nursing babies should not take tolbutamide. During pregnancy, insulin is required to control a woman's diabetes properly. If you become pregnant while taking tolbutamide, contact your doctor immediately.

DOSAGE AND STORAGE

Your doctor will determine how often you should take tolbutamide and at what time of day you should take it. Carefully follow the instructions on your prescription label and ask your doctor or pharmacist to explain any part of the instructions you do not understand.

Tolbutamide comes in tablets and should be taken exactly as prescribed by your doctor. This medicine begins to work about three to six hours after you take it. However, you may have to take this medicine every day for one to two weeks before it is fully effective in controlling your diabetes.

Keep in close touch with your doctor while you are taking tolbutamide, particularly during the first few weeks of therapy. Your doctor may need to adjust your dose to fit your particular needs.

At the time your doctor prescribes tolbutamide, ask him what you should do if occasionally you forget to take a dose at the right time. Write down his instructions and refer to them if you forget to take a dose.

Keep tolbutamide in the container it came in, and store the container in a cool place. Keep this medicine out of the reach of children. Do not allow anyone else to take your tolbutamide.

Tolazamide

(tole az' a mide)

Brand name: Tolinase

Tolazamide helps to lower blood sugar by increasing the amount of insulin produced by the pancreas. Tolazamide is used to treat adult-onset sugar diabetes in those people whose diabetes cannot be controlled by diet alone or who cannot tolerate insulin injections. Tolazamide is not used to treat juvenile-onset diabetes.

UNDESIRED EFFECTS

Tolazamide may cause diarrhea, headache, heartburn, loss of appetite, nausea, vomiting or general stomach upset. If you experience any of these problems and they are severe, contact your doctor. He may want you to take less of this medicine or to take it in several small doses a day rather than in a larger, single dose.

Stop taking tolazamide and contact your doctor if you develop a skin rash or itching. This medicine also may make some people more sensitive to sunlight than they normally are. Protect your skin when you are in sunlight until you know how you will react to tolazamide.

Although they are not common with tolazamide, liver or blood problems will require medical attention if they occur. Contact your doctor if you have dark urine, itching of the skin, light-colored stools, yellowing of the eyes or skin, fatigue, fever and sore throat, or unusual bleeding or bruising.

Tolazamide may cause your blood sugar level to drop too low, particularly if you skip or delay meals, exercise more than usual or drink significant amounts of alcohol. Symptoms of low blood sugar are drowsiness, nervousness, headache, excessive hunger, warmth, sweating, and numbness of the fingers, lips and nose. If you experience any of these symptoms, drink orange juice or eat something sweet and contact your doctor immediately. If you think you are going to faint, instruct someone with you to take you to your doctor or to a hospital right away.

PRECAUTIONS

Before you start to take tolazamide, tell your doctor if you have kidney disease, liver disease, thyroid disease or a severe infection. Tolazamide may make these conditions worse or may not have the desired effect when these conditions are present.

Tolazamide may affect the way your body responds to certain other drugs. Tell your doctor what other prescription or nonprescription drugs you are taking, particularly anticoagulants (blood thinners), aspirin or other salicylates, chloramphenicol, cortisonelike medicines, dextrothyroxine, epinephrine, guanethidine, insulin, MAO inhibitors, oxyphenbutazone, oxytetracycline, phenytoin (medicine for seizures), probenecid, propranolol, sulfonamides, thiazide diuretics (water pills) and medicine for your thyroid. If you do not know the names of the drugs or what they were prescribed for, bring them in their labeled containers to your doctor or pharmacist.

While you are taking tolazamide do not take any other medicine, including nonprescription medicine, unless you have your doctor's permission.

Before having any kind of surgery, including dental surgery, tell the doctor or dentist in charge that you are taking tolazamide.

Diet is extremely important in the treatment of diabetes. Tolazamide will work properly only if you follow your doctor's instructions concerning diet and exercise. Maintaining a proper diet and exercise schedule also will help you avoid the problems of a severe drop in blood sugar.

It is better not to drink alcoholic beverages while you are taking tolazamide. Alcohol can cause a severe drop in blood sugar and produce the symptoms described earlier. Contact your doctor if you have any of these symptoms.

You may have to take insulin rather than tolazamide if you develop diabetic coma or ketoacidosis, have a severe injury or burn, develop a severe infection or need to have surgery. If you have any questions about this, check with your doctor or pharmacist.

Women who are pregnant or who are nursing babies should not take tolazamide. During pregnancy insulin is required to control a woman's diabetes properly. If you become pregnant while taking tolazamide, contact your doctor immediately.

DOSAGE AND STORAGE

Your doctor will determine how often you should take tolazamide and at what time of day you should take it. Carefully follow the instructions on your prescription label and ask your doctor or pharmacist to explain any part of the instructions you do not understand.

Tolazamide comes in tablets and should be taken exactly as prescribed by your doctor. This medicine begins to work about four to six hours after it is taken. However, it may be necessary for you to take it every day for one to two weeks before it is fully effective in controlling your diabetes. Keep in close touch with your doctor, particularly during the first few weeks you are taking this medicine. Your doctor may need to adjust your dose to your particular needs.

Before you start to take tolazamide, ask your doctor what you should do if occasionally you forget to take a dose at the right time. Write down his instructions so you can refer to them later.

Keep tolazamide in the container it came in, and store it in a cool, dry place. Keep this medicine out of the reach of children. Do not allow anyone else to take your tolazamide.

GLAUCOMA

DRUGS USED TO TREAT GLAUCOMA

GLAUCOMA

Glaucoma is a disease in which the pressure inside the eyeball is greatly increased. This is the result of a fluid buildup inside the eyeball caused by infection, injury or other, unknown factors.

This increased pressure inside the eyeball damages the retina and the optic nerve. For this reason, glaucoma is one of the most common causes of blindness.

Glaucoma has two major forms. Open-angle glaucoma is a chronic hereditary disease that progresses slowly and often is not diagnosed until significant damage to the eyes causes changes in vision. Open-angle glaucoma is the most common type of glaucoma and occurs predominantly in people over 40. Because this type of glaucoma produces no symptoms until significant damage has already occurred, it is important to have periodic eye exams, particularly if you have a family history of glaucoma.

Closed-angle glaucoma is a rapid increase in pressure inside the eyeball. Closed-angle glaucoma causes severe pain, nausea, vomiting and visual disturbances.

People with such symptoms (particularly if there is a family history of glaucoma) should seek treatment at once. This form of glaucoma is treated with drugs or with surgery.

Acetazolamide
(a set a zole' a mide)

Brand name: Diamox

Acetazolamide is used to remove excess fluid from body tissues in order to help the heart work more efficiently in the treatment of heart failure and may be used in some patients with chronic lung disease. It is also used against glaucoma to decrease pressure in the eyeball and against certain kinds of epilepsy. Sometimes acetazolamide is used to change the acidity of the urine for short periods of time.

UNDESIRED EFFECTS

Acetazolamide can cause nausea, vomiting or loss of appetite. To decrease the chance of stomach upset, take this medicine with food or after meals.

Some people become dizzy or less alert than normal when they take acetazolamide. Be sure you know how this drug will affect you before you drive a car or operate dangerous machinery.

Other side effects, which tend to decrease or disappear as your body adjusts to acetazolamide, include tingling of the fingers and toes, increased urination, rash, confusion, fatigue and dryness of the mouth. If these effects are severe or give you great discomfort, contact your doctor. He may want to decrease the amount of acetazolamide you are taking.

Serious side effects do not happen often when you take acetazolamide, but they require medical attention when they do occur. Contact your doctor at once if you develop a severe headache, blurred vision or other disturbances of vision, convulsions, fever, itching, urine in the blood or black stools.

PRECAUTIONS

If you are allergic to sulfa drugs, you should not take acetazolamide because you may be allergic to this medicine also. Before you start to take acetazolamide tell your doctor if you have ever had an unusual reaction to a sulfa drug.

Acetazolamide makes the urine alkaline, and this may affect the way other drugs are cleared from your body. Tell your doctor what prescription or non-prescription drugs you are taking, including lithium, amphetamines, medicine for irregular heartbeat, medicine for depression, methenamine compounds, diuretics (water pills), medicine for diabetes, digitalis, cortisonelike medicine, amphotericin B, phenytoin and primidone. If you do not know the names of the drugs or what they were prescribed for, bring them in their labeled containers to your doctor or pharmacist.

Because acetazolamide can make some medical conditions worse, tell your doctor if you have liver disease, cirrhosis of the liver, kidney disease, a breathing disorder or lung disease, or diabetes.

Take acetazolamide exactly as prescribed by your doctor. If you think you need more acetazolamide to relieve your symptoms, contact your doctor.

Your doctor will want to determine how you are responding to this medicine. *Remember to keep all your appointments with him for checkups and for blood tests.*

Acetazolamide may have a bad effect on the fetus during the first few months of pregnancy. Be sure to tell your doctor if you are pregnant or think you may become pregnant while you are taking this drug.

DOSAGE AND STORAGE

Your doctor will determine how much acetazolamide you should take and how often you should take it. Carefully follow the instructions on your prescription label and ask your doctor or pharmacist to explain any part of the instructions you do not understand.

Acetazolamide comes in tablets and in long-acting capsules, which are taken several times a day at evenly spaced intervals.

If you forget to take a dose of acetazolamide, take it as soon as you remember and then take any remaining doses for that day at evenly spaced intervals. If you do not remember a missed dose until it is time for you to take another, omit the missed dose entirely and take only the regularly scheduled dose. *Do not take a double dose to make up for a missed dose.*

Keep acetazolamide in the container it came in, and keep it out of the reach of children. Do not allow anyone else to take your acetazolamide.

Carbachol

(kahr′ bah coal)

Brand names: Carbacel, Isopto Carbachol, Miostat, Murocarb

Carbachol is applied directly to the eye to treat glaucoma, an eye disease that increases the intra-ocular pressure. This medicine reduces the pressure and helps to prevent loss of vision and damage to the optic nerve.

UNDESIRED EFFECTS

The most common side effects of carbachol are eye pain, blurred vision, decreased vision for distance and poor vision in dim light (night blindness). Do not drive a car or operate dangerous machinery until you know how carbachol will affect you.

Other side effects are twitching of the eyelids, stinging or burning of the eyes, production of tears, eye pain or headache, unusual sensitivity to light and seeing floating shapes before the eyes. Contact your doctor if these effects are severe or give you a great deal of discomfort.

When you use carbachol for a long period of time, it can be absorbed into the body. Stop using this medicine and contact your doctor if you develop nausea, vomiting, diarrhea, abdominal pain, stomach pain and cramps, frequent urination, unusual paleness or difficulty breathing.

PRECAUTIONS

Before you start to take carbachol, tell your doctor if you have asthma, intestinal disease, an obstruction of the urinary tract, an ulcer, heart or blood vessel disease, an overactive thyroid, high blood pressure, seizures or Parkinson's disease.

Because some drugs can affect the way carbachol works, tell your doctor what prescription or nonprescription drugs you are taking, including other medicine for glaucoma, cortisone medications, antihistamines, medicines for allergies and colds, medicine for Parkinson's disease, prescription medicine for pain, medicine for ulcers and medicine for depression. If you do not know the names of the drugs or what they were prescribed for, bring them in their labeled containers to your doctor or pharmacist.

Use carbachol exactly as prescribed by your doctor. Do not use more or less; do not use it more often or for a longer period of time than instructed by your doctor.

Do not stop using this medicine until your doctor tells you to. If you still have the symptoms of glaucoma after you begin using carbachol, contact your doctor.

Tell your doctor if you are pregnant or think you may be. The safe use of carbachol in pregnant women has not been established.

DOSAGE AND STORAGE

Your doctor will determine how often you should use carbachol. To be effective, this medicine should be used at regularly spaced intervals. Carefully follow the instructions on your prescription label and ask your doctor or pharmacist to explain any part of the instructions you do not understand.

Carbachol comes in eyedrops which should be used as follows: First, check the eyedrops in the bottle. The solution should be clear and the end of the dropper should not be cracked or chipped. Next, wash your hands thoroughly with soap and water.

Stand in front of a mirror and tilt your head back until you are looking at the ceiling. With one hand, pull the lower lid of your eye downward to form a kind of pocket. Hold the eyedropper in your other hand, as close as possible to your eye without touching it, and drop the prescribed number of drops into the pocket. Try to keep the eyedropper pointed downward all the time you are using it so that the drops do not flow back into the bulb of the eyedropper.

Put the eyedropper back into the bottle. Now press your finger against the inner corner of your eye (the corner next to your nose) for one minute. This is important because it prevents the drops from going into your nose and throat, where they might be absorbed into your system and cause problems.

Close your eye gently and wipe away any liquid around the eye with a tissue. Wash your hands again with soap and water.

Keep carbachol in the container it came in, and store the container in a cool place. Keep this medicine out of the reach of children. Do not allow anyone else to use your carbachol.

Physostigmine
(fye so stig' meen)

Brand name: Isopto Eserine

Physostigmine, in the form of eyedrops or ointment, is applied to the eye to treat glaucoma. Physostigmine helps relieve the excess pressure in the eye and therefore helps prevent the eye damage glaucoma can cause.

UNDESIRED EFFECTS

Eye pain, blurred vision, decreased vision for distance and poor vision in dim light (night blindness) are common side effects of physostigmine. Until you know how this medicine will affect you, do not drive a car or operate dangerous machinery.

Other side effects, which usually do not require medical attention, include twitching of the eyelids, stinging or burning of the eyes, tearing, headache, unusual sensitivity to light and seeing floating shapes before the eyes. However, if you experience these effects and they are severe or give you a great deal of discomfort, contact your doctor.

More serious side effects result from the absorption of physostigmine into your body. If you develop nausea, vomiting, diarrhea, abdominal pain, stomach pain and cramps, frequent urination, unusual paleness or difficulty breathing, stop using this medicine and contact your doctor.

Tell your doctor what prescription or nonprescription drugs you are taking, including other medicine for glaucoma, cortisonelike medicine, antihistamines, medicines for allergies and colds, medicine for Parkinson's disease, prescription medicine for pain, medicine for ulcers and medicine for depression. If you do not know the names of the drugs or what they were prescribed for, bring them in their labeled containers to your doctor or pharmacist.

Your doctor will want to examine your eyes periodically to make sure that physostigmine is controlling your glaucoma. *Be sure to keep all your appointments for these checkups.*

Use physostigmine exactly as prescribed by your doctor. Do not use more or less of it and do not use it more often or for a longer period of time than instructed by your doctor.

Do not stop using this medicine until your doctor tells you to. If you still have the symptoms of glaucoma after you begin using this medicine, contact your doctor.

Before you have any kind of surgery, including dental surgery, tell the doctor or dentist in charge that you are taking physostigmine.

If you are pregnant or think you may become pregnant while taking this medicine, tell your doctor. The safe use of physostigmine in pregnant women has not been established.

DOSAGE AND STORAGE

Your doctor will determine how often you should use physostigmine. Carefully follow the instructions on your prescription label and ask your doctor or pharmacist to explain any part of the instructions you do not understand. This medicine should be used at regularly spaced intervals to be effective.

Physostigmine comes in eyedrops to be used during the day and in ointment form, which usually is put into the eye at night.

Before you use the eyedrops, check the color of the solution. If it has turned red, blue or brown, throw away the solution. It is no longer effective and may irritate your eyes.

To apply the eyedrops, follow the instructions with your medicine or proceed in the following way: First, check the end of the eyedropper to make sure it is not chipped or cracked. Next, wash your hands thoroughly with soap and water.

Stand in front of a mirror and tilt your head back until you are looking at the ceiling. With one hand, pull the lower eyelid downward to form a kind of pocket. Hold the eyedropper in your other hand, as close as possible to your eye without touching it. Drop the prescribed number of drops into the pocket. Try to keep the eyedropper pointed downward all the time you are using it so that the drops do not flow back into the bulb of the eyedropper.

Put the eyedropper back into the bottle. Now press your finger against the inner corner of your eye (the corner next to your nose) for one minute. This is important because it prevents the drops from going into your nose and throat, where they might be absorbed into your body and cause problems.

Close your eye gently and wipe away any liquid around the eye with a tissue. Wash your hands again with soap and water.

Keep this medicine in the container that it came in, and store the container in a cool place. Keep physostigmine out of the reach of children. Do not allow anyone else to use your physostigmine.

Pilocarpine
(pie low car' peen)

Brand names: Adsorbocarpine, Almocarpine, Isopto Carpine, Ocusert, Pilocar, Pilocel, Pilomiotin, Pilo-M, Piloptic, P.V. Carpine

Pilocarpine is one of the primary drugs used in the treatment of glaucoma because pilocarpine is relatively free of side effects, particularly serious side effects. It is applied directly to the eye to reduce the pressure.

Pilocarpine also is frequently used prior to certain types of eye surgery.

UNDESIRED EFFECTS
Pilocarpine affects the ability of some patients to see well, especially at night. Do not drive a car or operate dangerous machinery until you know how this medicine will affect you.

Other side effects that may occur after you use pilocarpine are twitching of the eyelids, stinging, burning, tearing, headache and eye pain. These effects usually are mild. However, if they are severe or cause you great discomfort, contact your doctor.

Contact your doctor if you experience excessive sweating, nausea, fainting or confusion.

PRECAUTIONS
Before you start to use pilocarpine, tell your doctor if you have asthma, intestinal disease, obstruction of the urinary tract, ulcer, heart or blood vessel disease, an overactive thyroid, high blood pressure, seizures or Parkinson's disease.

Tell your doctor what prescription or nonprescription drugs you are taking, including other medicines for glaucoma, cortisonelike medicines, antihistamines, medicines for allergies and colds, medicine for Parkinson's disease, prescription medicine for pain, medicine for ulcers and medicine for depression. If you do not know the names of the drugs or what they were prescribed for, bring them in their labeled containers to your doctor or pharmacist.

Use pilocarpine exactly as prescribed by your doctor. Do not use more or less of it and do not use it more often or for a longer period of time than instructed by your doctor. Do not stop using this medicine until your doctor tells you to.

If you still have the symptoms of glaucoma after you begin using pilocarpine, contact your doctor. The amount of pilocarpine you use and the frequency with which you use it may need to be adjusted to your particular needs.

Tell your doctor if you are pregnant or think you may become pregnant while you are using pilocarpine. Safe use of this medicine in pregnant women has not been established.

DOSAGE AND STORAGE

Your doctor will determine how often you should use pilocarpine. To be effective, this medicine should be used at regularly spaced intervals. Carefully follow the instructions on your prescription label and ask your doctor or pharmacist to explain any part of the instructions you do not understand.

Pilocarpine comes in eyedrops and in controlled-release systems, which put the drug into your eye over a seven-day period. If your doctor has prescribed the controlled-release system, be sure you understand exactly how to use it. Check with your doctor or pharmacist if you have questions.

Directions for the use of eyedrops usually are included with the prescription. The eyedrops should be used in this way: First, check the eyedrops in the bottle. The solution should be clear and the end of the eyedropper should not be cracked or chipped. Next, wash your hands thoroughly with soap and water.

Stand in front of a mirror and tilt your head back until you are looking at the ceiling. With one hand, pull the lower lid of your eye downward to form a kind of pocket. Hold the eyedropper in your other hand, as close as possible to your eye without touching it, and drop the prescribed number of drops into the pocket. Try to keep the eyedropper pointed downward all the time you are using it so that the drops do not flow back into the bulb of the eyedropper.

Put the eyedropper back into the bottle. Now press your finger against the inner corner of your eye (the corner next to your nose) for one minute. This is important because it prevents the drops from going into your nose and throat, where they might be absorbed into your body and cause problems.

Close your eye gently and wipe away any liquid around the eye with a tissue. Wash your hands again with soap and water.

Try to keep the eyedropper from touching anything. If it does touch the eye or any other surface, rinse the eyedropper thoroughly with tap water before you put it back into the bottle.

Keep pilocarpine in the container it came in, and store the container in a cool place. Keep this medicine out of the reach of children, and do not allow anyone else to use your pilocarpine.

THYROID DISEASE

DRUGS USED TO TREAT THYROID DISEASE

Thyroid Disease

The thyroid gland is located in the neck just below the voice box. The thyroid gland produces hormones that regulate all the metabolism in the body.

When the thyroid gland is overactive (hyperthyroidism), excessive hormone levels cause the body's metabolism to speed up. This results in weight loss, excessive growth (particularly in children), rapid heartbeat, increased blood pressure and respiratory rate, diarrhea, excitement and muscle tremors. An underactive thyroid (hypothyroidism) causes just the opposite.

The causes of thyroid disease are, for the most part, unknown. Hyperthyroidism occurs more commonly in young adult women and in cold climates and is hereditary. In addition to the symptoms mentioned earlier, hyperthyroidism causes the thyroid gland to increase in size, and in most people it causes the eyes to bulge.

Hypothyroidism also causes a great increase in the size of the thyroid gland. In severe cases, the body retains additional fluid and the result is a swollen, bloated appearance.

Treatment of hyperthyroidism is aimed at decreasing the amount of thyroid hormone produced. This is accomplished by using drugs that decrease thyroid hormone output, or through surgery. Hypothyroidism is corrected by administering additional thyroid, which is produced from animals or made synthetically.

DRUGS FOR OVERACTIVE THYROID
Methimazole
(meth im′ a zole)

Brand name: Tapazole

Methimazole is used to treat hyperthyroidism, a condition that occurs when the thyroid gland produces too much of the thyroid hormone. Methimazole also may be given to people before they have surgery for goiter.

UNDESIRED EFFECTS

Methimazole can cause skin rash. Rashes over a small area of skin may disappear without treatment. However, if the rash lasts more than a few days or covers a lot of your body, contact your doctor.

Other side effects, which tend to disappear as your body adjusts to methimazole, are itching, dizziness, pain in joints, loss of taste and stomach pain. If you experience these effects and they are severe or cause you great discomfort, contact your doctor.

More serious side effects, when they occur, will require medical attention.

Stop taking this medicine and contact your doctor immediately if you have fever and chills, sore throat, loss of hearing, swelling of the lymph nodes in the neck, severe skin rash, unusual bleeding or bruising, an unusual increase or decrease in urination, backache, swelling of the feet and lower legs or yellowing of the eyes and skin.

PRECAUTIONS

Before you start to take methimazole, tell your doctor if you have blood disease, any kind of infection or liver disease.

Tell your doctor what prescription or nonprescription drugs you are taking, including anticoagulants (blood thinners). If you do not know the names of the drugs or what they were prescribed for, bring them in their labeled containers to your doctor or pharmacist.

Take methimazole exactly as prescribed. Do not take more or less of it and do not take it more often or for a longer period of time than your doctor has ordered.

To work properly, methimazole must be taken every day in regularly spaced doses. Be sure you have enough of this medicine on hand at all times to permit you to take all the doses that have been prescribed for you. Check your supply before vacations, holidays and other times when it may be difficult for you to get more. You must take this medicine as often as your doctor tells you to, even if you have to get up during the night to take it.

Food in your stomach affects the way methimazole works. To be sure that you always get the same effect from each dose, take the prescribed doses *always* with meals or *always* on an empty stomach.

Your dosage of methimazole may have to be increased or decreased to obtain the desired effect. *Be sure to keep all your appointments for checkups* so that your doctor can monitor the effect this medicine is having on you.

Before you have any kind of surgery, including dental surgery, be sure to tell the doctor or dentist in charge that you are taking methimazole. Check with your doctor right away if you have an injury, infection or illness of any kind; he may want you to stop taking this medicine.

If you are pregnant or are nursing a baby, you should not take methimazole. Be sure to tell your doctor if you are pregnant or think you may be. If you get pregnant while taking this medicine, contact your doctor at once.

DOSAGE AND STORAGE

Your doctor will determine how much methimazole you should take and how often you should take it. Carefully follow the instructions on your prescription label and ask your doctor or pharmacist to explain any part of the instructions you do not understand.

Methimazole comes in tablets. You may need to take this medicine for one or two weeks before you feel that it is working. Even if you do not see benefits immediately, continue to take this medicine as instructed.

If you forget to take a dose of methimazole, take it as soon as you remember, and then take any remaining doses for that day at evenly spaced intervals. If you do not remember a missed dose until it is time for you to take another, omit the missed dose completely and take only the regularly scheduled dose. *Do not take two doses at one time.*

Keep methimazole in the container it came in, and store the container away from direct sunlight. Keep this medicine out of the reach of children. Do not allow anyone else to take your methimazole.

Propylthiouracil
(proe pill thye oh yoor' a sill)

Brand name: Propacil

Propylthiouracil is used to treat conditions in which the thyroid gland produces too much thyroid hormone. Propylthiouracil also may be used in preparation for surgery for goiter. When given before surgery, this medicine is usually combined with a strong iodine solution.

UNDESIRED EFFECTS

Propylthiouracil can cause skin rash, which may disappear in a few days without treatment if only a small area of the skin is involved. However, you should contact your doctor if you have a rash that lasts more than a few days or covers a lot of your body.

Side effects, which tend to disappear as your body adjusts to propylthiouracil, include itching, dizziness, joint pain, loss of taste and stomach pain. If these effects are severe or cause you a great amount of discomfort, contact your doctor.

More serious side effects include blood problems, severe allergic reactions, kidney problems and liver problems. Stop taking propylthiouracil and contact your doctor immediately if you have fever and chills, sore throat, loss of hearing, swelling of the lymph nodes in the neck, severe skin rash, unusual bleeding or bruising, an unusual increase or decrease in urination, backache, swelling of the feet and lower legs or yellowing of the eyes and skin.

PRECAUTIONS

To help your doctor select the treatment best for you, tell him if you have blood disease, any kind of infection or liver disease. Propylthiouracil can make these conditions worse.

Before you start taking propylthiouracil, tell your doctor what prescription or nonprescription drugs you are taking, particularly anticoagulants (blood thinners). If you do not know the names of the drugs or what they were prescribed for, bring them in their labeled containers to your doctor or pharmacist.

Take propylthiouracil exactly as prescribed. Do not take more or less of it and do not take it more often or for a longer period of time than your doctor has ordered.

This medicine must be taken every day in regularly spaced doses if it is to work properly. Be sure you have enough propylthiouracil on hand at all times to permit you to take all the doses that have been prescribed for you. Check your supply before holidays, vacations and other times when it may be difficult for you to get more. You must take this medicine as often as your doctor tells you to, even if you have to get up during the night to take it.

Food in your stomach affects the way propylthiouracil works. To be sure you always get the same effect from each dose, take the prescribed doses *always* with meals or *always* on an empty stomach.

Your dosage of this medicine may have to be increased or decreased to obtain the desired effect. *Be sure to keep all your appointments for checkups* so that your doctor can monitor this medicine's effect on you.

Before you have any kind of surgery, including dental surgery, be sure to tell the doctor or dentist in charge that you are taking propylthiouracil. If you get an injury, infection or illness of any kind, check with your doctor right away; he may want you to stop taking this medicine.

If you are pregnant or are nursing a baby, you should not take propylthiouracil. Be sure to tell your doctor if you are pregnant or think that you may be. If you get pregnant while taking this medicine, contact your doctor at once.

DOSAGE AND STORAGE

Your doctor will determine how much propylthiouracil you should take and how often you should take it. Carefully follow the instructions on your prescription label and ask your doctor or pharmacist to explain any part of the instructions you do not understand.

Propylthiouracil comes in tablets to be taken orally. You may need to take this medicine for one or two weeks before you feel that it is working. Even if you do not see benefits immediately, continue to take propylthiouracil as instructed.

If you forget to take a dose of propylthiouracil, take it as soon as you remember. Then take the remaining doses for that day at evenly spaced intervals. If you do not remember a missed dose until it is time for you to take another, omit the missed dose entirely and take only the regularly scheduled dose. *Do not take two doses at one time.*

Keep this medicine in the container it came in, and keep it out of the reach of children. Store propylthiouracil away from direct sunlight. Do not allow anyone else to take your propylthiouracil.

DRUGS FOR UNDERACTIVE THYROID
Iodine
(eye′ o dyne)

Other names: Lugol's solution, potassium iodide

Iodine, also called strong iodine solution, is used alone or with other antithyroid medicine to treat certain types of goiter or in preparation for goiter surgery.

UNDESIRED EFFECTS

Strong iodine solution can cause allergic reactions. Stop taking the medicine and contact your doctor immediately if you experience swelling of the larynx (voice box), skin rash, swelling of the salivary glands or increased salivation.

PRECAUTIONS

If you have ever reacted to strong iodine solution in any of the ways described above, you should not take this medicine. Before you start to take iodine, tell your doctor if you have tuberculosis—strong iodine solution can make this condition worse.

Tell your doctor what prescription or nonprescription drugs you are taking. If you do not know the names of the drugs or what they were prescribed for, bring them in their labeled containers to your doctor or pharmacist.

DOSAGE AND STORAGE

Your doctor will determine how much of this medicine you should take and how often you should take it. Carefully follow the instructions on your prescription label and ask your doctor or pharmacist to explain any part of the instructions you do not understand.

Strong iodine solution comes in liquid form and usually is taken mixed with water three times a day after meals. If you forget to take a dose of this medicine, take it as soon as you remember. If you do not remember a missed dose until it is almost time for you to take another, take both doses together and return to your regular schedule. If you have any questions about this, check with your doctor or pharmacist.

Keep this medicine in the container it came in and store it in a cool, dark place, but do not refrigerate it. If the liquid turns yellowish-brown, discard it and get a fresh supply. Do not allow anyone else to take your iodine.

Thyroid Hormone Preparations
(thye′ roid)

Brand names:

thyroid USP: Armour Thyroid, S-P-T, Thyrar

levothroxine: Letter, Levoid, Levothroid, Synthroid, Titroid

liothyronine: Cytomel

liotrix: Euthroid, Thyrolar

thyroglobulin: Proloid

Thyroid is a hormone produced by the body that regulates the body's metabolism. When too little of this important hormone is produced by the thyroid gland, the result usually is poor growth, slow speech, lack of energy, weight gain, hair loss, dry and thick skin or increased sensitivity to cold. To treat these symptoms, your doctor will prescribe thyroid hormone, either that extracted from the thyroid glands of animals or made in the laboratory. Thyroid hormone, when taken correctly, can reverse all the symptoms of hypothyroidism.

UNDESIRED EFFECTS

Side effects of thyroid hormone preparations include rapid heart rate, weight loss, chest pain, tremor, headache, diarrhea, nervousness, insomnia, sweating and heat intolerance. If any of these effects occur, stop taking the medicine and contact your doctor immediately. In most cases a reduction in dose is all that is necessary.

Thyroid hormone preparations may take a few weeks to begin relieving the symptoms of hypothyroidism that were described earlier. If these symptoms persist longer than a few weeks or if they become worse after you begin to take a thyroid hormone preparation, contact your doctor.

When you begin to take a thyroid hormone preparation, it may take several weeks to get your dosage correctly adjusted. If your dose is too low, some of the symptoms of hypothyroidism will remain. If, on the other hand, your dose is too high, you may experience nervousness, diarrhea, weight loss, fever, muscle tremors or cramps and insomnia. Check with your doctor if any of these effects occur.

PRECAUTIONS

Because thyroid hormone preparations can make certain medical conditions worse, tell your doctor if you have diabetes, hardening of the arteries, heart disease, high blood pressure, a history of an overactive thyroid gland, kidney disease, liver disease, an underactive adrenal gland or an underactive pituitary gland.

Tell your doctor what prescription or nonprescription drugs you are taking, including anticoagulants (blood thinners), cholestyramine, cough syrup or cold medicine, medicine for diabetes, phenytoin and medicine for depression. If you do not know the names of the drugs or what they were prescribed for, bring them in their labeled containers to your doctor or pharmacist.

Take this medicine exactly as prescribed. Do not take more or less of it and do not take it more often than your doctor has ordered. For the best effect, try to take your thyroid hormone preparation at the same time each day.

Since your condition is due to a lack of thyroid hormone, you may have to take this medicine for the rest of your life. However, your doctor may have to adjust the dose from time to time to fit your body's needs. *Be sure to keep all appointments with him for checkups.*

Do not stop taking your thyroid hormone preparation without your doctor's permission. Be sure you have enough medicine on hand at all times to take the doses you need. Check your supply before vacations, holidays and other times when it may not be possible for you to get more.

Before you have any kind of surgery, including dental surgery or emergency treatment, tell the doctor or dentist in charge that you are taking this medicine.

Before you start to take any other medicine, particularly an "over the counter" medicine, check with your doctor or pharmacist to make sure the other medicine will not interfere with the way your thyroid hormone preparation works.

DOSAGE AND STORAGE

Your doctor will determine how much thyroid hormone preparation you should take and how often you should take it. Carefully follow the instructions on your prescription label and ask your doctor or pharmacist to explain any part of the instructions you do not understand.

If your doctor tells you to take this medicine once a day, it may be easier for you to remember to take it if you take it at the same time you do something else each day, such as brushing your teeth in the morning or eating dinner at night.

Thyroid hormone preparations come in tablets and capsules. If you forget to take a dose of this medicine, take it as soon as you remember. However, if you do not remember a missed dose until it is time for you to take another, omit the missed dose completely and take only the regularly scheduled dose. *Do not take two doses at one time.*

Keep this medicine in the container it came in. Keep it out of the reach of children. Do not let anyone else take your thyroid hormone preparation.

GOUT

DRUGS USED TO TREAT GOUT

GOUT

Gout is caused by excess uric acid in the blood. The excess uric acid accumulates in different tissues throughout the body to produce pain and inflammation. Although arthritis is the most common form of gout, gout also can appear in skin, and in the kidney to produce kidney stones.

Most frequently, gout causes inflammation, swelling and pain in the joints, particularly in the feet and ankles. A gout attack can be precipitated by factors such as surgery, excessive alcohol consumption, dietary excess, emotional stress or even excessive walking.

Several different types of medications are used to treat gout. Colchicine and phenylbutazone are used to relieve pain and inflammation. Usually these drugs begin to relieve these symptoms within six to 12 hours. Other medications such as probenecid and sulfinpyrazone are used to increase the amount of uric acid passed in the urine, thereby preventing or relieving a buildup of uric acid in the bloodstream.

Another drug used to treat gout is allopurinol. It acts to prevent the formation of uric acid in the blood.

The choice of these medications depends on a variety of factors, including your response to a particular medication, other health problems and other medication you may be taking.

With any treatment, it is important that you continue to take the medications as prescribed. They control gout only as long as they are taken regularly. Your doctor probably will want to perform some blood tests periodically to measure your response to treatment. *Be sure to keep all such appointments.*

Allopurinol
(al oh pure′ i nole)

Brand name: Zyloprim

Allopurinol is used to treat chronic gout. Allopurinol also is used to keep the body from producing too much uric acid, which could lead to or aggravate various medical problems.

UNDESIRED EFFECTS

Skin rash is the most common side effect of allopurinol. If you develop a rash, stop taking the medicine and contact your doctor.

Allopurinol makes some people drowsy or dizzy. Do not drive a car or operate dangerous machinery until you know how this medicine will affect you. Allopurinol also can cause stomach upset, stomach pain or diarrhea. If allopurinol upsets your stomach, you may take it after meals. Contact your doctor if stomach upsets continue.

Rarely, allopurinol will cause nerve, blood or liver problems, which will require medical attention. Contact your doctor if you have numbness, tingling, pain or weakness in the hands or feet; sore throat and fever; unusual bruising or bleeding; unusual weakness or tiredness; or yellowing of the eyes or skin.

PRECAUTIONS
Before you start to take allopurinol, tell your doctor if you have kidney disease or if you or any member of your immediate family has a disease known as idiopathic hemochromatosis.

Tell your doctor what prescription or nonprescription drugs you are taking, particularly ampicillin, anticoagulants (blood thinners), azathioprine, cyclophosphamide, diuretics (water pills), medicine to make the urine more acid, or mercaptopurine. If you do not know the names of the drugs or what they were prescribed for, bring them in their labeled containers to your doctor or pharmacist.

Do not drink alcoholic beverages and do not take vitamin C while you are taking allopurinol. Too much alcohol can lessen the effect of allopurinol, and too much vitamin C can increase the chance of your developing kidney stones. If you have any questions about this, check with your doctor or pharmacist.

To help prevent kidney stones you should drink at least 10 to 12 full (eight-ounce) glasses of fluids a day while you are taking allopurinol. If you are giving this medicine to a child, ask your doctor how much water or other fluids the child should drink every day.

Allopurinol is used to help prevent gout attacks, but it will not relieve a gout attack that has already started. Even if you take another medicine for gout attacks, continue to take allopurinol as well. Check with your doctor if you have any questions about this.

Be sure to keep in touch with your doctor while you are taking allopurinol so that he can check on the way this medicine is affecting you.

Your doctor should be told if you are pregnant or are nursing a baby, although no harm to the fetus or nursing baby has been reported as a result of using allopurinol. This will help your doctor choose the best and safest treatment for you and your baby.

DOSAGE AND STORAGE
Your doctor will determine how often you should take allopurinol and how much you should take at each dose. Carefully follow the instructions on your prescription label and ask your doctor or pharmacist to explain any part of the instructions you do not understand.

Allopurinol comes in tablets that are usually taken once a day. They should be taken with meals if this medicine upsets your stomach.

Allopurinol only controls the conditions for which it is prescribed; it does not cure them. Therefore it is important to follow the schedule prescribed by your doctor. Do not stop taking allopurinol unless your doctor tells you to.

If you forget to take a dose of allopurinol, take it as soon as you remember it. Take any remaining doses for that day at evenly spaced intervals. If you miss two or more doses in a row, contact your doctor.

Keep allopurinol in the container it came in, and keep it out of the reach of children. Do not allow anyone else to take your allopurinol.

Colchicine
(kol′ chi seen)

Brand name: none

Names of preparations containing colchicine: Acetycol, ColBenemid, Colsalide, Darth with Colchicine, Neocylate, Salamide with Colchicine, Salpaba, Tolsylate-K

Colchicine relieves inflammation, pain and swelling caused by attacks of gout and gouty arthritis. Colchicine is used to treat and to prevent these attacks. It is prescribed alone or in combination preparations with medicine for pain.

UNDESIRED EFFECTS

The most common effects of colchicine are diarrhea, nausea, vomiting and stomach pain. These effects are signs the medicine is beginning to poison your body. If any of them occur, stop taking colchicine immediately and contact your doctor.

If you take this medicine over a long period of time, you may develop skin rash or numbness, tingling, pain or weakness in your hands or feet; you may have symptoms of serious blood problems, such as sore throat and fever, unusual bruising or bleeding, unusual tiredness or weakness. Stop taking colchicine and contact your doctor if you have any of these effects.

PRECAUTIONS

Because colchicine may make some medical problems worse, tell your doctor if you have blood disease, heart disease, intestinal disease, kidney disease, liver disease, stomach ulcers or other stomach problems.

Before you start to take colchicine, tell your doctor what other prescription or nonprescription drugs you are taking. If you do not know the names of the drugs or what they were prescribed for, bring them in their labeled containers to your doctor or pharmacist.

Do not drink alcoholic beverages while you are taking colchicine, unless you have your doctor's permission to do so. Drinking too much alcohol can lessen the effectiveness of this medicine.

Colchicine may affect the results of certain kinds of urine tests. If you are to have a urine test while you are taking this medicine, tell the doctor or laboratory personnel that you are taking colchicine.

If you take this medicine for a long period of time, your doctor will want to check your progress with complete blood counts and other tests at regular intervals. *Be sure to keep all appointments with your doctor.*

DOSAGE AND STORAGE

Colchicine comes in tablets to be taken orally and in an injectable form. Your doctor will prescribe the form best for you and will determine how often you should take this medicine and how much you should take at each dose. Carefully follow the instructions on your prescription label and ask your doctor or pharmacist to explain any part of the instructions you do not understand.

If you are taking colchicine to relieve symptoms of gout attack, take colchicine at the first sign of pain. This medicine will not be fully effective if you do not take it when you first start to feel pain. Relief usually will be felt in 24 to 48 hours. Take a dose of colchicine every two hours until the pain is relieved or until you begin to have nausea, vomiting or diarrhea.

If you are taking colchicine regularly to reduce the number and severity of attacks, follow your doctor's instructions for taking this medicine.

When you are taking colchicine to relieve symptoms of a gout attack, the medicine should be taken according to the dosage schedule your doctor has recommended. If you forget to take a dose, take it as soon as you remember it. However, if you do not remember it until it is almost time for you to take another dose, omit the missed dose entirely and take only the regularly scheduled dose. *Do not take a double dose.*

If you are taking colchicine to prevent a gout attack and you forget to take a dose, omit that dose completely. *Do not take an extra dose the next day to make up for the missed dose.* If you take this medicine every day or once every few days, you may find it easier to remember to take your doses if you take them at the same time you do something else every day, such as brushing your teeth in the morning or going to bed at night.

Keep colchicine in the container it came in, and keep it out of the reach of children. Do not allow anyone else to take your colchicine.

Probenecid
(proe ben' e sid)

Brand names: Benemid, Probalan, Probenimead, Robenecid

Probenecid is used to prevent attacks of gout and to treat other medical problems that cause too much uric acid to be produced by the body. Probenecid acts on the kidneys to help the body eliminate uric acid by passing it in the urine. Probenecid also is used to make certain antibiotics more effective because it prevents the body from passing them in the urine.

UNDESIRED EFFECTS

The most common side effects of probenecid are headache, loss of appetite, nausea and vomiting. To help prevent stomach upset, take probenecid with solid food or milk. If this is not effective, take it with an antacid. Contact your doctor if stomach upsets continue in spite of your precautions.

Other effects, which may disappear as you continue to take probenecid and as your body adjusts to it, are dizziness, flushing or redness of the face, a frequent urge to urinate and sore gums. If these effects continue or are severe, contact your doctor.

Probenecid can cause the formation of uric acid stones, particularly after you begin to take this medicine. Contact your doctor if you have bloody urine, pain in the lower back or painful urination.

Rarely, probenecid will cause an allergic reaction or blood problems, which will require medical attention. Contact your doctor if you have difficulty breathing, skin rash or itching, unexplained fever, sore throat and fever, unusual bleeding or bruising, or unusual tiredness or weakness.

PRECAUTIONS

Because probenecid can make certain medical conditions worse, tell your doctor if you have blood disease, kidney stones, stomach ulcers or a history of stomach ulcers.

Tell your doctor what prescription or nonprescription drugs you are taking, including aminosalicylic acid, antibiotics, aspirin or other salicylates, dapsone, diuretics (water pills), indomethacin, methotrexate, nitrofurantoin, oral medicine for diabetes and sulfa drugs.

While you are taking probenecid, drink at least six to eight eight-ounce glasses of water or fruit juice each day, unless your doctor tells you to limit the amount of fluids you drink.

Do not drink alcoholic beverages or take aspirin or any medication containing aspirin while you are taking probenecid. Both alcohol and aspirin can affect the way your body responds to probenecid. If you need to take something to relieve minor pain or fever, ask your doctor or pharmacist to recommend a substitute for aspirin.

Take probenecid exactly as prescribed by your doctor. This medicine must be taken regularly to be effective. Do not stop taking it unless your doctor tells you to. Your doctor may want you to start with a small dose and then gradually increase the amount you take. Keep in touch with your doctor so he can adjust your dose of probenecid to meet your needs.

Be sure you have enough probenecid on hand at all times to permit you to take all the doses prescribed for you. Check your supply before vacations, holidays and other occasions when you may not be able to obtain more.

If you have diabetes, probenecid can cause inaccurate results in certain types of tests for urine sugar. Check with your doctor or pharmacist if you have any questions about this.

Children under the age of two years should not take probenecid.

Probenecid has been used in pregnant women with no reported problems. However, it is best to tell your doctor if you are pregnant or are nursing a baby.

DOSAGE AND STORAGE

Your doctor will determine how often you should take probenecid and how much you should take at each dose. Carefully follow the instructions on your prescription label and ask your doctor or pharmacist to explain any part of the instructions you do not understand.

Probenecid comes in tablets. Probenecid should be taken at meals or with a snack to avoid stomach upset.

If you forget to take a dose of probenecid, take it as soon as you remember. If you do not remember a missed dose until it is almost time for you to take another, omit the missed dose entirely and take only the regularly scheduled dose. *Do not take a double dose to make up for a missed one.*

Keep probenecid in the container it came in, and keep it out of the reach of children. Do not allow anyone else to take your probenecid, which was prescribed for your particular problem.

Sulfinpyrazone
(sul fin pye′ ra zone)

Brand name: Anturane

Sulfinpyrazone acts on the kidneys to help the body eliminate uric acid by passing it in the urine. Sulfinpyrazone is used to prevent attacks of gout and to treat other medical conditions that cause the body to produce too much uric acid.

UNDESIRED EFFECTS

Sulfinpyrazone frequently causes indigestion, nausea, or pain in the stomach or intestines. To lessen stomach upset, take this medicine with solid food or milk; contact your doctor if stomach upsets continue in spite of your taking this precaution.

Other side effects, which may go away as you continue to take sulfinpyrazone and as your body adjusts to it, are dizziness, fainting, ringing or buzzing in the ears, and swelling of the feet or legs. If these effects continue or are severe, contact your doctor.

Sulfinpyrazone may cause the formation of uric acid stones, Contact your doctor if you have bloody urine, pain in the lower back or painful urination.

Although serious side effects are rare when you are taking sulfinpyrazone, they require medical attention if they do occur. Contact your doctor if you have difficulty breathing, skin rash or itching, unexplained fever, sore throat and fever, unusual bleeding or bruising, or unusual tiredness or weakness.

PRECAUTIONS

You should not take sulfinpyrazone if you have ever had an unusual reaction to oxyphenbutazone or to phenylbutazone. Check with your doctor or pharmacist if you have questions about this. Before you start to take sulfinpyrazone, tell your doctor if you have blood disease, kidney disease, a stomach ulcer or a history of stomach ulcer, or inflammation or ulceration of the intestines. Sulfinpyrazone may make these conditions worse.

Tell your doctor what prescription or nonprescription drugs you are taking, including aminosalicylic acid, antibiotics, aspirin or other salicylates, dapsone, diuretics (water pills), indomethacin, methotrexate, nitrofurantoin, oral medicine for diabetes, sulfonamides, anticoagulants (blood thinners), colchicine and insulin. If you do not know the names of the drugs or what they were prescribed for, bring them in their labeled containers to your doctor or pharmacist.

While you are taking sulfinpyrazone, drink at least six to eight eight-ounce glasses of water or fruit juice each day, unless your doctor tells you to limit the amount of fluids you drink.

Do not drink alcoholic beverages or take aspirin or any medication containing aspirin while you are taking sulfinpyrazone. Both alcohol and aspirin can affect the way your body responds to sulfinpyrazone. If you must take something to relieve minor pain or fever, ask your doctor or pharmacist to recommend a substitute for aspirin.

Take this medicine exactly as prescribed by your doctor. Sulfinpyrazone must be taken regularly to be effective. Do not stop taking it unless your doctor tells you to. Your doctor may want you to start with a small dose and then gradually increase the amount you take.

Keep in touch with your doctor while you are taking this medicine so he ca 1 adjust the amount you take to meet your needs and can check on your response to the medicine.

Be sure you have enough sulfinpyrazone on hand at all times to permit you to take all the doses prescribed for you. Check your supply before vacations, holidays and other occasions when you may not be able to obtain more.

Although sulfinpyrazone has been used in pregnant women with no reported problems, it is best to tell your doctor if you are pregnant.

DOSAGE AND STORAGE

Your doctor will determine how often you should take sulfinpyrazone and how much you should take at each dose. Carefully follow the instructions on your prescription label and ask your doctor or pharmacist to explain any part of the instructions you do not understand.

Sulfinpyrazone comes in tablets and capsules. Sulfinpyrazone should be taken at meals or with a snack to avoid stomach upset.

If you forget to take a dose of this medicine, take it as soon as you remember. If you do not remember a missed dose until it is almost time for you to take another, omit the missed dose entirely and take only the regularly scheduled dose. *Do not take a double dose to make up for a missed one.*

Keep sulfinpyrazone in the container it came in, and keep it out of the reach of children. Do not allow anyone else to take your sulfinpyrazone.

PAIN

DRUGS USED TO TREAT PAIN

Pain

Pain probably is the most common of all symptoms, yet its causes are not well understood. Most of the time, pain is caused by a combination of physical and psychological factors. It is well known that anxiety and depression will increase the sensation of pain. As a result, the perception of pain varies widely among individuals, making it difficult for doctors to evaluate.

Pain has a number of characteristics that help determine its cause. These include:

- Severity
- Type—dull and aching, sharp
- Location—pain may be located in a specific place (for example, a joint), or may be more diffuse
- Time of appearance—pain may appear only at certain times of the day (for example, before or after meals or upon awakening)
- Factors that affect its appearance—some types of pain may be worse in certain types of weather, or may be affected by foods or movement.

All of these characteristics provide clues to the underlying cause or causes of pain.

Drugs used to relieve pain are called analgesics. Certain analgesics, such as aspirin and other salicylates, reduce inflammation and fever as well as relieve pain. Because of their ability to decrease inflammation they are commonly used to treat arthritis.

Acetaminophen and phenacetin relieve pain and fever but do not reduce inflammation. All of the nonprescription analgesics are used for headache and other minor aches and pains, and are safe and effective when used according to instructions. The biggest danger associated with these medications is accidental overdosage. Because of its widespread use, aspirin causes more accidental poisonings in children than any other drug. It is important to store these products out of the reach of children and keep them in childproof containers.

The narcotic analgesics are reserved for use in treating severe pain. They are usually prescribed in small quantities following tooth extractions, treatment of fractures or surgery. Although narcotics are very effective pain relievers, they have other effects that make them unsuitable for long-term use. These effects include depression of the central nervous system and high potential for addiction. Because of these effects, narcotics usually are used only for short periods of time.

NONPRESCRIPTION ANALGESICS
Acetaminophen
(a seat a mee' noe fen)

Brand names: Datril, Liquiprin, Phenaphen, SK-Apap, Tapar, Tempra, Tylenol, Valadol and others

Acetaminophen is used to relieve pain and reduce fever. It does *not* relieve the stiffness, redness and swelling of arthritis.

Acetaminophen and preparations containing acetaminophen are available without a prescription. Many cough and cold products also contain acetaminophen. *Carefully read the label on the container for a nonprescription medicine to determine if the medicine contains acetaminophen.*

UNDESIRED EFFECTS

When taken as directed for short periods of time, acetaminophen is almost free of side effects. Rarely, this medicine can cause dizziness, which tends to disappear as your body adjusts to the drug.

Liver problems, allergic reactions and blood disorders are rare side effects, but they require medical attention if they occur. If you experience unusual weakness or tiredness, yellowing of the skin and eyes (symptoms of liver problems), itching or skin rash (symptoms of an allergic reaction), sore throat and fever or unusual bleeding or bruising (symptoms of blood problems), contact your doctor.

Very large doses of this medicine can cause acetaminophen poisoning. Some signs of overdose are diarrhea, nausea or vomiting, and stomach cramps or pain. Contact your doctor immediately if any of these occur.

PRECAUTIONS

Before you start to take acetaminophen or a product containing this drug, tell your doctor or pharmacist if you have ever had an unusual reaction to this medicine or to phenacetin, if you have kidney disease, or if you have liver disease or cirrhosis of the liver.

Take only as much acetaminophen as directed by your doctor or as recommended on the package label. Taking too much of this medicine for too long a time can cause liver damage.

Children up to 12 years of age should not take acetaminophen for more than five days in a row; adults should not take it for more than 10 days in a row. If the symptoms of the condition for which acetaminophen was prescribed still exist after these periods of time, contact your doctor.

If you take acetaminophen to lower a fever, contact your doctor if the fever lasts for more than three days, or if it returns.

Check the labels on all the prescription or nonprescription medicines you are taking. If any of them contains acetaminophen, ask your doctor or pharmacist about taking acetaminophen with medicine containing acetaminophen you are now taking. You will avoid taking an overdose this way.

DOSAGE AND STORAGE

Acetaminophen comes in tablets, in liquid form and in rectal suppositories. The liquid should be measured in a specially marked spoon to be sure of an accurate dose. Liquid drops for infants and children should be measured with the dropper that comes with the bottle. Drops may be placed directly into the child's mouth or mixed with water or juice.

To use one of the rectal suppositories, remove the wrapper and dip the tip of the suppository in water. Then lie on your side, draw your top knee up to your chest and insert the suppository well into the rectum with your finger. Hold it there for a few moments, then get up and resume your usual activities. Try not to have a bowel movement for at least an hour after inserting the suppository.

Keep acetaminophen in the container it came in. Be sure to keep this medicine out of the reach of children. An overdose of acetaminophen is very dangerous in young children. Do not allow anyone else to use your acetaminophen.

Aspirin

(as′ pir in)

Brand names: ASA, Aspergum, Bayer Aspirin, Ecotrin, Empirin, Measurin and others

Some common brand names of products containing aspirin and an antacid: Alka-Seltzer, Arthritis Pain Formula, Ascriptin, Bufferin

Aspirin belongs to the group of medicines known as salicylates. Aspirin also is called acetylsalicylic acid. Aspirin is used to relieve mild to moderate pain, to reduce fever caused by infection and to relieve redness and swelling caused by arthritis. Aspirin also helps prevent blood from clotting.

Because aspirin is available without a prescription and is so widely used, it is important to know what problems it can cause and what precautions you should take when using it. *Carefully read the label on the container for a nonprescription medicine to determine if the medicine contains aspirin.*

UNDESIRED EFFECTS

The most common side effects of aspirin are nausea, vomiting and stomach pain. To prevent these effects, take aspirin with meals or with a full eight-ounce glass of water, with a meal or snack, or with an antacid. If these measures do not help and stomach upsets continue, contact your doctor.

Less common effects, but ones that require medical attention if they occur, are loss of hearing, bloody or black stools, wheezing, tightness in the chest and shortness of breath. If you experience any of these effects, stop taking aspirin and contact your doctor.

Taking large doses of aspirin, taking aspirin over a long period of time or giving aspirin to young children who are dehydrated by fever can cause aspirin poisoning. Some signs of aspirin poisoning are dizziness or mental confusion, rapid breathing, a continuous ringing or buzzing in the ears, and severe or continuing headache. Contact your doctor if these effects occur.

Aspirin also can cause allergic reactions. Some symptoms of allergic reaction are itching, hives, runny nose, swelling of the throat, chest pains and fainting. If you have any of these symptoms, contact your doctor at once.

PRECAUTIONS

Before you take aspirin, tell your doctor or pharmacist if you have ever had a reaction to aspirin or other salicylates, including methyl salicylate (oil of wintergreen).

If you have certain medical conditions you should not take aspirin except on the advice of your doctor. These conditions include anemia, asthma, allergies, history of nasal polyps, gout, hemophilia or other bleeding problems, Hodgkin's disease, kidney disease, liver disease, and ulcers or other stomach problems.

Your doctor should supervise your use of aspirin if you are taking any of the following medications on a regular basis: anticoagulants (blood thinners), medicine for gout, medicine for inflammation (such as the inflammation of arthritis), methotrexate, oral medicine for diabetes and medicine to make your urine more or less acidic. Tell your doctor or pharmacist what prescription or nonprescription drugs you are taking. If you do not know the names of the drugs or what they were prescribed for, bring them in their labeled containers to your doctor or pharmacist.

Children under 12 should not take aspirin for more than five days in a row; adults should not take this medicine for more than 10 days in a row.

Do not take more aspirin than is recommended on the package label unless so directed by your doctor. Contact your doctor if your symptoms do not improve, if they become worse or if your fever lasts for more than three days.

If you are taking aspirin on a regular schedule to treat a chronic illness such as arthritis, the medicine will be effective only if you carefully follow your medication schedule. It is also important that your doctor check your response to aspirin at regular visits when you take this medicine over a long period of time.

If you have diabetes, regular use of eight or more aspirin tablets a day may cause inaccurate results of tests for your urine sugar. If you have any questions about this, check with your doctor.

If you are taking large doses of aspirin or taking aspirin for a long period of time, drinking alcoholic beverages may increase the possibility or severity of stomach problems.

Aspirin is an ingredient in many prescription and nonprescription drugs. *Do not take other medication while you are taking aspirin unless you first check the ingredients with your doctor or pharmacist.*

If you are pregnant, use aspirin sparingly. Do not take it at all if you are within two or three months of delivery or if you are breast-feeding. If you have any questions about this, check with your doctor.

DOSAGE AND STORAGE

Aspirin comes in chewable tablets, tablets to be swallowed and rectal suppositories. Chewable tablets may be chewed, dissolved in liquid, crushed or swallowed whole. Tablets to be swallowed should be taken with meals, with a full glass of water or with antacids.

To use one of the suppositories, remove the foil wrapper and dip the tip of the suppository in water. Then lie on your side, bring your top knee up to your chest and insert the suppository well into your rectum. Hold it there for a few moments; then get up and resume your normal activities. Try not to have a bowel movement for at least an hour after inserting the suppository.

Keep aspirin in a tightly closed bottle (preferably one with a childproof cap), and keep it out of the reach of children. Overdose with aspirin is especially dangerous in young children.

Store aspirin in a cool, dry place. Do not keep it in the bathroom or in a bathroom medicine cabinet, because the dampness may cause aspirin to lose its effectiveness. Throw away any aspirin that smells like vinegar.

Phenacetin
(fen a see' tin)

Some common brand names of products containing phenacetin with other drugs: APC, Apectol, ASA Compound, Aspirin Compound, Buff-A Comp, Buffadyne, Darvon Compound, Emprazil, Emprazil-C, Fiorinal, Monacet with Codeine, Norgesic, Norgesic Forte, PAC Compound, Propoxyphene Compound, Sinubid, Sinus Compound, SK-65 Compound, Soma Compound, Synalgos, Synalgos-DC

Phenacetin is similar to acetaminophen and is used to relieve pain and reduce fever. Although phenacetin can be given alone, usually it is combined with aspirin and caffeine (APC). Many nonprescription products contain phenacetin, often combined with other medicines for pain and/or decongestants and/or antihistamines. *Carefully read the label on the container for a nonprescription medicine to determine if the medicine contains phenacetin.*

UNDESIRED EFFECTS
Phenacetin is almost free of side effects when it is taken as directed for short periods of time. Although this effect is rare, phenacetin can cause dizziness that tends to disappear as your body adjusts to the medicine.

Taking larger doses of phenacetin than recommended or taking it over an extended period of time can cause liver problems, allergic reactions or blood disorders. These effects, although rare, require medical attention. Stop taking phenacetin and contact your doctor if you experience unusual weakness or tiredness, yellowing of the skin or eyes (symptoms of liver problems), itching or skin rash (symptoms of allergic reaction), sore throat and fever or unusual bleeding or bruising (symptoms of blood).

Taking very large doses of phenacetin can cause drug poisoning. Contact your doctor if you have signs of overdose such as diarrhea, nausea or vomiting, or stomach cramps or pain.

PRECAUTIONS

If you have ever had an unusual reaction to phenacetin or acetaminophen, you should not take any product containing phenacetin. If you have kidney disease, liver disease, cirrhosis of the liver or anemia, you should take phenacetin *only* under medical supervision. If you have any questions about this, check with your doctor or pharmacist.

Take only as much phenacetin as directed by your doctor or as recommended on the package label. *Taking too much phenacetin for too long can cause liver or kidney damage.*

Children up to 12 years of age should not take phenacetin for more than five days in a row; adults should not take it for more than 10 days in a row. If you have taken phenacetin for the safe period of time and still have symptoms of the condition for which it was prescribed, contact your doctor.

If you are taking phenacetin to bring down a fever and the fever lasts for more than three days, or if it returns, contact your doctor.

Because many prescription and nonprescription drugs contain phenacetin or acetaminophen, check the labels of the medicines you are taking so you will avoid taking an overdose. Check with your doctor or pharmacist if you have any questions about this.

If you have diabetes, phenacetin can cause inaccurate positive test results in some types of tests for sugar in your urine. Do not change your diet or your medicine for diabetes unless you first check with your doctor.

DOSAGE AND STORAGE

Carefully follow the instructions on your prescription label or the package label. The instructions tell you how often to take phenacetin and how much to take at each dose. Phenacetin comes in tablets and capsules, which are best taken with a full eight-ounce glass of water.

Keep this medicine in the container it came in. Be sure to keep products containing phenacetin out of the reach of children. An overdose of phenacetin is very dangerous in young children.

PRESCRIPTION ANALGESICS
Codeine
(keo' deen)

Names of pain medicines containing codeine: A.P.C. with Codeine, Acetaco, Acetaminophen with Codeine, Ascriptin with Codeine, Bancap with Codeine, Capital with Codeine, Codalan, Colrex Compound, Empirin with Codeine, Empracet with Codeine, Fiorinal, G-3, Maxigesic, Phenaphen with Codeine, SK-Apap with Codeine, Soma Compound with Codeine, Tabloid brand A.P.C. with Codeine, Tylenol with Codeine

In addition to its use as a cough suppressant, codeine is prescribed in higher doses to relieve pain. It is often combined with other medicines for pain and then is available only by prescription.

(See **codeine**, page 233, in the section for cough suppressants for undesired effects and precautions in using preparations containing codeine.)

Ethoheptazine
(eth o hep' ta zeen)

Names of preparations containing ethoheptazine: Equagesic and Meprogesic (with meprobamate and aspirin), Zactirin (with aspirin), Zactirin Compound (with aspirin, phenacetin and caffeine)

Ethoheptazine is used to relieve mild to moderate pain; ethoheptazine is not effective against severe pain. When it is combined with aspirin, ethoheptazine is used to relieve the pain of arthritis and other muscle or bone conditions.

UNDESIRED EFFECTS

The most common side effects of ethoheptazine are nausea, vomiting and stomach upset. To prevent these effects, take this medicine with meals or a light snack. If stomach upsets continue or are severe, contact your doctor.

When you start to take ethoheptazine you may become dizzy. Do not drive a car or operate dangerous machinery until you know how this drug will affect you. These effects tend to decrease or disappear as you continue to take ethoheptazine and as your body adjusts to it. Contact your doctor if they continue or bother you.

Very large doses of ethoheptazine can cause headaches, vision problems, continuing dizziness, nervousness and fainting. If any of these effects occur, stop taking the medicine and contact your doctor.

PRECAUTIONS

Because ethoheptazine usually is combined with other drugs, the precautions for these drugs should be considered. (See **aspirin**, page 415; **phenacetin**, page 417; and **meprobamate**, page 302.)

Take any preparation containing ethoheptazine exactly as prescribed by your doctor. Do not take more of it, do not take it more often and do not take it for a longer period of time than instructed by your doctor.

Be sure to tell your doctor about any other medical conditions you may have. Ethoheptazine may increase the drowsiness caused by alcohol and by other medications such as medications to help you sleep, tranquilizers, medications for seizures, antidepressants and other medications for pain. Be sure to tell your doctor or pharmacist what medications you are taking. If you do not know the names of the medications or what they were prescribed for, bring them in their labeled containers to your doctor or pharmacist.

DOSAGE AND STORAGE

Your doctor will determine how often you should take any preparation containing ethoheptazine and how much you should take at each dose. Carefully follow the instructions on your prescription label and ask your doctor or pharmacist to explain any part of the instructions you do not understand.

Ethoheptazine preparations come in tablets. You may take them with meals or a snack if this medicine upsets your stomach.

If you forget to take a dose, take it as soon as you remember. However, if it is almost time for you to take another dose, take only the regularly scheduled dose. Omit the missed dose entirely. *Do not take a double dose to make up for a missed one.*

Keep preparations containing ethoheptazine in the containers they came in. Keep out of the reach of children. Do not allow anyone else to take your ethoheptazine.

Meperidine
(me per' i deen)

Brand names: Demerol, Mepergan

Meperidine is a narcotic used to relieve moderate to severe pain. Meperidine is available only by a doctor's prescription and, because the law prohibits refilling a prescription containing a narcotic, you will have to obtain a new prescription each time you need this medicine.

The injectable form of meperidine also is used to make a person drowsy before an operation, to supplement a general anesthesia during surgery and to relieve the pain of childbirth.

UNDESIRED EFFECTS

Meperidine may cause nausea or vomiting, especially after you take the first few doses. If you lie down for a while, these effects usually will disappear.

Meperidine makes some people drowsy or less alert than usual. Do not drive a car or operate dangerous machinery until you know how this medicine will affect you.

While you are taking meperidine, you may experience dizziness, lightheadedness or fainting when you get up from a lying or a sitting position. Getting up slowly should help lessen these effects.

Other effects that may occur when you start to take meperidine include redness or flushing of the face, unusual increase in sweating, blurred vision, constipation, difficult urination or a frequent urge to urinate, dry mouth, unusual tiredness or weakness and an unusually fast or pounding heartbeat. These effects tend to decrease or disappear as you continue to take meperidine and as your body adjusts to it. If they continue or are severe, contact your doctor.

More serious side effects as a result of taking meperidine are shortness of breath, difficult breathing and an unusually slow heartbeat, all signs that this medicine is having a bad effect on your central nervous system. Stop taking meperidine and contact your doctor at once if any of these effects occurs.

PRECAUTIONS

Before you start to take meperidine, tell your doctor if you have a history of emphysema, asthma, chronic lung disease, an enlarged prostate, problems with urination, gallbladder disease, gallstones, kidney disease, liver disease, an underactive adrenal gland (Addison's disease), an underactive thyroid, or an unusually slow or irregular heartbeat. Meperidine can make these conditions worse.

Tell your doctor what prescription or nonprescription drugs you are taking, including antihistamines or other medicine for hay fever, allergies or colds; barbiturates, other narcotics or other prescription medicine for pain; sedatives, tranquilizers or medicine to help you sleep; medicine for seizures; medicine for depression; and prescription medicine for stomach cramps or spasms. Also tell him if you are now taking or have taken MAO inhibitors within the past two weeks.

If you do not know the names of the drugs you are taking or what they were prescribed for, bring them in their labeled containers to your doctor or pharmacist.

Do not drink alcoholic beverages while you are taking meperidine and do not start to take any of the drugs listed above without first consulting your doctor or pharmacist. All of these drugs can increase the possibility and the severity of side effects.

Because meperidine can be habit-forming, do not take more of it, do not take it more often and do not take it for a longer time than directed by your doctor.

If you will be taking meperidine for several months, your doctor will want to check regularly on your response to this medicine. *Be sure to keep all your appointments with your doctor.*

Before you have any kind of surgery, including dental surgery, tell the doctor or dentist in charge that you are taking meperidine.

Although meperidine is used to relieve the pain of childbirth, it is not known whether it is safe to use early in pregnancy. To help your doctor select the best and safest treatment for both you and your baby, tell him if you are pregnant or are breast-feeding.

DOSAGE AND STORAGE

Your doctor will determine how often you should take meperidine and how much you should take at each dose. Carefully follow the instructions on your prescription label and ask your doctor or pharmacist to explain any part of the instructions you do not understand.

Meperidine comes in two forms to be taken orally—tablets and liquid. Take the liquid with one-half glass of water to lessen the numbing effect on your mouth and throat.

Keep meperidine in the container it came in. Keep it out of the reach of children. Do not let anyone else take your meperidine.

Oxycodone

(ox i koe' done)

Brand names of products containing oxycodone: (with aspirin, phenacetin and caffeine) Percobarb, Percobarb-Demi, Percodan, Percodan-Demi; (with acetaminophen) Percogesic, Tylox

Oxycodone is a narcotic used to relieve moderate pain, such as that associated with bursitis, dislocations, simple fractures and nerve problems. Oxycodone also is used to relieve pain following surgery, tooth extraction and childbirth.

Oxycodone is available only in combination with aspirin, phenacetin and caffeine (A.P.C.) or with acetaminophen. These combination products can be obtained only with a doctor's prescription, and the prescription cannot be refilled. You must get another prescription if you continue to take a product containing oxycodone.

UNDESIRED EFFECTS

Oxycodone can cause nausea and vomiting, especially after the first few doses. You may take the medicine with food or milk, or lie down for a while to relieve nausea or vomiting. If this does not make you more comfortable or if these effects are very uncomfortable, contact your doctor.

Some people become drowsy or less alert than usual when they take oxycodone. Do not drive a car or operate dangerous machinery until you know what effect this medicine will have on you.

If you experience dizziness, lightheadedness or fainting when you get up from a lying or a sitting position, get up slowly. This should help decrease these effects. If they continue or are severe, contact your doctor.

When you start to take oxycodone, you may have redness or flushing of the face, unusual increase in sweating, blurred vision, constipation, difficult urination or a frequent urge to urinate, dry mouth, unusual tiredness or weakness, or unusually fast or pounding heartbeat. These effects may decrease as you continue to take oxycodone and as your body adjusts to it, but if they do not, you should contact your doctor.

More serious side effects of oxycodone are shortness of breath, difficult breathing and an unusually slow heartbeat. These are signs the medicine is having a bad effect on your central nervous system, and they require medical attention. Alert family members or some other person who is likely to be nearby to call your doctor immediately if you have difficulty breathing.

(Be sure to check the side effects of **aspirin**, page 415, and **phenacetin**, page 417, if you are taking a preparation that combines oxycodone with A.P.C. Side effects for **acetaminophen**, page 414, should be checked if you are taking a combination of oxycodone and acetaminophen.)

PRECAUTIONS

Before you start to take oxycodone, tell your doctor if you have any history of emphysema, asthma, chronic lung disease, an enlarged prostate, problems with urination, gallbladder disease, gallstones, kidney disease, liver disease, an underactive adrenal gland (Addison's disease), an underactive thyroid, or an unusually slow or irregular heartbeat. Oxycodone can make these conditions worse.

Certain medications, when taken with oxycodone, can increase the possibility and severity of side effects. These include antihistamines or other medicine for hay fever, allergies or colds; sedatives, tranquilizers or medicine to help you sleep; barbiturates, other narcotics or other prescription medicine for pain;

medicine for seizures; medicine for depression; prescription medicine for stomach cramps or spasms; and MAO inhibitors.

Tell your doctor what prescription or nonprescription medicines you are taking (or in the case of MAO inhibitors, have taken within the past two weeks). If you do not know the names of the drugs or what they were prescribed for, bring them in their labeled containers to your doctor or pharmacist.

Do not drink alcoholic beverages while you are taking oxycodone, and do not take any of the drugs listed above without first checking with your doctor or pharmacist.

Oxycodone can be habit-forming. Be sure you do not take more of it, do not take it more often and do not take it for a longer time than directed by your doctor.

Before you have any kind of surgery, including dental surgery, with a general anesthetic, tell the doctor or dentist in charge that you are taking oxycodone.

The safe use of oxycodone in pregnancy has not been established. Be sure to tell your doctor if you are pregnant so he can select the best treatment for you and your baby.

Check the precautions for aspirin, phenacetin and acetaminophen when you are taking oxycodone combined with any of these drugs.

DOSAGE AND STORAGE

Preparations containing oxycodone come in capsules and tablets. Your doctor will determine how often you should take this medicine and how much you should take at each dose. Carefully follow the instructions on your prescription label and ask your doctor or pharmacist to explain any part of the instructions you do not understand.

Keep oxycodone in the container it came in, and keep it out of the reach of children. Do not allow anyone else to take your oxycodone.

Pentazocine

(pen taz' oh seen)

Brand names: Talwin, Talwin Compound (pentazocine combined with aspirin)

Pentazocine is used to relieve moderate to severe pain caused by many types of medical problems. The injectable form of this medicine is used to supplement anesthesia during surgery, to treat pain following surgery and to relieve the pain of childbirth.

Pentazocine is available only with a doctor's prescription, and a prescription for pentazocine may not be refilled. If you continue to take this medicine, you will need a new prescription each time.

UNDESIRED EFFECTS

With the first few doses of pentazocine, you may experience nausea or vomiting. If you lie down for a while, these effects usually will disappear.

Some people who take pentazocine become drowsy, dizzy or lightheaded or get a false sense of well-being. Do not drive a car or operate dangerous machinery until you know how this drug will affect you.

Other effects that may occur when you start to take pentazocine are flushing, sweating, itching, constipation, difficulty urinating, headache, tremor or shakiness, numbness, blurred vision and ringing in the ears. These effects tend to decrease or disappear as your body adjusts to the medicine. However, contact your doctor if they continue or are severe.

Contact your doctor if you have any signs of an allergic reaction to pentazocine such as hives, skin rash, chills or fever.

More serious side effects also can occur, and they will require medical attention if they do occur. Stop taking this medicine and contact your doctor if you have difficulty breathing, changes in mood, mental confusion, a feeling that something wrong is about to happen, depression or hallucinations (seeing, hearing or feeling things that are not there).

PRECAUTIONS

Before you start to take pentazocine, tell your doctor if you have emphysema, asthma, chronic lung disease, an enlarged prostate, problems with urination, gallbladder disease, gallstones, a history of convulsions or seizures, kidney disease, liver disease, or dependence on or addiction to narcotics. Pentazocine may make these medical problems worse.

Certain other medications, when taken with pentazocine, can increase the possibility of or severity of side effects. Tell your doctor if you are taking any of the following: meperidine; methadone or other narcotics to treat dependence on or addiction to narcotics; morphine; prescription medicine for stomach cramps or spasm; antihistamines or other medicine for hay fever, allergies or colds; barbiturates, narcotics or other prescription medicine for pain; sedatives, tranquilizers or medicine to help you sleep; medicine for seizures; medicine for depression; or MAO inhibitors (even if you stopped taking them recently).

If you do not know the names of the drugs you are taking or what they were prescribed for, bring them in their labeled containers to your doctor or pharmacist.

Do not drink alcoholic beverages while you are taking pentazocine, and do not start to take any of the medicines listed above without first checking with your doctor or pharmacist.

Pentazocine can be habit-forming. Therefore, be sure you do not take more of it, take it more often or take it for a longer period of time than directed by your doctor. If the amount prescribed does not relieve your pain, contact your doctor. He may want to adjust your dose or change your medication.

If you will be taking pentazocine for several weeks or months, your doctor will want to check your progress at regular intervals. *Be sure to keep all your appointments with him.*

Do not have surgery, including dental surgery, with general anesthesia unless you tell the doctor or dentist in charge that you are taking pentazocine.

Pentazocine should not be taken by children under 12 years of age or by pregnant women. Before you start taking pentazocine, tell your doctor if you are pregnant. If you become pregnant while taking this medicine, contact your doctor immediately.

DOSAGE AND STORAGE
Your doctor will determine how often you should take pentazocine and how much you should take at each dose. Carefully follow the instructions on your prescription label and ask your doctor or pharmacist to explain any part of the instructions you do not understand.

Pentazocine comes in tablets to be taken orally. (If you are taking a combination of pentazocine and aspirin, check **aspirin**, page 415, for side effects, precautions and special instructions on the use of aspirin.)

Keep pentazocine in the container it came in. Keep it out of the reach of children. Do not allow anyone else to take your pentazocine.

Propoxyphene
(proe pox′ i feen)

Brand names: Darvon, Dolocap, SK-65

Propoxyphene is used for the relief of mild or moderate pain. Propoxyphene is prescribed alone or in combination with aspirin, A.P.C. (aspirin, phenacetin and caffeine) or acetaminophen. (If you are taking one of these combination preparations, check **aspirin**, page 415; **phenacetin**, page 417; and **acetaminophen**, page 414, for additional side effects and precautions.)

UNDESIRED EFFECTS
Nausea and vomiting may occur, particularly after the first few doses. If you lie down for a while, these effects usually will disappear. Contact your doctor if these effects continue after you lie down.

Propoxyphene makes some people drowsy, dizzy or lightheaded or gives them a false sense of well-being. Do not drive a car or operate dangerous machinery until you know how this medicine will affect you.

Other effects, which tend to decrease or disappear as your body adjusts to propoxyphene, include blurred vision, constipation, headache, stomach pain or unusual weakness or tiredness. If these effects continue or are severe, contact your doctor.

Itching or skin rash indicates you are allergic to this medicine. If you have either of these effects, stop taking propoxyphene and contact your doctor.

Taking more propoxyphene than prescribed or taking it with alcohol or other narcotics can cause symptoms of overdosage, including weakness, difficult breathing, confusion, anxiety, and severe drowsiness and dizziness. You may become unconscious. If any of these symptoms occur, call your doctor or arrange to have someone call your doctor to obtain emergency help immediately.

PRECAUTIONS
Certain medications should not be taken with propoxyphene. These include carbamazepine (medicine for seizures); antihistamines or medicine for hay fever, other allergies or colds; barbiturates, narcotics and other prescription medicine

for pain; sedatives, tranquilizers or medicine to help you sleep; medicine for seizures; and medicine for depression. Anyone who is taking MAO inhibitors or who has taken them within the past two weeks should not take propoxyphene.

Before you start to take propoxyphene, tell your doctor what prescription or nonprescription medicines you are taking. If you do not know the names of the drugs or what they were prescribed for, bring them in their labeled containers to your doctor or pharmacist.

Take propoxyphene only as directed by your doctor. Do not take more of it, do not take it more often and do not take it for a longer time than your doctor has ordered. If you take too much of this medicine, it can be habit-forming or may result in an overdose.

Do not drink alcoholic beverages while you are taking propoxyphene because you may have serious side effects. Do not start to take any of the drugs listed above unless you have permission from your doctor.

If you will be taking this medicine for several weeks or months, your doctor will want to check your response at regular intervals. *Be sure to keep all your appointments with him.*

If you are going to have surgery, including dental surgery, with a general anesthetic, be sure the doctor or dentist in charge knows you are taking propoxyphene.

Tell your doctor if you are pregnant or think you may become pregnant while taking this medicine. Propoxyphene is passed by the mother to her unborn child and may lead to withdrawal symptoms in the newborn baby.

DOSAGE AND STORAGE

Propoxyphene comes in tablets and capsules. Your doctor will choose the form best for you and will determine how often you should take this medicine and how much you should take at each dose. Carefully follow the instructions on your prescription label and ask your doctor or pharmacist to explain any part of the instructions you do not understand.

Keep propoxyphene in the container it came in. Keep this medicine out of the reach of children. Overdose is very serious in young children. Do not allow anyone else to take your propoxyphene.

MUSCLE PAIN

Muscle ache and pain is a frequent problem in our society, where people do not regularly perform strenuous work or exercise. Muscles that are unaccustomed to vigorous activity become strained easily, resulting in pain and stiffness in them. Muscle pain also can follow prolonged periods of staying in one position or result from anxiety or from exposure to dampness and cold.

In most cases, the discomfort of muscle strain will disappear within a few days. Nonprescription analgesics, such as aspirin and acetaminophen, and topical liniments, gels and lotions are helpful in relieving pain during that time. When muscle strains are more severe, the prescription drugs described in this section are used to help relax the muscles.

In addition to therapy with drugs, application of heat is an effective means of relaxing muscles. Moist heat is more effective than dry heat because moist heat penetrates to muscles better than dry heat does. The easiest method to apply moist heat is to use towels soaked in hot water. Steam packs and moist electric heating pads also are available.

Dry heat can be applied by heating pad, heat lamp or hot water bottle. Any type of heat treatment, dry or moist, should be used cautiously in order to avoid burns. Never go to sleep while using a heating pad or a heat lamp.

MUSCLE RELAXANTS
Diazepam

Brand name: Valium

Diazepam is used primarily to treat patients who are anxious or tense. However, diazepam also acts as a muscle relaxant and frequently is used for this purpose. (For a complete description for **diazepam**, see page 314, in the section for drugs used to treat anxiety.)

Methocarbamol
(meth oh kar' ba mole)

Brand names: Metho-500, Robaxin, Romethocarb

Methocarbamol relaxes certain muscles of the body. Methocarbamol is used along with rest, physical therapy, medicine for pain and other measures to relieve the pain and discomfort of strains, sprains, injury, bursitis or surgery.

UNDESIRED EFFECTS

The most common side effects of methocarbamol are blurred or double vision, dizziness, drowsiness or lightheadedness. Do not drive a car or operate dangerous machinery until you know how this medicine will affect you. These effects tend to decrease or disappear as you continue to take methocarbamol and as your body adjusts to it. However, if they continue or are severe, contact your doctor.

Less often, methocarbamol will cause a fever, headache or nausea. Contact your doctor if these effects bother you.

The most serious side effect of methocarbamol is an allergic reaction. Stop taking this medicine and contact your doctor at once if you get a skin rash, itching, stuffy nose and red or bloodshot eyes.

Do not be concerned if your urine has a brown, black or green color. This effect is harmless.

PRECAUTIONS

Before you start to take methocarbamol, tell your doctor if you have epilepsy or kidney disease. The injectable form of this medicine may make these conditions worse.

Tell your doctor what prescription or nonprescription drugs you are taking, including antihistamines or medicine for hay fever, allergies or colds; barbiturates, narcotics or prescription medicine for pain; sedatives, tranquilizers or medicine to help you sleep; medicine for seizures; medicine for depression and MAO inhibitors (even if you stopped taking them two weeks ago).

If you do not know the names of the drugs or what they were prescribed for, bring them in their labeled containers to your doctor or pharmacist.

Do not drink alcoholic beverages while you are taking methocarbamol. Do not start to take any of the drugs listed above unless you have your doctor's permission to do so. All of these can increase the possibility or severity of side effects. If you have any questions about this, ask your doctor or pharmacist.

To help your doctor select the best treament for you and your baby, tell him if you are pregnant or if you are breast-feeding. Safe use in pregnancy and during breast-feeding has not been established.

Children under the age of 12 should not take methocarbamol. Safe use in this age group has not yet been established.

DOSAGE AND STORAGE

Your doctor will determine how often you should take methocarbamol and how much you should take at each dose. Carefully follow the instructions on your prescription label and ask your doctor or pharmacist to explain any part of the instructions you do not understand.

If you forget to take a dose of this medicine, take it as soon as you remember. If you remember a missed dose at the time you are scheduled to take another, omit the missed dose entirely and take only the regularly scheduled dose. *Do not take a double dose.*

Keep methocarbamol in the container it came in. Keep it out of the reach of children. Do not allow anyone else to take your methocarbamol.

Orphenadrine
(or fen' a dreen)

Brand names: Disipal, Estamul, Norflex

Other products containing orphenadrine: Norgesic (with aspirin, phenacetin and caffeine)

Orphenadrine helps to relax muscles and reduce muscle spasm. Orphenadrine is used to relieve the pain and discomfort of strains, sprains and other muscle injuries. It also is used to treat the symptoms of Parkinson's disease.

UNDESIRED EFFECTS

Dryness of the mouth is a common side effect of orphenadrine. Sucking hard candy, chewing gum or drinking fluids will help to relieve the dryness.

Orphenadrine makes some people dizzy, lightheaded or drowsy. Do not drive a car or operate dangerous machinery until you know how this medicine will affect you.

Other effects that may occur when you start to take orphenadrine and then decrease as your body adjusts to the medicine are blurred vision, constipation, difficulty urinating, fainting, headache, nausea or vomiting, nervousness or restlessness, stomach upset or trembling. If these effects are persistent or severe, contact your doctor.

More serious side effects, although they occur infrequently, may require medical attention. If you experience mental confusion, unusually fast or pounding heartbeat, skin rash or itching, stop taking orphenadrine and contact your doctor.

PRECAUTIONS

Before you start to take orphenadrine, tell your doctor if you have any disease of the digestive tract (such as esophagus disease, ulcers or intestinal blockage), an enlarged prostate, glaucoma, heart disease, myasthenia gravis, an unusually fast or irregular heartbeat or urinary tract blockage. Orphenadrine may make these conditions worse.

Tell your doctor what prescription or nonprescription drugs you are taking, particularly antihistamines or medicine for hay fever, other allergies or colds; barbiturates, narcotics or prescription medicines for pain; sedatives, tranquilizers or medicine to help you sleep; medicine for seizures; medicine for depression; and MAO inhibitors (even if you stopped taking them within the past two weeks).

If you do not know the names of the drugs you are taking or what they were prescribed for, bring them in their labeled containers to your doctor or pharmacist.

Do not drink alcoholic beverages while you are taking orphenadrine. Do not start to take any of the drugs listed above unless you have your doctor's permission. All of these can increase the possibility of and severity of side effects.

Orphenadrine should not be given to children under six years of age. Its safe use in this age group has not been established.

To help your doctor select the best treatment for you and your baby, tell him if you are pregnant or plan to become pregnant while taking this medicine. If you become pregnant while taking orphenadrine, contact your doctor.

DOSAGE AND STORAGE

Your doctor will determine how often you should take orphenadrine tablets and how much of this medicine you should take at each dose. Carefully follow the instructions on your prescription label and ask your doctor or pharmacist to explain any part of the instructions you do not understand.

If you forget to take a dose of orphenadrine, take it as soon as you remember and then take any remaining doses for the day at regularly spaced intervals. If you do not remember a missed dose until it is almost time for the next dose, omit the missed dose entirely and take only the regularly scheduled dose. *Do not take a double dose to make up for a missed dose.*

Keep this medicine in the container it came in. Keep orphenadrine out of the reach of children. Do not allow anyone else to take your orphenadrine.

MISCELLANEOUS

MISCELLANEOUS DRUGS

Estrogen and Progestogen Combinations

(ess' tro jen) (proe jes' to jen)

Brand names: Brevicon, Demulen, Enovid, Loestrin, Lo-Ovral, Modicon, Norinyl, Norlestrin, Norquen, Oracon, Ortho-Novum SQ, Ovcon, Ovral, Ovulen

Birth-control pills contain estrogen and progestogen, two female hormones. During pregnancy your body manufactures these two hormones to prevent your ovaries from releasing eggs. Therefore, when you take these hormones regularly, they will keep you from getting pregnant by preventing the release of eggs from your ovaries.

Recent attempts to improve the effectiveness and decrease the side effects of birth-control pills have led to the development of two variations on the original combination birth-control pills. These are the sequential pills (estrogen alone for 14 to 16 days, followed by progestogen for six days) and low-estrogen combinations (containing less than 35 micrograms of estrogen). Norquen, Oracon and Ortho-Novum SQ are sequential pills; Loestrin and Lo-Ovral are low-estrogen combinations.

UNDESIRED EFFECTS

The most common side effects of birth-control pills are similar to those experienced during early pregnancy such as tenderness of the breasts, weight gain or loss, nausea and vomiting, and spotted darkening of the skin. These effects usually are mild but should be reported to your doctor if they are bothersome.

Spotting or bleeding between menstrual periods is not uncommon during the first few months of taking birth-control pills. However, you should contact your doctor if such bleeding continues after the second month. You may need a change in your medication.

While serious side effects such as blood clots, stroke and liver problems are rare when you take birth-control pills, be on the alert for symptoms of these problems. Contact your doctor if you develop a sharp pain in the chest or shortness of breath or cough up blood (symptoms of blood clots in the lungs); crushing pain or heaviness in the chest (possibly a heart attack); pain in the calf of the leg (possibly a blood clot); sudden severe headache or vomiting, dizziness or fainting, disturbance of vision or speech, or weakness or numbness in an arm or a leg (symptoms of a stroke); sudden partial or complete loss of vision (possibly a blood clot in the eye); severe pain in the abdomen or yellowing of the skin (symptoms of liver problems); breast lumps; or severe depression.

PRECAUTIONS

You should not take birth-control pills if you have or have ever had blood clots in the legs or lungs; have had a stroke, heart attack or angina pectoris (heart pain); have known or suspected cancer of the breast or sex organs; or have unusual vaginal bleeding that has not been diagnosed.

You should use another type of contraception if you have scanty or irregular periods or are a young woman without a regular menstrual cycle. If you use birth-control pills you may have difficulty getting pregnant or may fail to have menstrual periods after you stop taking this medicine.

To make your taking birth-control pills as safe as possible, tell your doctor if you have a family history of breast cancer, have breast nodules or cysts, diabetes, high blood pressure, a high cholesterol level, migraine headaches, heart or kidney disease, epilepsy, mental depression, fibroid tumors of the uterus or gallbladder disease, or smoke cigarettes.

Before you start to take birth-control pills, tell your doctor what prescription or nonprescription drugs you are taking, including rifampicin, ampicillin, tetracycline, barbiturates, phenylbutazone and phenytoin.

Oral contraceptives must be taken daily for at least 10 days before they can be considered fully effective in preventing unwanted pregnancy. To prevent pregnancy during the first few weeks in which you take birth control pills, use some other form of birth control as well.

See your doctor regularly (every six to 12 months) for a complete physical examination, particularly breast and pelvic examinations and a Pap smear. Follow your doctor's instructions for examining your own breasts between checkups.

Before you start to take birth-control pills, tell your doctor if you are pregnant or think you may be pregnant. If you are pregnant, you should not take birth-control pills because they may damage your developing child. If you miss one menstrual period and have been taking your tablets as directed, continue taking them. However, if you miss one period and have not taken your tablets as directed, notify your doctor, and use another method of birth control until you can determine if you are pregnant.

DOSAGE AND STORAGE

Oral contraceptives come in tablets. They are available in packets of 21 tablets or 28 tablets. In the 28-tablet packet, the last seven tablets are colored. Your menstrual period should begin while you are taking these colored tablets. If you are using the 21-tablet packet, your menstrual period should begin after you take the last tablet.

Counting the first day of your period as day one, oral contraceptives are taken from day five through 26 of your menstrual cycle. Be sure you carefully follow your doctor's instructions. Always have your prescription refilled often enough so that when you finish one pack of tablets you have another pack ready to start.

Be sure to take one tablet regularly each day. It is a good idea to take a tablet at the same time every day and at a time when you do something else each day, such as brushing your teeth in the morning or eating dinner in the evening.

If you forget to take one tablet at the scheduled time, take it as soon as you remember it. Take the next one at the regular time, even though you may be taking two tablets in one day. If you miss two tablets, take two tablets a day for the next two days. Also, use another method of birth control until you have taken one tablet each day for seven consecutive days.

If you miss three tablets, do not take them when you remember. Throw away any remaining tablets and wait four days. Then start a new pack (this will be on the eighth day after you took your last pill), even if you have had your period or are still bleeding. Use another method of birth control until your next period begins.

Keep this medicine out of the reach of children. Do not allow anyone else to take it.

Estrogen
(ess' tro jen)

Brand names: Amnestrogen, Conestron, Premarin and others

Estrogen is a hormone produced by the body that is needed by women to bear children and for other natural functions. Additional estrogen is prescribed for women to relieve certain symptoms of menopause, such as "hot flashes," sweating, irritability, anxiety, depression and other discomforts.

Estrogen also is used to help promote normal physical growth in young women who are not maturing at the usual rate. Certain types of cancer, including cancer of the breast and of the prostate, are treated with estrogen.

UNDESIRED EFFECTS
Nausea is the most frequent side effect of estrogen. If you take this medicine with milk or a light snack, you may avoid this problem. The nausea should disappear as your body adjusts to estrogen. If it does not, contact your doctor. You may notice tenderness and fullness of the breast while you are taking estrogen. This side effect is harmless and will disappear when you stop taking estrogen.

More serious side effects will require medical attention if they occur. Contact your doctor if you have puffiness of the hands or ankles, weight gain, leg cramps, bleeding or discharge from the vagina, or pain and tenderness of the calf or groin.

PRECAUTIONS
If you or any member of your family has ever had lumps in the breast or breast cancer, you should not take estrogen. Tell your doctor about this and any other medical condition that may be made worse by estrogen, such as diabetes, asthma, epilepsy, migraine headaches, heart or kidney disease, bone disease, liver disease, or an underactive or an overactive thyroid.

Estrogen may affect the way your body responds to any other medicine you are taking. Before you begin to take estrogen, tell your doctor what prescription or nonprescription drugs you are taking. If you do not know the names of the drugs or what they were prescribed for, bring them in their labeled containers to your doctor or pharmacist.

It is important that your doctor check the way you are responding to estrogen. *Be sure to keep all your appointments for checkups.* You may have to take estrogen for several weeks before its full effects can be determined.

Do not stop taking estrogen unless your doctor specifically tells you to do so. Before you have any kind of laboratory test, tell the doctor in charge that you are taking estrogen.

To help your doctor select the best treatment for you and your baby, tell him if you are pregnant or are breast-feeding. If you become pregnant while taking this medicine, contact your doctor.

Dosage and Storage
Your doctor will determine how much estrogen you should take and how often you should take it. Carefully follow the instructions on your prescription label and ask your doctor or pharmacist to explain any part of the instructions that you do not understand.

Estrogen comes in tablets to be taken orally and as a cream to be inserted in the vagina. If you are to use the estrogen cream, your doctor or pharmacist will tell you how to insert it. You may wish to wear a sanitary napkin after inserting the cream to avoid staining your clothes.

If you forget to take a tablet, take it as soon as you remember it. If you remember a missed dose when it is time for you to take another, omit the missed dose entirely and take only the regularly scheduled dose.

Keep estrogen in the container it came in, and keep it out of the reach of children. Do not allow anyone else to take your estrogen.

Doxylamine and Pyridoxine
(dox il' a meen) (peer i dox' een)

Brand name: Bendectin

The combination of doxylamine (an antihistamine) and pyridoxine (vitamin B_6) is used to treat nausea and vomiting. Frequently doxylamine and pyridoxine are prescribed for the nausea and vomiting of pregnancy ("morning sickness").

Undesired Effects
Doxylamine and pyridoxine make some people drowsy, dizzy or less alert than normal. Do not drive a car, operate dangerous machinery or perform tasks that require you to be alert until you know how this medicine will affect you.

Contact your doctor if doxylamine and pyridoxine make you nervous or disoriented, or give you a headache, heart palpitations or diarrhea.

Precautions
This medicine can make some medical conditions worse. Before you start to take it, tell your doctor if you have heart disease, high blood pressure, increased pressure in the eye, an enlarged prostate, an overactive thyroid, a stomach ulcer or blockage of the urinary tract.

Tell your doctor what prescription or nonprescription drugs you are taking, including other antihistamines, medicine for allergies or colds, barbiturates, medicine for seizures, narcotics, prescription medicine for pain, sedatives, tranquilizers, medicine to help you sleep, medicine for depression and MAO inhibitors (even if you stopped taking them in the past two weeks).

If you do not know the names of the drugs or what they were prescribed for, bring them in their labeled containers to your doctor or pharmacist.

Do not drink alcoholic beverages while you are taking doxylamine and pyridoxine. Alcohol can increase the chance of and severity of side effects. Do not start to take any of the drugs listed above unless you first check with your doctor.

Since this medication is used to prevent or relieve nausea and vomiting, it should be taken only when necessary and only as directed. Do not take more of it and do not take it more often than your doctor has directed.

DOSAGE AND STORAGE

Doxylamine and pyridoxine come in tablets to be taken orally. Take this medicine with solid food or a glass of water or milk to decrease stomach irritation. If you are taking doxylamine and pyridoxine for the nausea and vomiting of pregnancy, take it at bedtime. The special coating on the tablet delays the medicine's action until the morning hours.

Keep this medicine in the container it came in, and keep it out of the reach of children. Do not allow anyone else to take your doxylamine and pyridoxine.

Ferrous Sulfate
(fer' us sul' fate)

Brand names: Feosol, Fer-in-Sol, Fero-Gradumet, Ferolix, Ferralyn, Fesotyme, Ferospace, Mol-Iron and others

Ferrous sulfate provides the body with the extra amounts of iron needed to produce red blood cells. It is used to treat iron-deficiency anemia, a condition that occurs when the body has fewer red blood cells than it needs. Iron-deficiency anemia is usually the result of poor diet, excess bleeding or certain medical problems.

UNDESIRED EFFECTS

Stomach upset, nausea and vomiting are common side effects of taking ferrous sulfate. If you experience these effects, disregard instructions to take this medicine on an empty stomach and take it with meals or a snack.

If this medicine makes you constipated, drink extra fluids and add foods such as bran and prunes to your diet. If you have questions about foods that can help prevent constipation, check with your doctor or pharmacist.

Ferrous sulfate can cause darkening of the stools. This side effect is harmless. It also can darken the teeth of children. This is a harmless effect, and if it occurs, the child's teeth can be cleaned once a week with tooth powder or baking soda.

PRECAUTIONS

Because ferrous sulfate can make some medical conditions worse, tell your doctor if you have hemochromatosis (an anemia caused by something other than iron deficiency), a stomach ulcer, or inflammation or ulcerative disease of the bowel.

Before you start to take ferrous sulfate, tell your doctor what prescription or nonprescription drugs you are taking, particularly antacids, tetracycline, chloramphenicol and pencilliamine (medicine for rheumatoid arthritis). If you do not know the names of the drugs or what they were prescribed for, bring them in their labeled containers to your doctor or pharmacist.

Take ferrous sulfate exactly as your doctor has prescribed. It may take several days or weeks before you begin to see the full benefit of this medicine. Be sure to take ferrous sulfate as long as your doctor tells you to. Your doctor may want to perform blood tests to determine if this medication is working. *Be sure to keep all appointments with him for checkups.*

DOSAGE AND STORAGE

Your doctor will determine how much ferrous sulfate you should take and how often you should take it. Carefully follow the instructions on your prescription label and ask your doctor or pharmacist to explain any part of the instructions you do not understand.

Ferrous sulfate comes in tablets and in liquid form to be taken orally and in drops for small children. This medicine should be taken on an empty stomach (at least two hours after meals), unless it upsets your stomach; then it may be taken with meals or a snack.

Over a period of time liquid ferrous sulfate may change color from pale green-blue to light yellow. This does not affect the strength of the drug, and you may continue to take it if this change occurs.

If you are giving drops to a child, you may place the drops directly into the child's mouth or mix them into water or fruit juice. Be sure to measure the drops carefully and give your child only the amount the doctor has prescribed.

If you forget to take a dose of this medicine, take it as soon as you remember it. If you do not remember a missed dose until it is time for your next dose, omit the missed dose entirely and take only the regularly scheduled dose. *Do not take a double dose.*

Keep ferrous sulfate in the container it came in, and keep it out of the reach of children. This is very important, because an overdose of ferrous sulfate can be fatal to a small child. Do not let anyone else take your ferrous sulfate.

Phentermine
(fen′ ter meen)

Brand names: Adipex, Fastin, Ionamin, Unifast, Wilpo

Because phentermine suppresses the appetite, it is used in combination with diet to help a person lose weight. However, this appetite-decreasing effect is only temporary, and phentermine is useful only for the first few weeks of dieting until new eating habits are established. Drugs such as phentermine are not effective for long-term diet control.

UNDESIRED EFFECTS

Common side effects of phentermine are dryness of the mouth and an unpleasant taste. To help relieve these problems, chew gum or drink fluids.

This medicine makes some people dizzy, drowsy, lightheaded or less alert than they usually are. Do not drive a car or operate dangerous machinery until you know how phentermine will affect you.

Phentermine also can cause irritability, nervousness or trouble falling asleep. If these effects occur and they are severe or continue over a long period of time, contact your doctor.

Contact your doctor if you have more serious side effects, such as mood changes, skin rash or hives, heart palpitations or severe irritability.

PRECAUTIONS

Tell your doctor if you have ever had an unusual reaction to an amphetamine, dextroamphetamine, ephedrine, epinephrine, isoproterenol, metaproterenol, methamphetamine, norepinephrine, phenylephrine, phenylpropanolamine, pseudoephedrine or terbutaline. If you have, you may have a bad reaction to phentermine.

Before you start to use phentermine, tell your doctor if you have diabetes, glaucoma, heart or blood vessel disease, high blood pressure or an overactive thyroid.

Phentermine should not be taken when you are taking certain other medicines. Tell your doctor what prescription or nonprescription drugs you are taking, including medicine for diabetes, guanethidine, phenothiazines, caffeine, medicine for hyperactivity (in children), medicine for narcolepsy, other medicine for appetite control and MAO inhibitors (even if you stopped taking them during the past two weeks).

Because phentermine can be habit-forming, take this medicine exactly as prescribed by your doctor. Do not take more of it, do not take it more often and do not take it for a longer period of time than your doctor has ordered. Do not stop taking this medicine without first checking with your doctor. He may want you gradually to decrease the amount you take before you stop taking it completely.

Be sure to follow your diet while you are taking phentermine. However, if you have diabetes the combination of phentermine and a low-calorie diet may affect your levels of blood sugar. Check with your doctor if you notice changes in the results of your tests for urine sugar or if you have any questions about this.

DOSAGE AND STORAGE

Your doctor will determine how much phentermine you should take and how often you should take it. Carefully follow the instructions on your prescription label and ask your doctor or pharmacist to explain any part of the instructions that you do not understand.

Phentermine comes in tablets and in extended-release capsules. If you are taking the short-acting (tablet) form of this medicine, take the last dose for the day four to six hours before bedtime to help prevent sleeping problems. If you are taking the long-acting (extended-release) form of phentermine, take the daily dose in the morning or at least 10 to 14 hours before bedtime so it will affect your sleep less.

If you forget to take a dose of phentermine, omit the missed dose completely and take only the regularly scheduled dose.

Keep phentermine in the container that it came in, and keep it out of the reach of children. Do not allow anyone else to take your phentermine.

APPENDIX
CANADIAN BRAND NAMES

Many brand names under which drugs are sold in Canada differ from those used in the United States. Canadian readers who do not know the generic names of the drugs that have been prescribed for them can refer to this Appendix; Canadian brand names are followed here by the names of the generic drugs to which they refer. The pages of this book on which discussions of each of these generic drugs can be found are listed in the Index.

A

Acetazolam — acetazolamide
Acetophen — aspirin
Achromycin — tetracycline hydrochloride
Achromycin V — tetracycline hydrochloride
Actidil — triprolidine hydrochloride
Adeflor — fluoride vitamin preparations
Adrenalin — epinephrine
Aerosporin — polymyxin B sulfate
Aldactone — spironolactone
Aldomet — methyldopa
Algoverine — phenylbutazone
Allerdryl — diphenhydramine hydrochloride
Alloprin — allopurinol
Alupent — metaproterenol sulfate
Amcill — ampicillin
Amersol — ibuprofen
Aminophyl — aminophylline
AmoxICAN — amoxicillin
Amoxil — amoxicillin
Amphojel — aluminum hydroxide gel
Ampicin — ampicillin
Ampilean — ampicillin
Amytal — amobarbital
Ancasal — aspirin
Anevral — phenylbutazone
Antazone — sulfinpyrazone
Antilirium — physostigmine salicylate
Anturan — sulfinpyrazone

Aparkane — trihexyphenidyl hydrochloride
Apo-Asen — aspirin
Apo-Haloperidol — haloperidol
Apo-Oxazepam — oxazepam
Apo-Propranolol — propranolol hydrochloride
Apo-Sulfinpyrazone — sulfinpyrazone
Apresoline — hydralazine
Aristocort — triamcinolone
Aristospan hexacetonide — triamcinolone
Artane — trihexyphenidyl hydrochloride
Astrin — aspirin
Atarax — hydroxyzine hydrochloride
Atasol — acetaminophen
Atasol Forte — acetaminophen
Athrombin-K potassium — warfarin
Atromid-S — clofibrate
Aureomycin — chlortetracycline
Aventyl — nortriptyline hydrochloride
Ayercillin — penicillin G

B

Baciguent — bacitracin
Bacitin — bacitracin
Bactopen — cloxacillin sodium
Balminil D.M. Syrup — dextromethorphan hydrobromide

Balminil Expectorant—glyceryl guaiacolate
Banlin—propantheline bromide
Barriere—simethicone
Basaljel—aluminum hydroxide gel
Beben—betamethasone
Benadryl—diphenhydramine hydrochloride
Benemid—probenecid
Bensylate—benztropine mesylate
Bentylol—dicyclomine hydrochloride
Benuryl—probenecid
Benzedrine—amphetamine sulfate
Betacort—betamethasone
Betaderm—betamethasone
Betnelan—betamethasone
Betnesol—betamethasone
Betnovate—betamethasone
Bicillin—penicillin G
Biosan—ampicillin
Bleph-10—sulfacetamide
Bonamine—meclizine hydrochloride
Brevicon—estrogen and progestogen combinations
Bricanyl—terbutaline sulfate
Broncho-Grippol-DM—dextromethorphan hydrobromide
Bronkaid Mistometer—epinephrine
Butagesic—phenylbutazone
Butazolidin—phenylbutazone
Butisol Sodium—butabarbital

C

Calcilean calcium—heparin
Calciparine subcutaneous calcium—heparin
Campain—acetaminophen
Carbolith—lithium carbonate
Cardioquin—quinidine polygalacturonate
Catapres—clonidine hydrochloride
Cefracycline—tetracycline hydrochloride
Celestoderm—betamethasone
Celestone—betamethasone
Celontin—methsuximide
Ceporex—cephalexin monohydrate
Cetamide—sulfacetamide
Chloralvan—chloral hydrate
Chloromide—chlorpropamide

Chloromycetin—chloramphenicol
Chloronase—chlorpropamide
Chloroptic—chloramphenicol
Chlorprom—chlorpromazine
Chlor-Promanyl—chlorpromazine
Chlor-Tripolon—chlorpheniramine maleate
Cidomycin—gentamicin sulfate
Claripex—clofibrate
Climestrone Tablets—estrogens
Cloxilean—cloxacillin sodium
Cogentin—benztropine mesylate
Colace—dioctyl sodium sulfosuccinate
Coldecon—phenylpropanolamine hydrochloride
Colisone—prednisone
Coly-Mycin (as colistimethate sodium)—colistin
Conjugated Estrogens—estrogens
Constiban—dioctyl sodium sulfosuccinate
Corax—chlordiazepoxide hydrochloride
Coronex—isosorbide dinitrate
Corophyllin—aminophylline
Cortamed—hydrocortisone
Cortate—hydrocortisone
Cort-Dome—hydrocortisone
Cortef—hydrocortisone
Cortenema—hydrocortisone
Corticreme—hydrocortisone
Cortiment—hydrocortisone
Cortril—hydrocortisone
Corutol DH—hydrocodone bitartrate
Corutol Expectorant—glyceryl guaiacolate
Coryphen—aspirin
Coumadin sodium—warfarin
Cremocort—triamcinolone
Crystapen—penicillin G
C-Tran—chlordiazepoxide hydrochloride
Cyclospasmol—cyclandelate
Cytomel—liothyronine sodium

D

Dalacin C—clindamycin
Dalmane—flurazepam hydrochloride
Dantoin—phenytoin
Darbid—isopropamide iodide

Darvon-N—propoxyphene napsylate
Day-Barb—butabarbital
Decadron—dexamethasone
Declomycin—demeclocycline
Deltasone—prednisone
Demer-Idine—meperidine
Demerol—meperidine
Demo-Cineol Antitussive Syrup—
   dextromethorphan hydrobromide
Demi-Cineol Expectorant Syrup—
   glyceryl guaiacolate
Demulen—estrogen and progestogen
   combinations
Deprex—amitriptyline hydrochloride
Depronal SA—propoxyphene
   hydrochloride
Dermalar—fluocinolone acetonide
Dermophyl—fluocinolone acetonide
Deronil—dexamethasone
Detensol—propranolol hydrochloride
Dexasone—dexamethasone
Dexedrine—dexamphetamine
Diabinese—chlorpropamide
Diamox—acetazolamide
Dilantin—phenytoin
Dimetane—brompheniramine maleate
Diprosone—betamethasone
Disipal hydrochloride—orphenadrine
Diuchlor H—hydrochlorothiazide
Dixarit—clonidine hydrochloride
DM Syrup—dextromethorphan
   hydrobromide
Dopamet—methyldopa
Doriden—glutethimide
D-Tran—diazepam
Duretic—methyclothiazide
Dynapen—dicloxacillin sodium
   monohydrate
Dyrenium—triamterene
Dysne-Inhal hydrochloride—epinephrine

E

Ecotrin—aspirin
Edecrin—ethacrynic acid
EES-200—erythromycin
EES-400—erythromycin
Elavil—amitriptyline hydrochloride
Eltor—pseudoephedrine hydrochloride

Eltroxin—levothyroxine sodium
Emcinka—erythromycin
Emo-Cort—hydrocortisone
E-Mycin—erythromycin
Enovid—estrogen and progestogen
   combinations
Entrophen—aspirin
E-Pam—diazepam
Epifrin hydrochloride—epinephrine
Epitrate bitartrate—epinephrine
Equanil—meprobamate
Ergomar—ergotamine tartrate
Erythrocin ethyl succinate, stearate, or
   lactobionate—erythromycin
Erythromid—erythromycin
Esidrix—hydrochlorothiazide
Eskabarb—phenobarbital
Estinyl—estrogens
Estrace—estrogens
Etibi—ethambutol hydrochloride
Exdol—acetaminophen

F

Falapen—penicillin G
Fastin—phentermine
Fenicol—chloramphenicol
Fer-In-Sol—ferrous sulfate
Fero-Grad—ferrous sulfate
Fesofor—ferrous sulfate
Flagyl—metronidazole
Flozenges—fluoride
Fluoderm—fluocinolone acetonide
Fluolean—fluocinolone acetonide
Fluorac—fluoride vitamin preparations
Fluorinse—fluoride
Fluotic—fluoride
Formulex—dicyclomine hydrochloride
Fulvicin-U/F—griseofulvin
Furacin—nitrofurazone
Furatine—nitrofurantoin
Furoside—furosemide

G

Gantanol—sulfamethoxazole
Gantrisin—sulfisoxazole
Garamycin—gentamicin sulfate

Gardenal—phenobarbital
gBh—gamma benzene hexachloride
Geopen Oral—carbenicillin
Gesterol—progesterone
Glaucon—epinephrine
Gonio-Gel—methylcellulose
Grisovin-FP—griseofulvin
Gynergen—ergotamine tartrate

H

Haldol—haloperidol
Hepalean—heparin
Herisan Antibiotic—neomycin sulfate
Herplex—idoxuridine
Herplex-D Liquifilm—idoxuridine
Hexadrol—dexamethasone
Histalon—chlorpheniramine maleate
Histantil—promethazine hydrochloride
Hycodan—hydrocodone bitartrate
Hyderm—hydrocortisone
Hydro-Aquil—hydrochlorothiazide
Hydro-Cortilean—hydrocortisone
Hydrocortone—hydrocortisone
HydroDiuril—hydrochlorothiazide
Hygroton—chlorthalidone

I

Ilosone estolate—erythromycin
Impril—imipramine hydrochloride
Inapsine—droperidol
Inderal—propranolol hydrochloride
Inderal-LA—propranolol hydrochloride
Indocid—indomethacin
Insulin Lente—insulin zinc suspension
Insulin Semilente—insulin zinc
    suspension
Insulin Ultralente—insulin zinc
    suspension
Intal—cromolyn sodium
Intrabutazone—phenylbutazone
Ionamin ion-exchange resin complex—
    phentermine
Ismelin—guanethidine sulfate
Isobec base—amobarbital
Isomnal—diphenhydramine
    hydrochloride

Isopto Carbachol—carbachol
Isopto Carpine hydrochloride—
    pilocarpine
Isopto Cetamide—sulfacetamide
Isopto Fenicol—chloramphenicol
Isopto Tears—methylcellulose
Isordil—isosorbide dinitrate
Isotamine—isoniazid
Isuprel—isoproterenol

K

Kalium Durules—potassium chloride
Kaochlor—potassium chloride
Kaochlor-20 Concentrate—potassium
    chloride
Kaon—potassium gluconate
Kay Ciel—potassium chloride
KCL 20%—potassium chloride
Keflex—cephalexin monohydrate
Kenacort—triamcinolone
Kenalog—triamcinolone
Kenalog-E acetonide—triamcinolone
K-Long—potassium chloride
K-Lor—potassium chloride
K-Med—potassium tartrate
K-Sol—potassium gluconate
K-10—potassium chloride
Kwellada—gamma benzene hexachloride

L

Lacril—methylcellulose
Lanoxin—digoxin
Largactil—chlorpromazine
Larodopa—levodopa
Lasix—furosemide
Laxagel—dioctyl sodium sulfosuccinate
Ledercillin VK potassium—
    phenoxymethyl penicillin
Lente Insulin—insulin zinc suspension
Levate—amitriptyline hydrochloride
Librium—chlordiazepoxide hydrochloride
Lincocin—lincomycin hydrochloride
    monohydrate
Lithane—lithium carbonate
Lithizine—lithium carbonate

Loestrin—estrogen and progestogen combinations
Lomin C—dicyclomine hydrochloride
Lomotil—diphenoxylate hydrochloride
Lo-Ovral—estrogen and progestogen combinations
Luminal—phenobarbital

M

Macrodantin—nitrofurantoin
Malgesic—phenylbutazone
Manticor—hydrocortisone
Maxidex—dexamethasone
Medicycline—tetracycline hydrochloride
Medihaler-Epi bitartrate—epinephrine
Medihaler-Ergotamine—ergotamine tartrate
Medihaler-Iso—isoproterenol
Medilium—chlordiazepoxide hydrochloride
Medimet-250—methyldopa
Meditran—meprobamate
Megacillin Suspension—penicillin G
Megacillin Tablets—penicillin G
Mellaril—thioridazine hydrochloride
Menospasm—dicyclomine hydrochloride
Menrium—estrogens
Meprospan-400—meprobamate
Meravil—amitriptyline hydrochloride
Methidate—methylphenidate hydrochloride
Meval—diazepam
Micatin—miconazole nitrate
Microcort—hydrocortisone
Miltown—meprobamate
Minihep—heparin
Minocin—minocycline hydrochloride
Miocarpine hydrochloride—pilocarpine
Miostat—carbachol
Mobenol—tolbutamide
Modicon—estrogen and progestogen combinations
Motrin—ibuprofen
Moxilean trihydrate—amoxicillin
Murocel—methylcellulose
Myambutol—ethambutol hydrochloride
Mycifradin—neomycin sulfate
Myciguent—neomycin sulfate

Mycostatin—nystatin
Mydfrin—phenylephrine hydrochloride
Mysoline—primidone

N

Nadopen-V—phenoxymethyl penicillin
Nadostine—nystatin
Nadozone—phenylbutazone
Nafrine—oxymetazoline hydrochloride
Nalcrom—cromolyn sodium
Nalfon calcium—fenoprofen
Naprosyn—naproxen
Nati-K—potassium tartrate
Natrimax—hydrochlorothiazide
Navane—thiothixene
Nefrol—hydrochlorothiazide
NegGram—nalidixic acid
Neo-Barb—butabarbital
Neo-Calme—diazepam
Neocin—neomycin sulfate
Neo-Codema—hydrochlorothiazide
Neo-Renal—furosemide
Neo-Synephrine—phenylephrine hydrochloride
Neo-Tetrine—tetracycline hydrochloride
Neo-Tran—meprobamate
Neo-Tric—metronidazole
Neo-Zoline—phenylbutazone
Nephronex—nitrofurantoin
Nifuran—nitrofurantoin
Nilstat—nystatin
Nitrol—nitroglycerin
Nitrong—nitroglycerin
Nitrostabilin—nitroglycerin
Nitrostat—nitroglycerin
Noctec—chloral hydrate
Noludar—methyprylon
Norflex citrate—orphenadrine
Norinyl—estrogen and progestogen combinations
Norlestrin—estrogen and progestogen combinations
Norpramin—desipramine
Norquen—estrogen and progestogen combinations
Novamoxin trihydrate—amoxicillin
Nova-Phase—aspirin
Nova-Pheno—phenobarbital

Novasen—aspirin
Novobetamet—betamethasone
Novobutamide—tolbutamide
Novobutazone—phenylbutazone
Novochlorhydrate—chloral hydrate
Novochlorocap—chloramphenicol
Novocloxin—cloxacillin sodium
Novocolchine—colchicine
Novodipam—diazepam
Novoferrosulfa—ferrous sulfate
Novofibrate—clofibrate
Novoflupam—flurazepam hydrochloride
Novoflurazine—trifluoperazine
Novofuran—nitrofurantoin
Novohexidyl—trihexyphenidyl
   hydrochloride
Novohydrazide—hydrochlorothiazide
Novolexin—cephalexin monohydrate
Novomedopa—methyldopa
Novomepro—meprobamate
Novomethacin—indomethacin
Novonidazol—metronidazole
Novopen-G—penicillin G
Novopen-VK—phenoxymethyl penicillin
Novopheniram—chlorpheniramine
   maleate
Novophenytoin—phenytoin
Novopoxide—chlordiazepoxide
   hydrochloride
Novopramine—imipramine hydrochloride
Novopropamide—chlorpropamide
Novopropanthil—propantheline bromide
Novopropoxyn—propoxyphene
   hydrochloride
Novopyrazone—sulfinpyrazone
Novoridazine—thioridazine
   hydrochloride
Novorythro base, stearate, or estolate—
   erythromycin
Novosemide—furosemide
Novosoxazole—sulfisoxazole
Novotetra—tetracycline hydrochloride
Novothalidone—chlorthalidone
Novotriptyn—amitriptyline hydrochloride
Nyaderm—nystatin

O

Ocusert Pilo-20—pilocarpine
Ocusert Pilo-40—pilocarpine

Oestrilin—estrogens
Ogen Tablets—estrogens
Opticrom—cromolyn sodium
Optosulfex—sulfacetamide
Oracon—estrogen and progestogen
   combinations
Orbenin—cloxacillin sodium
Orinase—tolbutamide
Ortho-Novum—estrogen and progestogen
   combinations
Ovcon—estrogen and progestogen
   combinations
Ovol—simethicone
Ovral—estrogen and progestogen
   combinations
Ovulen—estrogen and progestogen
   combinations
Ox-Pam—oxezepam
Oxybutazone—oxyphenbutazone

P

Paracort—prednisone
Paveral—codeine phosphate
Penamox trihydrate—amoxicillin
Penbec-V potassium—phenoxymethyl
   penicillin
Penbritin—ampicillin
Penioral 500—penicillin G
Pentamycetin—chloramphenicol
Pen-Vee potassium or benzathine—
   phenoxymethyl penicillin
Periactin—cyproheptadine hydrochloride
Peritrate—pentaerythritol tetranitrate
Persantine—dipyridamole
Pertofrane—desipramine
P-50—penicillin G
Phenazine—perphenazine
Phenazo—phenazopyridine hydrochloride
Phenbuff—phenylbutazone
Phenbutazone—phenylbutazone
Phenergan—promethazine hydrochloride
Phenoptic—phenylephrine hydrochloride
Phyllocontin—aminophylline
Pitrex—tolnaftate
Polaramine—dexchlorpheniramine
   maleate
Polymox trihydrate—amoxicillin
Poly-Vi-Flor—fluoride vitamin
   preparations

Potassium Rougier—potassium gluconate
Prefrin Liquifilm—phenylephrine
  hydrochloride
Premarin—estrogens
Pro-Banthine—propantheline bromide
Progestasert (intrauterine)—progesterone
Progestilin—progesterone
Program Tablets—estrogens
Proloid—thyroglobulin
Proloprim—trimethoprim
Pronestyl—procainamide hydrochloride
Pronidin—phentermine
Propanthel—propantheline bromide
Propyl-Thyracil—propylthiouracil
Pro-65—propoxyphene hydrochloride
Prostaphlin—oxacillin sodium
Pseudofrin—pseudoephedrine
  hydrochloride
Purinol—allopurinol
P.V. Carpine nitrate—pilocarpine
PVF benzathine—phenoxymethyl
  penicillin
PVF K potassium—phenoxymethyl
  penicillin
Pyopen—carbenicillin
Pyribenzamine hydrochloride or citrate—
  tripelennamine
Pyridium—phenazopyridine
  hydrochloride

Q

Questran—cholestryamine resin
Quietal—meprobamate
Quinaglute—quinidine gluconate
Quinate—quinidine gluconate
Quinidex Extentabs—quinidine sulfate

R

Regulex—dioctyl sodium sulfosuccinate
Relaxil—chlordiazepoxide hydrochloride
Relium—chlordiazepoxide hydrochloride
Reserfia—reserpine
Reserpanca—reserpine
Resyl—glyceryl guaiacolate
Rifadin—rifampin
Rimactane—rifampin

Rimifon—isoniazid
Ritalin—methylphenidate hydrochloride
Rival—diazepam
Robaxin—methocarbamol
Robidex—dextromethorphan
  hydrobromide
Robidone—hydrocodone bitartrate
Robidrine—pseudoephedrine
  hydrochloride
Robigesic—acetaminophen
Robimycin—erythromycin
Robitussin—glyceryl guaiacolate
Rofact—rifampin
Rogitine hydrochloride or mesylate—
  phentolamine
Roucol—allopurinol
Rounox—acetaminophen
Rouqualone-"300"—methaqualone
  hydrochloride
Roychlor—potassium chloride
Royonate—potassium gluconate
Rynacrom—cromolyn sodium

S

Sal-Adult—aspirin
Sal-Infant—aspirin
S-Cortilean—hydrocortisone
Secogen sodium—secobarbital
Seconal Sodium—secobarbital
Sedatuss—dextromethorphan
  hydrobromide
Sedatuss Expectorant—glyceryl
  guaiacolate
Seral—secobarbital
Serax—oxazepam
Serpasil—reserpine
Sertan—primidone
Sinequan—doxepin hydrochloride
642—propoxyphene hydrochloride
Slow-Fe—ferrous sulfate
Slow-K—potassium chloride
Sodium Amytal—amobarbital
Sodium Sulamyd—sulfacetamide
Solazine—trifluoperazine
Solium—chlordiazepoxide hydrochloride
Solu-Cortef—hydrocortisone
Somnium—diphenhydramine
  hydrochloride

Somophyllin—aminophylline
Sopamycetin—chloramphenicol
Spasmoban—dicyclomine hydrochloride
Stabinol—chlorpropamide
Staphcillin sodium—methicillin
Stelazine—trifluoperazine
Stemetil—prochlorperazine
Stoxil—idoxuridine
Stress-Pam—diazepam
Sudafed—pseudoephedrine hydrochloride
Sudodrin—pseudoephedrine
    hydrochloride
Sulf-10—sulfacetamide
Sulf-30—sulfacetamide
Sumycin—tetracycline hydrochloride
Supasa—aspirin
Supeudol—oxycodone
Surfak—dioctyl calcium sulfosuccinate
Sus-Phrine—epinephrine
Symmetrel—amantadine hydrochloride
Synalar—fluocinolone acetonide
Synamol—fluocinolone acetonide
Synthroid—levothyroxine sodium

T

Talwin—pentazocine
Tandearil—oxyphenbutazone
Tapazole—methimazole
T-Caps—tetracycline hydrochloride
Teething Syrup—benzocaine
Tegopen—cloxacillin sodium
Tegretol—carbamazepine
Tempra—acetaminophen
Terfluzine—trifluoperazine
Terramycin—oxytetracycline
Tertroxin—liothyronine sodium
Tetracyn—tetracycline hydrochloride
Tetralean—tetracycline hydrochloride
Thioril—thioridazine hydrochloride
Tigan—trimethobenzamide hydrochloride
Tinactin—tolnaftate
Titralac—calcium carbonate
Tofranil—imipramide hydrochloride
Tolbutone—tolbutamide
Tolectin—tolmetin sodium
Tranxene—clorazepate dipotassium
Triaderm—triamcinolone
Triador—methaqualone hydrochloride
Trialean acetonide—triamcinolone

Triaphen-10—aspirin
Triflurin—trifluoperazine
Trikacide—metronidazole
Trilafon—perphenazine
Trilium—chlordiazepoxide hydrochloride
Trimacort acetonide—triamcinolone
Tri-Vi-Flor—fluoride vitamin
    preparations
Tri-Vi-Sol with fluoride—fluoride
    vitamin preparations
Trixyl—trihexyphenidyl hydrochloride
Tualone-300—methaqualone
    hydrochloride
Turbinaire Decadron Phosphate—
    dexamethasone
Tylenol—acetaminophen

U

Unicort—hydrocortisone
Unipen—nafcillin sodium
Uridon—chlorthalidone
Uritol—furosemide
Urozide—hydrochlorothiazide

V

Valisone Scalp Lotion—betamethasone
Valium—diazepam
Vallestril—estrogens
Vaponefrin—epinephrine
Vasodilan—isoxsuprine hydrochloride
V-Cillin K potassium—phenoxymethyl
    penicillin
VC-K 500 potassium—phenoxymethyl
    penicillin
Vibramycin—doxycycline
Vimicon—cyproheptadine hydrochloride
Vioform—iodochlorhydroxyquin
Viscerol—dicyclomine hydrochloride
Vitasol-F—fluoride vitamin preparations
Vivol—diazepam

W

Warfilone sodium—warfarin
Warnerin sodium—warfarin

Wel-K—potassium tartrate
Westcort—hydrocortisone
Winpred—prednisone
Wycillin 300—penicillin G
Wycillin 600—penicillin G

Z

Zarontin—ethosuximide
Zyloprim—allopurinol
Zynol—sulfinpyrazone

GLOSSARY

acid any chemical compound whose pH is less than 7, characterized by a sour taste; lemon juice, for example, is very acidic

acne an inflammatory disease of the skin characterized by the formation of pimples; acne often occurs during adolescence

alkaline the opposite of acidic; any chemical compound whose pH is greater than 7, characterized by a caustic and bitter taste

anemia a decrease in the number of red blood cells, which implies a lowered concentration of oxygen-carrying material in the blood; anemia is a symptom of various diseases and disorders

apathy lack of feeling or emotion; indifference

arrhythmia variation in the normal rhythm of the heartbeat; irregular heartbeat

artery a blood vessel that carries blood (primarily oxygenated blood) away from the heart

bacteria one-celled microorganisms of the class *Schizomycetes*, which often cause infection

blood clot a semisolid mass of blood

bone marrow the soft, organic material, made up of fat cells and maturing blood cells, that fills bone cavities

cholesterol the most abundant fat-soluble organic compound present in animal tissue; it is a precursor of a form of vitamin D, and has been implicated in the development of arteriosclerosis

chronic disease a disease of long duration and slow progress

clotting factor any of a number of agents that contribute to blood coagulation; a deficiency of any of these can lead to excessive bleeding

contraction (e.g., of the heart muscle) an increase in tension in muscle tissue; contracted muscles are generally shorter and thicker than in their relaxed state

dairy products foods containing principally milk, cream, butter or cheese

debilitated physically weakened; feeble

dehydrated having lost excessive body water; dehydration may occur when vomiting or diarrhea is present

eczema a skin inflammation marked by redness, itching and small, elevated lesions that weep, ooze and crust; this is followed by scaling, thickening and discoloration of the skin

electrolyte a liquid or solution capable of conducting an electric charge; the most important electrolytes in the human body are sodium, potassium, calcium, chloride and bicarbonate

extended-release tablet tablets that release medication slowly over a prolonged period of time

fungi a general term for mushrooms, yeasts, molds, etc.; all are marked by the absence of chlorophyll and the presence of a rigid cell wall

gallstone a solid mass formed in the gallbladder or bile duct

general anesthetic an agent that renders a patient unconscious and insusceptible to pain; general anesthetics may be administered by inhalation, by intravenous

[455]

or intramuscular injection or by other means

generic a nonproprietary drug name, usually describing the drug's chemical structure, which is not protected by a trademark

gram-negative a classification of bacteria determined by staining; bacteria not holding the dye are classified gram-negative

gram-positive a classification of bacteria determined by staining; bacteria holding the dye are classified gram-positive

hallucination a sensory perception that has no basis in external stimulation

heredity the genetic transmission of a particular quality or trait from parent to offspring; the genetic constitution of an individual

hypertension persistently high arterial blood pressure; the systemic condition accompanying high blood pressure

inherited disease a disease that is transmitted from parent to offspring

injection the forcing of liquid into some part of the body, generally intramuscular (into a muscle) or intravenous (into a vein)

insomnia inability to sleep; abnormal wakefulness

in vitro in an artificial environment, usually in a laboratory

jaundice yellowness of the skin, eyes and excretions, usually associated with liver disease or injury

lethargy a condition of drowsiness or indifference

maintenance dosage a specified dosage of a drug taken over a long period of time, usually for some chronic disease

meningitis inflammation of the membranes covering the brain and/or spinal cord

mucus a slippery secretion produced by the mucous membranes, which it moistens and protects

myasthenia gravis progressive paralysis of the muscular system unaccompanied by sensory disturbance

mycobacteria a genus of gram-positive, aerobic bacteria that includes those causing tuberculosis and leprosy

obstruction something that causes blocking or clogging; the state of being clogged

organism an individual living thing, whether plant or animal

parasiticide an agent that destroys parasites

pelvis the lower portion of the trunk of the body, bounded by the hip bones, the sacrum and the coccyx

pheochromocytoma a tumor of the adrenal medulla or sympathetic paraganglia; its symptoms, notably hypertension, reflect the increased secretion of epinephrine and norepinephrine

protozoa unicellular organisms ranging in size from submicroscopic to macroscopic (visible to the naked eye)

psoriasis a chronic skin disease characterized by red patches covered with white or silver scales

pulse the rhythmic expansion of an artery which may be felt with a finger

pus a thick, opaque, yellowish-white fluid made up of leukocytes (white blood cells), fluid and cellular debris

rickettsiae an order of microorganisms, usually found intercellularly, which are often parasitic to, and transmitted by, vertebrates and invertebrates

Rocky Mountain spotted fever a disease characterized by the sudden onset of headache, chills and fever, which last two to three weeks, and skin eruptions on the trunk and extremities, which appear on about the fourth day; delirium, shock and renal failure occur in severe cases; the disease is transmitted to humans by ticks

semisynthetic   related to, or produced by, natural materials

senility   physical and mental deterioration associated with old age

spasm   a sudden, violent, involuntary muscular contraction; a sudden, transitory constriction of a passage, canal or orifice

sputum   matter ejected from the trachea, bronchi and lungs through the mouth

sunscreen   an agent designed to block burning rays from the sun, especially ultraviolet rays

symptom   any subjective evidence of disease or of a patient's condition

synthetic   produced artificially

tissue   a group or layer of similarly specialized cells which together perform certain special functions

tolerance   an ability to endure without effect or injury; a decrease in susceptibility to the effects of a drug due to its continued administration

triglyceride   a neutral fat that is the usual form in which lipids are stored in animals

tumor   swelling; morbid enlargement; neoplasm; a new growth of tissue in which cell multiplication is uncontrolled and progressive

ulceration   the development of a break in the skin or mucous membrane, accompanied by the loss of surface tissue, the disintegration and death of epithelial tissues, and often by pus

venereal   due to or propagated by sexual contact

virus   a minute infectious agent, usually invisible under a light microscope, which replicates only within a host cell; a virus consists of DNA or RNA (but not both) and a protein shell

INDEX

(Note: The page numbers listed in this Index refer to the pages of the book on which discussions of a given drug or disease state begin. Also, Canadian readers may need to refer first to the Appendix, page 441, where the generic drugs to which Canadian brand names apply are listed; they can then check the Index to find where in the book discussions of each generic drug can be found.)

A

C

E

F

Fastin, see **Phentermine**, 438
Fatty acids, 49
Fedahist, see **Chlorpheniramine**, 211;
    pseudoephedrine, 230
Fedahist Expectorant, see **Guaifenesin**,
    232
Fedazril, see **Pseudoephedrine**, 230
Fenoprofen, 242
Fenylhist, see **Diphenhydramine**, 217
Feosol, see **Ferrous sulfate**, 437
Fer-in-Sol, see **Ferrous sulfate**, 437
Fernisone, see **Prednisone**, 255
Fero-Gradumet, see **Ferrous sulfate**, 437
Ferolix, see **Ferrous sulfate**, 437
Ferospace, see **Ferrous sulfate**, 437
Ferralyn, see **Ferrous sulfate**, 437
Ferrous sulfate, 437
Fesotyme, see **Ferrous sulfate**, 437
Fiogesic, see **Phenylpropanolamine**, 228
Fiorinal, see **Codeine**, 418;
    phenacetin, 417
Flagyl, see **Metronidazole**, 149
Fleet Mineral Oil Enema, see **Mineral
    oil**, 270
Fluocinolone, 179
Fluocinonide, 179
Fluonid, see **Fluocinolone**, 179
Flurandrenolide, 181
Flurazepam, 298
Flurosyn, see **Fluocinolone**, 179
4-Way Cold Tablets, see
    Chlorpheniramine, 211;
    phenylpropanolamine, 228
Fulvicin P/G, see **Griseofulvin**, 172
Fulvicin-U/F, see **Griseofulvin**, 172
Furacin, see **Nitrofurazone**, 169
Furadantin, see **Nitrofurantoin**, 138
Furalan, see **Nitrofurantoin**, 138
Furosemide, 20

G

Gantanol, see **Sulfamethoxazole**, 142
Gantrisin, see **Sulfisoxazole**, 144
Garamycin, see **Gentamicin**, 120
Garamycin Ophthalmic, see **Gentamicin**,
    160
Gas-X, see **Simethicone**, 265
GBH, see **Lindane**, 175
Gelusil, see **Aluminum hydroxide and
    magnesium hydroxide**, 261;
    simethicone, 265

Genoptic, see **Gentamicin**, 160
Gentamicin, 120, 160
Geocillin, see **Carbenicillin**, 81
Geopen, see **Carbenicillin**, 81
Gitaligin, see **Gitalin**, 6
Gitalin, 6
Glaucoma, 383
Glutethimide, 300
Glycerin suppositories, 269
Glyceryl guaiacolate, 232
Gout, 403
Grifulvin V, see **Griseofulvin**, 172
Grisactin, see **Griseofulvin**, 172
Griseofulvin, 172
Gris-PEG, see **Griseofulvin**, 172
G-3, see **Codeine**, 418
Guaiatuss, see **Guaifenesin**, 232
Guaifenesin, 232
Guaifensin-Dextromethorphan Syrup,
    see **Dextromethorphan**, 235
Guanethidine, 25
Guistrey, see **Chlorpheniramine**, 211;
    guaifenesin, 232
Gustalac, see **Calcium carbonate**, 262

H

Haldol, see **Haloperidol**, 332
Haley's M-O, see **Mineral oil**, 270
Haloperidol, 332
HC, see **Hydrocortisone**, 182
Heart attack, 3
Heartburn, 261
Heart pain, 39
Heb-Cort, see **Hydrocortisone**, 182
Hedulin, see **Phenindione**, 48
Herplex, see **Idoxuridine**, 161
Hetacillin, 87
Hexaderm, see **Hydrocortisone**, 182
Hexadrol, see **Dexamethasone**, 253
High blood pressure, 9
Hiprex, see **Methenamine**, 134
Histabid, see **Chlorpheniramine**, 211;
    phenylpropanolamine, 228
Hista-Clopine, see **Chlorpheniramine**, 211
Histadyl, see **Chlorpheniramine**, 211
Histadyl EC Syrup, see **Codeine**, 233
Histalet, see **Chlorpheniramine**, 211;
    dextromethorphan, 235;
    phenylpropanolamine, 228;
    pseudoephedrine, 230
Histalet X, see **Guaifenesin**, 232
Histapp, see **Brompheniramine**, 208
Histaspan, see **Chlorpheniramine**, 211

U

V